The ethics of animal and human experimentation

The ethics of animal and human experimentation

Edited by
P.P. De Deyn

Associate editors:
R. D'Hooge
A. Schafer

John Libbey
LONDON • PARIS • ROME

British Library Cataloguing in Publication Data

1. Ethics of Animal and Human Experimentation, The
I. De Deyn, Peter P.
174.28

ISBN: 0 86196 429 2

Published by
John Libbey & Company Ltd, 13 Smiths Yard, Summerley Street, London SW18 4HR, England.
Telephone: 0181-947 2777 – Fax: 0181-947 2664
John Libbey Eurotext Ltd, 127 avenue de la République, 92120 Montrouge, France
John Libbey – CIC s.r.l., via Lazzaro Spallanzani 11, 00161 Rome, Italy

Printed in Great Britain by Whitstable Litho Ltd, Whitstable, Kent, UK.

Contents

Foreword

Several historical and some more recent examples of scientific misconduct undoubtedly have contributed to suspicion towards research involving animal and human subjects. During the final preparation of this volume, one major historical series of abuse and misconduct related to human experimentation came to public attention: during the 1940s up until the late 1960s, the United States Government ordered radiation experiments on retarded children, pregnant women and convicts. Furthermore, a range of clandestine atomic-age projects became known. Already in 1986, the House energy committee of Rep. Edward Markey issued a report entitled 'American Nuclear Guinea Pigs: three decades of radiation on US citizens ' which the Reagan and Bush administrations did not pursue. The records of the U.S. Department of Energy at present partially released by Energy Secretary Hazel R. O'Leary and the Clinton administration, conjure up a nightmarish picture. These records show how successive radiation departments, determined at all costs to keep ahead of the former Soviet Union in the cold war nuclear arms race, placed thousands of uninformed and unsuspecting Americans at serious and lasting physical risks. Mentally retarded boys were fed radioactive milk in the 1940s and 1950s; pregnant women were dosed with radioactive iron in the late 1940s resulting in an increased incidence of cancer among their children; the testicles of inmates were exposed to high levels of radiation; and patients with apparently dangerous illnesses were injected with high doses of plutonium. Still on a larger scale, government scientists deliberately exploded atomic bombs over the US in order to examine the spread and effects of radioactive fall-out. The 'downwinders' who lived in Utah and who were repeatedly told that atomic tests just across the state border in Nevada were safe, were defenceless victims. At the Oak Ridge Institute for nuclear studies during the 1960s cancer patients were given total body irradiation in a project funded by the atomic energy commission and NASA without being informed about its potential lethal effect.

The radiation experiments conducted on the American civilians during the cold war are extremely disturbing for several reasons. First of all, they involved men, women and children who were uninformed or even lied to about the experimental nature of the procedures and their purposes and risks. Moreover, the experiments exposed the participating subjects to unacceptable risks. While several scientists involved expressed their concerns and ethical reservations regarding these research practices, some others considered them acceptable in view of the threat of a nuclear war and chose in a rather extreme way to 'serve many by sacrificing few'. The energy department was much more concerned with security and secrecy than with individual rights, illustrating that ethical values are not absolutes but can be influenced by or evolve side by side with changes in culture, necessities and opportunities.

While some unacceptable abuses and undeniable malpractice took place, a majority of bona fide scientists world-wide have been involved during the last decades in developing procedures and strategies to optimize biomedical research and to safeguard the well-being of all human and animal subjects involved. Progress has been made in, for example, prevention of infectious diseases as measles, poliomyelitis and in the treatment of infectious diseases such as tuberculosis and pneumonia, cardiac disease, gastrointestinal conditions, or metabolic disorders such as diabetes and renal failure, some cancers, epilepsy, stroke and Parkinson's disease. Among the major surgical advances one may recognize open heart surgery, hip prostheses, kidney and cornea transplantations. Virtually all medical and surgical procedures currently applied have been developed through long, elaborate and painstaking procedures involving in vitro as well as animal and human experimentation. Along with the increase of biomedical experimentation, institutional review boards and hospital ethics committees have been created and good laboratory and clinical practice guidelines have been developed.

In this book, we address several of the legitimate concerns related to the ethical acceptance and monitoring of biomedical research and hope to suggest some answers to a variety of questions.

One of the many questions raised is whether enhancement of human welfare justifies the occasional but unavoidable suffering of animal and human subjects. While most researchers believe that use of animals for biomedical research is justified, the acceptable level, modalities and extent of animal experimentation still remains to be defined. Although billions of animals are used world-wide for consumption by humans, while only some millions, mostly rodents, are used in biomedical experimentation, this fact does not reduce or alleviate our moral and ethical obligations towards experimental animals. The 3 Rs of reduction, refinement and replacement of animal experimentation, already proposed in 1959 by Russel and Burch, still remain an important guide. Where some promote and advance the development of alternatives in order to ensure protection of the health and safety of the public, others advocate a complete and unilateral ban of all animal use in biomedical research claiming that whole-animal experimentation is not contributory to biomedical sciences. It is obvious that animals can not be informed with regard to the proposed investigations or give their informed consent. Moreover, one could doubt whether well-informed and intelligible animals would be inclined to give informed consent to participation in experiments that almost invariably end with their sacrifice. In contrast to the animal subjects, human experimental subjects, patients or healthy volunteers, with the exception of so-called vulnerable populations, can give or deny a well-informed consent and thereby execute their rights to self-determination.

A second and equally important question concerns the guidelines, jurisdiction and control mechanisms regarding biomedical experimentation.

In order to provide some answers to the questions raised above as well as many others, a series of renowned clinical and laboratory researchers, lawyers, philosophers and statisticians performed a critical analysis of ethical aspects related to biomedical research and present their views in different sections and chapters of this book covering general and specific issues. The first section encompasses general reflections and considerations with regard to biomedical science. In a second section legislation regarding animal and human experimentation with special reference to the European guidelines and legislation is dealt with. Long standing controversies concerning animal research world-wide are discussed in a third section. Unfortunately, this section lacks a contribution from animals rights organisations. The spokesman from the Belgian animal liberation organisation GAIA was finally not found prepared to contribute a chapter. Nevertheless, we are confident that the seven chapters covering animal research will compensate for the 'missing' chapter. The two last sections focus on research involving human subjects. While section four describes a broad range of issues related to randomized clinical trials, the last section deals with specific clinical cases of special interest.

We invite the general public and all biomedical scientists to read this volume which aims at informing people about how ethically conducted research still can keep up with high scientific standard research. We hope that this collaborative effort will further contribute to a more ethically acceptable biomedical research at the benefit of human but also of animal welfare.

Special thanks go to Mr. Jos Caers, Ms. Frieda Franck and Ms. Sandra Van den Broeck who assisted in editing this book.

Peter P. De Deyn, MD PhD MMPR
Department of Neurology
General Hospital Middelheim and
Department of Neurochemistry and Behavior
Born Bunge Foundation
University of Antwerp
Antwerp, Belgium

Dedication:

This book is dedicated to the late Jos Caers, a well-respected friend, co-worker and warm-hearted person who helped in the preparation of this book and died unexpectedly at the age of 49.

Section I:
Biomedical science: general reflections and considerations

The ethics of animal and human experimentation, edited by P.P. De Deyn.

1

Ethical-philosophical aspects of human and animal experimentation

Etienne Vermeersch

University of Ghent, Sint-Pietersnieuwstraat 25, B-9000 Ghent, Belgium

Morally relevant conduct, as distinguished from behaviour in general, consists of activities that cause approval or disapproval. Such conduct can sometimes be governed by explicit maxims learned from others or formulated for ourselves; but mostly the rules are interiorized as 'values' or 'norms'. They may elicit either positive emotion or moral pain when we are confronted with the results of our actions, or they may provoke feelings of admiration or indignation when we observe the doings of others. Values and norms, which control the activities of individuals and groups, are of a factual nature: their presence or absence can be ascertained by empirical procedures.

Ethical research may consist of looking for information about the existence (or absence) of particular norms or values within a group, but it is concerned primarily with the question of how a *foundation* can be laid for them. Such foundational problems arise when generally accepted norms are suddenly challenged or when the need to introduce new ones imposes itself.

The reasons which are put forward in an ethical discourse to uphold or to change values, are of two types. (a) When one discusses conditional (hypothetical) norms (e.g. 'you should not smoke cigarettes *if* you do not want to get cancer'), a good reason can be the availability of scientific evidence that, if you act in a certain way, the desired (or undesired) situation will come about. (b) With unconditional (categorical) norms (e.g. 'I should do my duty, whatever the consequences'), it is not clear at first sight what a correct way of giving reasons could be. Some people think that no reasons are needed because the norms *are* categorical; others believe that we can rely on some general ethical principles (e.g. 'life is sacred') which should be accepted by everybody and from which more specific values and norms can be deduced.

Ultimately, such starting-points lead to a refusal of discussion: those who do not accept the norm as categorical are considered immoral and those who do not adhere to the general principles are, by that very fact, excluding themselves from the community in which the ethical discussion takes place. Providing a foundation for a value or norm would then amount to intellectually or morally (sometimes even physically) eliminating those who have the audacity to challenge it. Therefore it seems to be better to enter the discussion without any presuppositions concerning *absolute* ethical principles.

Indeed, whoever investigates the *history of morals*, will come to the conclusion that they develop spontaneously in the individual and social life of human beings. Every individual is endowed with some basic drives, which are genetically determined or formed during childhood. In the mutual contacts between individuals, who may have compatible drives but also conflicting ones, rules come into being which order their coexistence. In addition, in every society mechanisms develop which tend to guarantee the survival of the whole and which may or may not agree with the peculiar aspirations of its members. The interaction between these tendencies during the upbringing of the individual causes an interiorization of norms and values.

Depending on local needs and restraints, the development of moral usages has been observed which one would now consider totally immoral but which, given the necessities of a particular context, were then understandable and even acceptable. Thus it was considered normal in many societies to kill or expose disabled children or those whose bare existence threatened the survival of the family. Likewise, in some societies custom required that old people, who could no longer contribute to food gathering and became a burden to the community, be killed, sometimes by their own sons.

With the evolution of cultures, necessities and opportunities changed, as did the values and norms. The development of agriculture and trade, the concentration of people in cities, the formation of larger societies, etc. necessitated or favoured new values which made cooperation easier and promoted the peaceful coexistence of people who had no clear kinship or tribal relationships.

In short, values and norms arise from specific needs of societies, in interaction with the drives of individuals. They change as societies develop, and as societies become larger and more mutually dependent, their members get an increasing awareness of shared interests and tend more and more to adhere to similar values.

This way of approaching ethics and its foundations explains somewhat why this type of research is so difficult and controversial. (a) When you start from the historical or anthropological point of view, you almost inevitably come to the conclusion that the norms and values of a given society are determined by historical and cultural circumstances and consequently that they are of a *relativistic* nature. (b) For someone, however, who has been educated *within* a particular culture, lacking the knowledge of other possibilities, morals have an *absolute* character: he must follow them without discussion and the very act of challenging them would threaten to disrupt the whole value hierarchy and hence the society itself. (c) Nowadays, researchers have become aware of the relativistic aspect of norms and values, but at the same moment, we have the impression that, in the course of the previous centuries, a kind of ethical *progress* has taken place and that, with the growing unification of mankind, there also emerges a general agreement concerning a number of values, such as those expressed in 'declarations of human rights'. Now, if we are all members of the human community, we are supposed to respect these rights, and there seems to be no *outside* from which we could challenge them. But how then can they be in need of foundation when, being valid for all, including the moral philosopher, they are to be accepted without further ado?

The answer is that, notwithstanding our allegiance to them in practical life, we still have to realize that, from a scientific point of view, they have no absolute character. Like those of other cultures, they originated from specific conditions which include, amongst other things, the experiences of previous centuries and the growing scientific, technological and economic unification of mankind. Some of these values are probably the best possible ones at our disposal today, if we want to live in a peaceful and prosperous world, but they are not necessarily final.

It follows that the need for an ethical discourse, including the search for a 'foundation' of values and norms, is still there, and the more so because our world is continuously changing and new problems are emerging every year.

It is the task of the *ethicist* (in collaboration with many others), to make people conscious of the present-day system of norms and values. He should try to show the internal coherence of the value hierarchy and its relevance for the general welfare (or, if need be, its incoherence and lack of relevance). But he can also, especially with respect to controversial issues, argue for those solutions which, according to his insights, while fitting the core of our value system, are the most compatible with future evolution to a happy and peaceful humankind.

In such an ethical discourse, *rationality* is to be striven for; this means that logical coherence and reliance on factual evidence are of the utmost importance; but a *personal bias* in favour of particular values is inevitable and hence logical arguments can be accompanied by a more affective type of persuasion.

The topic at issue in this chapter, *the ethics of animal and human experimentation*, provides us with a good example of the need for such a way of tackling ethical problems. As far as human experimentation is concerned, a consensus has gradually been reached, especially since the Nuremberg trials, that a code of rules has to be followed and that certain procedures are totally unacceptable (Beaufort, 1985). In the field of animal experimentation, however, the discussions are still going on and neither in practice nor in theory has a consensus been reached.

In order to apply the general principles explained above, to the specific problems at stake here; (a) we will try to find a number of values which in the course of time have been or are being accepted to an increasing extent and which are directly or indirectly applicable in this domain; (b) by looking more closely at the distinctive characteristics of the activities we are concerned with (medical and biological research), we will try to find out whether there are particular reasons to fear that some of these values be put in jeopardy and, if necessary we will propose some rules of conduct which might reduce the dangers of derailment.

When studying the history of ethical attitudes and principles since the oldest civilizations which influenced Western thought (Egypt, Mesopotamia, Israel and the Greco-Roman world), one cannot but be struck by the impression of the ever growing importance and extension of the concept of *fellow human being.*

Anthropological studies suggest that people of palaeolithic and early neolithic tribes only identified with the members of the own tribe or clan: in many cultures the term 'human being' was not applied to others than kinsmen or members of one's own tribe.

With the growth of larger kingdoms (e.g. in Egypt and Mesopotamia), in which many tribes were united, the need for broader types of identification gradually arose. As a consequence, there developed an awareness that ethical obligations extend to all the inhabitants of the same kingdom. Somewhat paradoxically, at the time when new distinctions came into being (the rich and the poor, the mighty and the weak), a sense of solidarity was stimulated, which emphasized the equality of all people and which promoted feelings of charity, especially for the poor and the weak.

As an example taken from a great number of texts, we can refer to the Egyptian *Book of the Dead* (ca 1500 BC) where the deceased is supposed to protest his guiltlessness in a posthumous court: 'I have not committed evil against man; I have not mistreated cattle; I have not done violence to a poor man; I have not made anyone sick; I have not made anyone weep; I have not caused anyone suffering'; and further, 'I have given bread to the hungry, water to the thirsty, clothing to the naked'. In Mesopotamia we find analogous texts: on a tablet from the eighth century BC we read: 'unto your opponent do no evil, your evildoer recompense with good, unto your enemy let justice be done'. In the Bible also we notice that the concept of 'neighbour', which initially only referred to the closest relatives or friends, is extended to include all Israelites (Pritchard, 1955, pp. 34–36, 426, etc.).

Near the end of the first millenium BC, there is a growing tendency in a number of civilizations to widen these feelings of solidarity and identification to human beings in general (e.g. in Buddhism, Mazdeism, Christianity, Graeco-Roman Stoicism and, somewhat later, Islam). This attitude was crystallized in a moral norm, the so-called *Golden Rule*, the first formulation of which one finds with Confucius (ca. 500 BC): 'do unto others as you would have them do unto you' (Hersch, 1968).

Of course, this principle has undeniably been violated only too often in the concrete dealings of people and nations through the ages. Nevertheless, I would like to support the thesis that the growing complexity of human societies and the need of pacified relationships over ever larger domains, contributed to the spread of this moral attitude and its gaining in solidity and persuasiveness. In the 18th and 19th centuries this development led to a need for explicitation and systematization of this formerly rather vague cluster of attitudes and feelings.

Without going too much into detail, it seems to me that one can safely say that at least two important principles were clarified in the course of this process.

First of all, 'love of one's neighbour' or identifying with our fellow human being, signifies that we consider him as our *equal*. This notion of equality implies that we grant him the same rights as we claim for ourselves, especially the right to life, freedom and *self-determination*. In Kant's formulation, every person has the right to be treated as his own end and not merely as a means to another's ends.

In its second, no less important component, the Golden Rule refers to the idea of caring for those who *suffer*. Already in the Egyptian *Book of the Dead* the touching phrases: 'I have not made anyone weep, I have not caused anyone suffering' are supplemented with: 'I have not mistreated cattle', where a concern for suffering is present without any possible reference to self-determination (Pritchard, 1955, ibidem).

Even for those who are willing to accept these ethical principles, it is not an easy task to gain a clear insight into the exact field of their application, and into the problem of which choices to make when divergent values come into conflict. In order to answer these questions as fairly as possible, we should get a better look into the actual situations in which experiments on humans and animals are carried out, and try to get an insight into the specific difficulties generated by the confrontation of principle and practice.

As far as *human experimentation* is concerned, we assume that the ethical codes (Nuremberg, Helsinki, Tokyo), are by now widely accepted: the right to self-determination implies that no one may be subjected to a diagnosis, a therapy or a research project without his *informed consent* (Reich, 1978, Vol. 4, pp. 1764–1781). However, the existence of a broad consensus should not make us blind to the possibility that the specific context in which these activities take place might hinder, to some extent, the correct application of the norms accepted in principle.

In biomedical research one often has to deal with persons who are more or less in a state of *dependency*: a patient who is seeking the help of a doctor; an incompetent person facing a specialist; an individual confronted with a research team or a hospital association.

On the side of the specialists, this situation tends to engender a paternalistic attitude, because they think – with the best of intentions – that they know better than anyone else what is good for the persons they work with and what kind of information would be harmful rather than beneficial to them.

The quality of the 'informed consent' is even further affected when children, mentally handicapped persons, very old people, prisoners or poor people are involved. Either they are hardly able to understand the information, or their situation may raise doubts about the authenticity of their consent.

These risks are not always clearly realized by the researcher, due to the fact that people in the medical profession – researchers and therapists – tend to have a rather positive image of their activities. After all, as medical doctors they are assisting their suffering fellow man and as scientists they are engaged in the service of human well-being in general. The more they are thus convinced of their being on the right track, the more their commitment to the research project may tempt them to take less account of 'disturbing' factors, such as the requirements of informed consent or the imperative of maximal elimination of suffering.

A final hindrance to a clear assessment of the values involved in a particular type of activity can be reliance on the opinions, attitudes and procedures one learned and adopted from teachers or other predecessors and which are hence considered as perfectly sensible.

If I may refer to a personal experience, I remember that, 35 years ago, I attended a course in psychiatry, in which patients with severe mental disturbances were brought before an audience of more than a hundred students: people afflicted with depression, paranoia or schizophrenia, for whom the confrontation with this audience must have been a dreadful experience. At that moment, like the professor and most students, I considered this as absolutely normal and I am still ashamed now for not having understood the shocking inhumanity of this procedure.

Of course, my point is not to suggest that a great number of research workers are unaware of the ethical codes of their profession; I only submit that we should always remain conscious of the fact that the internal dynamics of our activities may result in making us less alert to the possibility of deviations.

Being acquainted with some classical examples of research procedures that we now consider as utterly immoral, we are inclined to place all of them exclusively in the past. There was the vivisection on criminals by Alexandrian physicians of the third century BC; there are the well-known cases of Jenner's and Cotton Mather's vaccination experiments and Walter Reed's research on yellow fever (Reich, 1978, Vol. 2, pp. 684–690).

After the Second World War, it was generally assumed that these aberrations had been definitely eradicated, but many years later it was found that experiments in the non-treatment of syphilitic patients were still going on in Tuskegee, and that mentally handicapped children had been contaminated with hepatitis virus in the Willowbrook school (Reich, 1978, Vol. 3, pp. 1319–1320). And although the Helsinki code was perfectly clear on the topic of informed consent, it did not prevent large-scale experiments being carried out in prisons in the United States, although it is difficult to understand what 'self-determination' can mean in these surroundings.

It certainly cannot be denied that science in general, and biomedical science in particular, has been extremely successful, and greatly contributed to the well-being of mankind. But the triumphalist self-image of many biomedical scientists as to being the best guardians of care and humanity, should be modified somewhat. A keen awareness of the risks involved in this profession (as of many others) is needed to guarantee that the ethical standards will be upheld, even and especially in borderline situations.

Only when these primary goods: the right to self-determination and the right not to be harmed, are continuously taken into account, are we entitled to wholeheartedly engage in the other good we intend to realize: the curing of many fellow human beings and the improvement of biomedical science in general.

These considerations lead us to the following principles regarding human experimentation.

(a) Every physician or researcher has the obligation always to take into account the right to *self-determination* of each human being. This principle implies that nobody may ever be submitted to experiment or therapy without their explicit consent and this consent should be the more informed, the more pain or risk are involved.

(b) Sometimes one is confronted with people who are not able or less able to give informed consent: small children, mentally disabled persons, comatose patients or people who can be put under pressure, the poor, prisoners, etc. These are the cases where the importance of the second moral value of our civilization comes into prominence: the right *not to suffer*. A decent application of this principle implies that all these people can only be subjected to therapy or research when their own well-being is directly aimed at and when, as best as one can, their minimal consent has been obtained; even then, suffering should be reduced to a minimum.

The importance and the indispensability of this second principle reveals itself in a pre-eminent way when one considers *experiments on animals*. Animals do not seem to have the potential, and hence have no right, to self-determination and this consideration has certainly influenced the fact that for centuries people in our civilization have made animals suffer needlessly or pointlessly without worrying much about it (Singer, 1975; Regan, 1983; Thomas, 1983).

This attitude was obviously influenced by the thesis that man – as God's image in the Christian tradition, or as the only creature with the gift of reason and consciousness in the philosophical tradition – had such a privileged position that a potential worth of animals and their capability to suffer was not thought of.

This point of view, however, was not a universal one. According to the Egyptian *Book of the Dead*, ill-treatment of cattle was prohibited, and in the Indian tradition – especially in Buddhism and Jainism – a very positive attitude towards animals was adopted. But in the Greek, Roman and Biblical traditions, which have thoroughly influenced Western culture, regard for animals was practically unknown and, as a consequence, the concern for their suffering is a relatively recent phenomenon in our civilization (Nash, 1990).

As far as Western biomedical science is concerned, it may certainly be considered a disgrace that for a long time and without much scruple, painful experiments on animals were carried out. We have to admit that considerable progress has been made in medical science by experiments on animals, but the fact that this, maybe indispensable, research was done frequently without caring about the suffering of animals will forever cast a shadow on this otherwise remarkable achievement.

Whoever is willing to consider seriously the second principle mentioned above which has developed in the course of our history, viz. that one should not cause suffering, inevitably gets confronted with the question of how we can advance a rationale for our intense involvement with the suffering of human beings on the one hand, and our unwillingness to extend this concern to the suffering of animals on the other.

The key problem in this respect comes to the fore when one examines the consequences of what I call 'the crucial hypothesis concerning animal suffering'. In the Western tradition the potential to suffer is often associated with the typically human form of consciousness: self-awareness. It is plausible indeed that the form of self-knowledge typical of human beings – that makes possible a simultaneous view of past, present and future – increases their potential to suffer because, amongst other things, an awareness of the duration of pain in the past, or the anticipation of it in the future, can arouse feelings of exhaustion or anxiety which, without this knowledge, could hardly be present to the same extent.

But as soon as human suffering has been associated with this typically human form of awareness, one cannot avoid the conclusion that whenever the level of consciousness is diminished or not yet present, as is the case with severely mentally handicapped people or with very young children, the *potential for pain* will be reduced to an equivalent degree.

If we assume, which is highly probable, that some higher animals possess a form of consciousness which exceeds that of these babies or mentally disabled, *the crucial hypothesis* inevitably forces itself upon us: *the potential of certain higher animals to suffer might be greater than that of certain human beings.*

Since we can never directly assess the quality of pain of other human beings, let alone of members of other species, this hypothesis certainly cannot be refuted. It is even a plausible one, because research of expressions (e.g. the detection of forms of anxiety) as well as the analysis of the central nervous system, show more complexity with certain animals than with the above-mentioned people (Sperlinger, 1981; Anstötz, 1993; Goodall, 1993; Patterson & Gordon, 1993; Ryder, 1993).

Considering the opinion which is gaining strength in our culture, that suffering is always *intrinsically wrong* and that we have to prevent it as much as possible, we have no right to discard the possibility that this crucial hypothesis may actually be true.

Considerations of this type have led some people, especially Peter Singer, to the opinion that a clear division between men and animals cannot be maintained and that in some cases more rights should be assigned to certain higher animals than to those people who are less liable to suffering (Singer, 1975).

I do not subscribe to this thesis. In my opinion, in the evolution of attitudes towards one's fellow man, it is a particularly valuable development that, when extending our neighbourly love, or in other words, when assigning certain fundamental rights, we do not introduce criteria according to which some people deserve such rights to a larger extent than others. The only means to maintain this principle in theory as well as in practice, is that we stick to a consensus which says that everyone born as a human being, alive and viable, has equal human rights. This means that every human being has the right to life and the right not to suffer and that every human being has the right to self-determination, except in case of non-competence.

It seems to me of the utmost importance that the consequences of the crucial hypothesis, however impressive they may be, should not affect this universal achievement.

But, as soon as these human rights are secured, one has to take into account all the implications of this hypothesis. This means that the suffering of animals must from now on be a real concern to us. As Bentham strikingly remarked, in this context the key question is not 'Can they *reason*? nor Can they *talk*? but Can they *suffer*'? (Bentham, 1789). If we care about the possible suffering of a newborn child, the reality or the quality of which is unknown to us, then we must be aware of the extreme inconsistency and incoherence of disregarding the suffering of animals, which, given the complexity of their facial and bodily expressions, seems almost unquestionable.

My conclusion would be the following. The principle that humans, because they are humans, have specific rights, is extremely valuable, but when this principle is used to introduce such a profound gap between men and animals that the suffering of the latter is disregarded, one can only consider this as an aberration.

It would, however, be a second misconception to argue that, concerning rights, the principle of equality, which is so valuable for human beings, must also be applied to animals in general. After all, there is no denying the fact that there *are* enormous differences between animals regarding the complexity of the central nervous system and the typical expressions that suggest suffering. It follows that our concern should increase in proportion to their potential for suffering.

Such an approach enables us to weigh the pros and cons of certain experiments in problematic cases. If a researcher holds that a specific animal experiment is vital for a substantial progress of science or an increase of human welfare (or possibly of animal welfare) he can take into account a number of considerations: the species of the animal and its liability to suffering, the importance of the research project, the fact that he has to kill the animal and that he may cause some harm to it. The significance of proper moral conduct – from this point of view – consists of the fact that such a decision *is not taken for granted*, but that it is only made after an authentic evaluation of the hierarchy of values and that even then no stone is left unturned to maximally reduce the suffering or even the discomfort of the animal.

Once such a responsible attitude is present – but only then – it seems to me that the use of experimental animals can be defended, even when some discomfort is caused, but alternatives should be more and more sought. It also follows that for purely economic aims or for reasons of human comfort (e.g. in the cosmetics industry), causing pain to animals is to be regarded as essentially immoral.

Finally, I have to point out again that the above-mentioned triumphalistic self image of the scientist as serving the progress of civilization and the conviction that traditional procedures and deontology offer a sufficient ethical basis, can prevent an adequate judgement of this ethical problem. A responsible scientist who wants to adhere to a coherent set of ethics in all his doings, must constantly keep in mind the two above-mentioned essential values of our civilization on the one hand, and the risks of too much confidence in his commitment and traditional attitudes on the other.

References

Anstötz, C. (1993): Profoundly intellectually disabled humans and the great apes: a comparison. In: *The Great Ape Project. Equality beyond Humanity*, eds. P. Cavalieri & P. Singer, pp. 158–172. London: Fourth Estate.

Beaufort, Inez Duconia de (1985): *Ethiek en Medische Experimenten met Mensen.* Maastricht: Van Gorcum.

Bentham, J. (1789): *An introduction to the principals of morals and legislation.* London: Athlone Press 1970 (reprinted).

Goodall, J. (1993): Chimpanzees – bridging the gap. In: *The Great Ape Project. Equality beyond Humanity*, eds. P. Cavalieri & P. Singer, pp. 10–18. London: Fourth Estate.

Hersch, J. (ed.) (1968): *Le droit d'être un homme.* Paris: Robert Laffont.

Nash, R. (1990): *The rights of nature. A history of environmental ethics.* Leichhardt NSW: Primavera Press.

Patterson, F. & Gordon, W. (1993): The case for the personhood of gorillas. In: *The Great Ape Project. Equality beyond Humanity*, eds. P. Cavalieri & P. Singer, pp. 58–77. London: Fourth Estate.

Pritchard, J.B. (ed.) (1955): *Ancient near Eastern texts relating to the old testament.* Princeton: University Press.

Regan, T. (1983): *The case for animal rights*. Berkeley: University of California Press.

Reich, W.T. (ed.) (1978): *Encyclopedia of bioethics*. 4 Vols.New York: The Free Press.

Ryder, R.D. (1989): *Animal revolution. Changing attitudes towards speciesism*. Cambridge, MA: Blackwell.

Singer, P. (1975): *Animal liberation: a new ethics for our treatment of animals*. New York: Random House.

Sperlinger, D. (ed.) (1981): *Animals in research. New perspectives in animal experimentation*. Chichester: John Wiley.

Thomas, K. (1983): *Man and the natural world: changing attitudes in England (1500–1800)*. Harmondsworth, UK: Allen Lane/Penguin Books.

The ethics of animal and human experimentation, edited by P.P. De Deyn.
©1994 John Libbey & Company Ltd., pp. 13–24.

2

The anthropological dimension of biomedical research

Evert van Leeuwen

Department of Metamedicine, Section of Philosophy and Medical Ethics, Faculty of Medicine, Free University, Van der Boechorststraat 7, 1081 BT Amsterdam, The Netherlands

Summary

Ethical review of biomedical research is nowadays accepted as an important part of the procedure which has to be followed in cases where human beings are involved in the research protocol. But nevertheless problems remain with regard to ways in which the ethical guidelines are interpreted in practice and with regard to new developments in the research itself.

In this chapter, those problems are brought into a relationship with philosophical views of man. The dichotomies of 19th century anthropology are still used in framing the moral questions with respect to biomedical research, while other perspectives have been developed in both science and philosophy. It is argued that these latter perspectives are more suitable to evaluate developments in biomedical research, while they still safeguard the freedom of choice and consent as preliminaries; moreover, that freedom is considered also as an essential stimulus of the biomedical research itself.

Introduction

The Declaration of Helsinki (Tokyo and Venice) has by now been widely accepted in matters concerning the ethics of biomedical research. The guidelines are considered essential to most of the research protocols and often it is explicitly stated that the protocol should only be carried out in keeping with the Declaration. Furthermore, Institutional Review Boards (IRBs) or Ethics Committees have been set up in many clinical centres to examine the protocols in an interdisciplinary manner. In the Netherlands such review boards also discuss experiments which are designed for general practice.

Apart from the guidelines, legal protection of human and animal subjects has been established in order to compensate for the possible damage. One could therefore say that, for example in many European countries as well as in the USA, an adequate social and moral framework has been established in order to tackle the different aspects of developments in biomedical research and technology. A broad consensus seems, moreover, to have been created between all the parties involved, enabling therapists, research-fellows and patients to discuss the ethical issues in a clear spirit and an unambiguous voice.

But the appearance of a clear sky conceals several dangers and risks. Solidification of the existing ethical procedures into binding rules might for instance create an institutional bureaucracy with its own 'free riders', to use a concept of Rawls (Rawls, 1971). Some areas of research or some influential scientists might be granted opportunities which are forbidden on moral grounds to others. Strict ethical ruling might on the other hand enlarge the distance between the daily practice in which protocols are carried out and the ethical considerations which accompany approval by the IRB. More rules, even enforceable ones, do not solve such a problem, since they do not necessarily lead to an improvement of a situation in which the scientist feels himself alienated from the meaning and content of the ethical rules.

Other problems arise with the progress in research. They are connected to the possibilities provided by medical technology. The moral evaluation of research on genetic modification for instance is only about to start. Experiments in this area are still controversial and have caught the attention of the general public. Administrators and politicians as well as philosophers and ethicists are now pondering public policies towards genetics. The ethics of carrying out experiments has become an issue, and the question is even debated whether or not those experiments should be designed at all. The IRBs do not have the capacity to evaluate these questions in local institutions and sometimes their integrity and independence is disputed in these matters. Legal frameworks and central commissions are therefore proposed, for instance in the Netherlands, to gain moral control of research developments. The danger of a moral straitjacket for scientific creativity reappears in this situation.

The danger of solidification and possible restrictions on research development jeopardize the present interaction of ethics and biomedical research. The problems are linked with the anthropology which underlies the moral and scientific outlook on biomedical research. The views on man which are at stake were created in 18th and 19th century philosophies and belong nowadays to the common sense of the Western democracies. The names of Locke, Hume, Rousseau and Kant are invariably connected to them. The anthropological thoughts of these philosophers were, however, accompanied by metaphysical views on science and epistemology, views that have nowadays become outdated in their basic philosophical dichotomies. Starting with these dichotomies we will try to show how they influence the present relationship between science and ethics. Then we will proceed by examining the central anthropological notions belonging to the moral guidelines and biomedical research. Finally we will suggest how the anthropological inheritance can be useful in order to meet the present demands of biomedical research.

Some philosophical dichotomies

The history of biomedical experiments is a lengthy one. Ethical issues of the last four decades, for instance concerning the use of prisoners or mentally handicapped persons as subjects, already bothered physicians and philosophers in Ancient Rome and Greece (Beecher, 1970). But the ways in which these issues are dealt with in history have changed radically over time, following the changes in the broader morality of Western culture and changes in the place and function of medicine in society. In other words, the history of biomedical experiments did not come up with a fixed morality pertaining to the use of human or animal subjects in the search for medical knowledge. The traditional medical ethics of the Hippocratic Oath alone constitutes an ambivalent ground for these actions.

The 'birth of the clinic' in the 19th century (Foucault, 1963) did not significantly change this situation. It moreover resulted in a sharp distinction between science and morality. The views of scientists like La Place, Sir Austin Bradford Hill, Bernard, Semmelweiss and Helmholtz were and still are influential in this matter. These pioneers of biomedical science and epidemiology mostly rejected every metaphysical understanding of living beings within science and they developed their interpretation of morality accordingly. Starting with some of the empirical concepts of the epistemology of the Enlightenment, a methodological difference between the natural sciences and the life sciences was denied and later a positive ideal of objective scientific theories was established. Science should restrict itself to delivering objective facts and definite laws or theories about observed living phenomena. To realize that positive ideal, a sharp distinction was made between scientific methods and other, like philosophical, religious or ethical methods of thinking. That distinction was corroborated by several dichotomies which made up the philosophical grounding for science during the Enlightenment but were heavily disputed in the metaphysics of the 19th century. Exclusion of this kind of metaphysics from science also meant that those dichotomies became considered as a self-evident part of 'common sense' knowledge on which scientific theories could be built. The following dichotomies are of interest here: mechanism–freedom; nature–nurture; animal–human; objective–subjective; fact–value; quantity–quality; organism–person; research–therapy.

Most of these dichotomies are nowadays overthrown by natural science as well as by the life-sciences and social sciences, but their self-evident, common sense character means that they still prevail in the philosophical and moral debates concerned with the applications of science and technology. That prevalence is perhaps due to the success of the scientific methodology behind which they stand, so that the philosophical critiques of, for instance, Husserl, Whitehead and Wittgenstein could not break their signifying strength.

What reasons can be given for that strength?

The principal reason seems nowadays to lie in the epistemology of Kantian idealism. Only rational procedures can account for the results of scientific reasoning and every external cause, coming either from the essence of the real thing or from some given morality, should be excluded. Not even human hopes or expectations should interfere with the process of gaining knowledge. Kant made this brilliantly clear in his distinction between the three functions of the human reason – the pure reason, the practical reason and the power of judgment – by connecting them to three questions with a definite order of priority: 'What can I know?', 'What should I do?', 'What can I hope for?' (Kant, 1956). This threefold distinction liberates the observing and knowing mind from external limitations and gives full priority to the freedom of research within the (metaphysically drawn) boundaries of the human capacity to know. By putting the question 'What can I know' first, Kant unquestionably made a major philosophical contribution to the advancement of science. He constructed a model in which knowledge could become the pure result of reason.

Within the context of a review board (IRB) this priority can still be recognized: firstly, the scientific claim must be examined, for without a genuine scientific problem with a suitable methodology, the experiment should not be performed at all ('What can we know?'). Then the procedure according to which the experiment is to be carried out must be examined, in order to prevent unnecessary risks and dangers ('What can we do?'). Finally the possible results have to be balanced against the possible burdens for the patient ('What can we hope for?'). Facts and values, objective results and subjective experiences, all have to be sharply delineated during the discussion about these matters.

But Kantian metaphysics are not being debated during the IRB deliberations. Instead, the aforementioned dichotomies are used in making distinctions and their strength seems to depend on that function: the way in which they serve to divide and to compartmentalize the questions involved so that they can gain a definite answer. In this way the dichotomies have taken over the fundamental position which metaphysics has in Kantian idealism: they are considered as the obvious notions belonging to ordinary language by means of which metaphysical questions can be evaded.

The use of the dichotomies enables us furthermore to give a rational account of otherwise incomparable things, such as the fruits of scientific insight versus the burden of pain for a patient, or the delay in his therapy. The dichotomies do not solve the ethical problems involved but their rhetorical function makes further distinctions possible that do not interfere with the process of gaining knowledge nor with that of moral deliberation. They only serve to partition the questions and provide a key for the ordering and weighting of these subsets. Of course these functions do make the dichotomies highly significant in the process of moral deliberation. Scientific interpretations become available without invoking underlying systems of religious, moral and cultural beliefs. If, for instance, a research protocol is designed for white males, scientific reasons can warrant the choice of the population as based on distinctions of natural fact, whereas in other circumstances the choice could be considered as resulting from a cultural flaw of racism or sexism. The difference between the option of a scientific selection and that of racism or sexism is made possible by the dichotomies of nature-nurture, organism–person and fact–value. From a Kantian point of view that would be impossible without questioning the dichotomies themselves. According to that view, the boundaries of the human capacity to know are metaphysically related to broader concepts of anthropology and morality. The exclusion of those metaphysical considerations implies that all kinds of interpretations become possible, even those which are flagrant contradictions of the Kantian ideal of human knowledge.

At this point we should reconsider the social function of the dichotomies in the ordering process which belongs to the ethical guidelines on biomedical research. The Declaration of Helsinki as well as the rules of Good Clinical Practice are essentially build upon the idea of objective knowledge that can be obtained on a solid basis of scientific procedures without harming anybody without his or her permission. This objective is congruent with the mentioned ideal of medical science as it emerged in the 19th century. But that is not all. We should not forget that most of the guidelines and rules have a more recent background in the tragic experiences of Nazi Germany and Japan, as well as in abuse in the United States and other countries (Beecher, 1966). Those negative experiences did not merely arise out of a personal lack of moral integrity or out of a malicious use of power. The Nuremberg Code which was drawn up after the Second World War, had a predecessor in Germany in 1931; a precise law which nonetheless was not obeyed. A horrifying ideology caused a twisting of the fundamental anthropological and metaphysical concepts which stood behind the legal ruling (Sass, 1988).

The codes or even laws concerning human experiments can therefore not in themselves prevent abuse or malpractice, they can only help someone to direct (guide) his thoughts and actions. They emphasize the human values at stake within the ordering of the scientific, therapeutic and moral topics and they stress the importance of balancing all the different items involved.

In this way they do not yield automatic results. They presuppose a perceptive scientist as well as an ideological climate in society that favours an interaction of scientific research and a discussion of basic human values. It is therefore necessary that those values are clearly stated in a way that is coherent with the development of biomedical research. That the dichotomies are not sufficient to serve this end as is shown not only by recent history as well as by the present pressures on biomedicine, related to genetics, fertility and other fields of innovative research, but also by economical and political demands. The anthropological views behind the guidelines and the ones implicated in biomedical research have therefore to be reexamined in order to see how these views can be linked together.

Guidelines and liberties

Moral guidelines, or moral codes in general, presuppose some kind of freedom. At least freedom in making decisions on reasonable grounds is preliminary. Honesty and integrity are also important virtues connected with responsible action. The guidelines are obviously addressed to people who possess such virtues in respecting other living beings.

The view that guidelines, as well as IRBs, should give moral directions in performing experiments, while granting freedom to scientists in making their decisions, has become part of the liberal view on man. This view suggests an equal capacity in every human being to reason without external constraints. That capacity is based on the concept of a free will. Every human being is supposed to be endowed with a free will, in contrast to animals or plants. The freedom of the will constitutes the ultimate ground for granting people a right in making decisions. While everybody is supposed to be endowed with the same free will, it follows that everybody has the same right in making decisions about his life and well being. Actions between two people should therefore be based on mutual agreement, on equal grounds. Equality has in this way become the cornerstone of the legal systems in democratic societies. The law exists to protect everyone's free will and to prosecute those who violate the rules which are made for the common benefit of all (Rawls, 1971; Broekman, 1991).

The concept of a free will which is at stake here is not without difficulties in daily practice, including the practice of medicine and biomedical research. Those difficulties are apparent even at the level of the legal aspects of the physician–patient relationship. The commitment from the medical professional towards his patient limits the concept of freedom in decision-making, while the patient has to entrust himself to the medical professional (Pellegrino & Thomasma, 1988). Dworkin (1993) showed recently which difficulties can be involved in a direct application of a legal system in matters of life and death.

These problems have to do with the philosophical background of the concept of a free will. Within the dichotomies, free will was opposed to mechanisms which are determined by laws of cause and effect. Only man was considered to be able to escape from these mechanisms by means of his reasoning capacity. The concept of a free will was regarded as the moral and philosophical basis to resist social pressure and repression and it became thus seen as a human fact underlying Western democracy. Problems connected with that view were originally debated in metaphysics, but are nowadays circumvented by considering the free will as a legal fact which has to be taken into consideration. Instead of a metaphysical dogma, a legal dogma has been created. The law has taken the place of metaphysics in this matter (Dworkin, 1986).

But if free will is conceived as a legal concept, stating a legal matter of fact, problems concerning the practice of medicine and of biomedical research still cannot be evaded by legal reasoning. These problems can be divided into three groups:

Problems connected to the question: how can it be verified that someone has free will?

This question is crucial to a scientific understanding of the dogma of legal reasoning. How is it to be answered? Remember William James who said: 'My first act of free will is to decide that I have a free will.' This statement makes clear that 'having a free will' is not an observable phenomenon or a scientific fact. It is a value created by a performative act and it has to be bestowed upon human beings by themselves or other human beings; or it has to be considered as a metaphysical token, characteristic of man in relation with the image of the Creator. The replacement of metaphysics by the law which has taken place in most Western societies has transformed those valuations into a matter of fact connected to the legal concept of a person. This means that someone who is above 18 years old and capable of a reasonable evaluation of his or her interests, is automatically endowed with a free will.

The transformation creates however a number of problems in biomedical research. If a free will is required, then experiments involving: fetuses, babies, children and adolescents under 18, comatose people, mentally handicapped, the insane and people suffering from dementia, and elderly people could not be accepted. Additional measures become therefore necessary within the legal system. A legal fact, however, cannot be misrepresented or disregarded, while on the other hand it leaves no room for multiple interpretations. Only reformulation of the fact or a circumventing procedure can solve the problem which is created by the juridification of the concept of free will.

Researchers from the Netherlands risk facing this situation at the present moment. Indeed, a proposed law which would systematically exclude all the abovementioned groups from biomedical experiments, because informed consent cannot be given, has been submitted to Parliament. Only a national Ethics Committee, consisting of at most 13 members, and falling under the direct control of the Minister of Justice, is allowed to give permission to perform an experiment with one of these groups (Tweede Kamer der Staten Generaal, 1992). With this proposal the acceptance of the ethical review by scientists is likely to be endangered and a bureaucratic process of alienation can be envisaged.

Problems concerning living beings to whom a free will is denied

Plants and animals are exempt from the possibility of having a free will. Until recent times these groups of living beings were consequently considered as possible subjects for all kinds of experiments. People like Schweitzer, who considered it an evil deed ('Grausames Tun') to make animals suffer for reasons of human interest were not taken seriously.

Owing to the ecological crisis, the general attitude of trivializing the suffering of animals has changed, however, and a new interest in the morality of experimenting with animals has emerged. But on what basis should these experiments be evaluated if the concept of a free will procedure is not applicable? All kinds of arguments come up in which animal and plant rights are defended. But these rights cannot be established as equal to human rights without disregarding the concept of a free will. Should ancient metaphysical and religious arguments about the essence of a natural being therefore be renewed, or are other strategies available?

An answer to the latter question is of great importance for developments in genetic research as well as in research on tissue transplantation. The type of moral judgement which could be relevant in these cases must not be based on emotional fears or on unwarranted beliefs that science will bring salvation. But within the context of genetics and transplantation, the ancient Aristotelian metaphysics will not suffice in the light of the theory of evolution, nor will the metaphysics of deterministic mechanisms.

Artificial life forms will now pose even more complex problems for which the present morality based on the legal concept of a free will has no solution (Edelman, 1987, 1992). In practice this means that moral judgements about developments in clinical genetics, genetic modification and cloning are left to moral and political struggles, or the experiments become legally forbidden, which in turn might create the risk of illegal research.

The third group concerns the explicit expression of the free will

Even if someone is supposed to have a free will, it does not imply that he will use it or will be asked to use it. A serious demand in democracies therefore is that people must give explicit consent on the basis of full information. But this can hamper some types of research, while it might cause a bias in others. Some people do not even want to have the knowledge which might result from the experiment. Epidemiology and population screening can in these cases be obstructed because of formal demands which are derived from legal statements and procedures (Van den Broecke, 1991; Brutel de la Riviere & Giard 1991).

These three groups of problems show that the legal concept of a free will, based on the liberal view of man, is not adequate for the development of moral arguments pro or contra biomedical research. We need an anthropological foundation which can be endorsed by the empirical findings of scientific research. Otherwise, the significance of the moral guidelines can be severely compromised by alien concepts which are dictated by law.

Biomedical research

What kind of anthropological view is implied in the attitude of the modern scientist? The ideal view of a positive science posed a detached scientist who pursues his search for truth even at the cost of his own life. The stories of Madame Curie and of many physicians show the scientific heroism and human tragedies to which this ideal could lead. The truth which these people pursued had a general form and lasted eternally. Newtonian mechanics was its paradigm until the end of the 19th century. At the core of that paradigm rested the metaphysical assumption that the universe is made up of rational, stable formulae which yield certainty and solid objectivity. The scientist should forget his vain and transitory doings on Earth in order to study those formulae.

The ethics involved in that view are still important: the scientist must be left alone in his creative job and not be obstructed by short-sighted morality or politics; rational critique must be possible at any time in any place; when everything has become clear in the end, the theory can be made understandable to everyone possessing normal rational capacities. Moral conditions on the application are then to be defined.

The ethical considerations of the ideal view of science are complementary to those of free will in the liberal view. Together they endorse the huge scientific progress which has been witnessed in this century. But nevertheless, the ideal view has been overthrown by science itself. In natural science, the indeterminacy of states has taken a place next to the certainty of eternal laws. Truth can only be eternal in some areas of scientific knowledge, but in many areas perhaps theories will always have a provisional character: they last until a better one comes up.

Within the life sciences the problems are even more substantial. The idea of an encompassing theory of life or its evolution is no longer pursued in the detached way of pure reasoning. Experimentation in laboratories has taken its place. The experiments require some involvement between the scientist and his experimental object when basic assumptions and expectations are formulated (Polanyi, 1962). The theoretical ideas behind the experiments mostly have a hypothetical character which can be denied or corroborated by the results of the experiment. In this way the life-sciences show a pattern of the type of open questioning as has been proposed by Sir Karl Popper (1972) in his epistemological writings.

The attitude of the experimenting scientist has also changed. Nowadays he is no longer detached, absent-minded, but energetic, alert and ready to make new observations. The scientist does not try to get to the bottom of things, but he hopes to gain successful results in his strategy of interrogating the phenomena of living beings. The scientist has become part of a world-wide systematic process of gaining knowledge in which all kinds of powers are at work.

What kind of anthropology is nowadays implied in the life sciences? Focusing on the experiments, the life sciences have left behind Kantian idealism and the dichotomies which belong to it. Living beings are supposed to give real answers in the experimental process of questioning. All living beings experiment continuously with their surroundings and are apt to change accordingly. Structural parts are not the result of eternal laws belonging to creation, but they follow slowly a pattern of evolution. With respect to mankind, for instance, morality can be considered as a structural and necessary part of social behaviour resulting from an adaptive process to a specific environment.

Scientific experiments can also be considered as a logical step in the evolution of intelligent life, while no sharp distinctions between man and several other forms of life exist any more. In other words, living beings, including scientists and ethicists, do all take part in a process of change in which no fixed a priori concepts or rules exist.

The changes in the attitude of the scientist which pertain to this view and the ways in which the object of research is conceived, make it tempting to say that it has become apparent that moral control over science has lost its meaning. The process can not be stopped or regulated, there is nobody in control while everybody has to participate (Latour, 1987). But this would be a false conclusion comparable to the naturalistic fallacy. The possibility of change presupposes two other aspects of living beings, namely their vulnerability and their finiteness in time. In order to cope with these latter aspects in relation to the possibility of change, the mere process of change must be transcended as has been done in morality or metaphysics. The ability to change and the vulnerability of living organisms must be reflected in the basic concepts of that morality as well as in the possible ways to modify them. This makes it possible to develop a concept of freedom which has a meaning broader than that of legal concept of a free will and which includes respect for different kinds of living beings, regardless of their capacities.

The concept of freedom which is mentioned here has to do with the plasticity and vulnerability of living beings as part of their capacity to create change (Hollis, 1977). That freedom is present in every living being and cannot be restricted to one species. It is not a legal fact, but one with roots in experience. It has therefore a broad and pluralistic meaning which science only touches in experiments and probabilistic models. But nonetheless the broader concept can be recognized even in the fundamental areas of research.

It follows from this concept that human beings do not have a specific advantage over other living beings, as is stated in the legal concept of a free will. One could still argue that when the possibility of creative change and adaptation grows, the vulnerability also does. But such a line of reasoning would not be sufficient. The main argument for separating human beings from other living beings remains the (metaphysical) perception that human beings are capable of transcending their behaviour in an act of self-consciousness. From this act follow the concepts of freedom and good or evil and the capacity of self-determination. Therefore special attention should be given to any living being who has this capacity.

Towards a reformulated anthropology

In the last two paragraphs we have tried to show how the moral guidelines in biomedical research have become dependent on the legal concept of free will, bestowed upon legal persons. This concept is accompanied by dichotomies which rest upon rejected metaphysical insights. It has moreover no direct equivalent in scientific experience and reasoning. Within the context of the life-sciences, another concept of freedom with an empirical content is possible regarding all living beings. The experience of human freedom can be considered as originating from that freedom by means of transcending intellectual insight and self-consciousness. It is therefore possible to formulate an anthropological view of man in biomedical research without giving up the basic concepts of the freedom of choice and of research. A proposal is made here in four steps.

1. The experimental view contains the basic solution. Until now a definition of experiment was not given: the common sense definition that an experiment involves systematic ways to discover facts and to test theories and hypotheses could suffice. By now this definition needs some extension: experiments are part of the ways in which living beings adapt themselves to their surroundings and to each other, a part which entails some kind of continuous learning. Scientific experiments are systematic and controlled ways of learning by using rational insights. They are no longer the tests or application of divine eternal truths, but they are part of the specific activities of human and other living beings in their environment. They constitute one of the latest stages in the open process of the evolution of living creatures (Van Leeuwen, 1990).
Experimentation can thus be considered to be an essential activity of every living being, while human beings have developed the capacity to obtain knowledge and insight into the basic general aspects of the processes involved.

2. Human values belong to the factual existence of human beings. They are necessary in structuring the ways in which human beings deal with themselves and other living beings. The capacity to discern right from wrong, to acknowledge and to justify laws has been part of the evolution of the species. This means that those values must be considered as a part of the experimenting process, while the values themselves are open to modification as a result of the experiments. Values and facts together are moments in the ongoing process of change (Van Peursen, 1992). Research and ethics have therefore an intrinsic relationship with respect to the future of mankind, but also with respect to other living beings.

3. The scientific concept of truth does not merely result from abstract logical reasoning but it has also a practical significance in human activities. It signifies what is believed to be real on rational grounds. The state of the art in research shows that what is true today, can be false tomorrow. This limits the concept of truth not only in time but also in its scope. Encompassing anthropological theories of the essence of being human seem no longer possible. Within different disciplines and specialisms, particular theoretical insights are developed and the accompanying experiments yield particular results. A holistic theory is therefore excluded from science and must be replaced by coincidental linkages of different strategies in different fields of research.

4. The question of what it is to be a living being or a human being has to be newly addressed in philosophy and metaphysics on the basis of those scientific insights. The anthropocentrism which gave man a place outside the cosmos and granted him a different moral position by means of the concept of free will has to be abandoned. All living beings are part of an open experimental process of change. New forms of life will perhaps appear when biological theories are for instance connected with those on artificial life (Pattee, 1988). It is our task to review the basic values of freedom and of being human. A new kind of metaphysics to fortify the relationship between ethics and research is needed to accommodate these developments.

Conclusion

The anthropological dimension which is contained in biomedical research is too one-sidedly focused on a supposed exclusiveness of man, expressed in the concept of the free will. If we consider human beings as a living species evolving in an open, creative process, it is possible to retain the basic conceptions of human freedom and creativity in a continuous process of experimentation. To stop that process by means of legal ruling not only endangers the future of research but possibly also that of future generations of human beings as well as that of other living beings. The moral problems involved have to be submitted to a careful process of moral reasoning and sincere experimentation in order to fortify the respect for the capacities of living beings. That respect cannot be restricted to those beings who are thought to be bestowed with a free will. Philosophical and ethical research is needed to provide a morality which accounts for the typical human aspects of self-consciousness and intellectual behaviour on the one hand while it retains on the other a fundamental respect for the experiential, vulnerable behaviour which mankind shares with all living creatures.

References

Beecher, H.K. (1966): Ethics and clinical research. *N. Engl. J. Med.* **274** , 1354–1366.

Beecher, H.K. (1970): *Research and the individual: human studies.* Boston: Little Brown.

Broekman, J.M. (1991): Recht en antropologie. Brussel, *E Story-Scientia*, pp. 299–305.

Brutel de la Riviere, G. & Giard, R.W.M. (1991): De meerwaarde van medische diagnostiek. *Ned. Tijdschr. Geneeskd.* **135**, 1049–1053.

Dworkin, R. (1986): *Law's Empire*, p. vii. London: Fontana.

Dworkin, R. (1993): *Life's Dominion*, pp. 118–148. New York: A. Knopf.

Edelman, G.M. (1987): *Neural darwinism. The theory of neuronal group selection.* New York: Basic Books.

Edelman, G.M. (1992): *Bright air, brilliant fire*, pp. 188 ff. New York: Basic Books.

Foucault, M. (1963): *La naissance de la clinique.* Paris: PUF.

Hollis, M (1977): *Models of man.* Cambridge: Cambridge University Press.

Kant, I. (1956): *Kritik der reinen Vernunft*, p. 728. Hamburg: F. Meiner.

Latour, B. (1987): *Science in action.* Oxford: Open University Press.

Levy, S. (1992): *Artificial life*, pp. 337 ff. New York: Pantheon.

Pattee, H.H. (1988): Simulations, realizations, and theories of Life. In: *Artificial life*, ed. C.G. Langton, pp. 63–79. Santa Fe: Addison-Wesley.

Pellegrino, E.D. & Thomasma, D.C. (1988): *For the patient's good*, pp. 51–61. New York: Oxford UniversityPress.

Polanyi, M. (1962): *Personal knowledge.* London: Routledge.

Popper, K. (1972): *Objective knowledge*, pp. 206–256. Oxford: Clarendon Press.

Putnam, H. (1993): Objectivity and science-ethics distinction. In: *The quality of life*, eds. M. C. Nussbaum & A. Sen, pp. 143–156. Oxford: Clarendon Press.

Rawls, J. (1971): *A theory of justice*, Cambridge, MA: Harvard University Press.

Sass, H.M. (1988): Comparative models and goals for the regulation of human research. In: *The use of human beings in research*, eds. S.F. Spicker & I. Alon, pp. 50–52. Dordrecht: Kluwer.

Tweede Kamer der Staten Generaal (1991): Regelen inzake medische experimenten (1991), 22588, Sdu Uitgeverij.

Van den Broecke, J.P. (1991): Wetenschappelijk onderzoek en Privacy. *Ned. Tijdschr. Geneeskd.* **135**, 1023–1024.

Van Leeuwen, E. (1990): Between scientific application and therapy: the ethical consideration. In: *Developments in biological standardization*, vol. 71, pp. 161–171. Basel: S. Karger.

Van Peursen, C.A (1992): *Verhaal en werkelijkheid: een deiktische ontologie*, pp. 156–160. Kampen, Kok Agora.

The ethics of animal and human experimentation, edited by P.P. De Deyn.
 pp. 25–34.

3

Ethical aspects of the statistical analysis of clinical data

Leonard Kaufman* Marie-Paule Derde* and Marc Despontin†

**Department of Biostatistics and Medical Informatics, Vrije Universiteit Brussel, Laarbeeklaan 103, B–1090 Brussels, Belgium;* †*Eenheid Statistiek en Operationeel Onderzoek, Vrije Universiteit Brussel, Pleinlaan 2, B–1050 Brussels, Belgium*

Summary

The necessity of protecting the conflicting interests of the individual participating in a clinical trial and the community which is expected to benefit from the results of the trial in the future makes it both extremely difficult and important to be very attentive to the ethical aspects of statistical practice.

Therefore, both the set-up of clinical trials and the analysis of their results should be performed according to the rules of good statistical practice. Besides the issues related to the reliability of data, among which are fraud, consistency checks, and auditing, good statistical practices include the detailed planning of the statistical analysis in terms of the data that will be considered, the variables that will be used to investigate the objectives of the trial, and the statistical techniques that will be used.

This paper focuses on each of these items, and on some broader issues of the relationship between ethics and the statistical analysis of data. Also, the basic hypotheses and paradigm of statistical testing are discussed.

Ethics and sample size determination

If we were able to observe an entire population, instead of a sample, no statistical inference would be necessary (for the sake of the argument we shall not consider experimental errors). One of the major reasons for using statistical inference consists in minimizing the costs *sensu lato*. These costs *sensu lato* include time, money and ethical considerations, and are mainly quantified by the sample size. One of the crucial points in the set-up of clinical trials is therefore an objective estimation of the sample size.

From a purely mathematical point of view, the only answer to the question 'how large should a sample be?' is 'as large as possible'. However, ethical considerations are certainly fundamental for applying statistical inference in clinical experimentation and for determining the sample size:

- in order to minimize the number of animals or humans subject to experimentation;
- in order to minimize the time before successes in experimentation can be applied on a larger scale, at the same time guaranteeing a reasonable chance of drawing the correct conclusions on the basis of the experiment.

Indeed, overestimation of the sample size is to be avoided since it unnecessarily exposes subjects to experimentation, and underestimation is to be avoided as well since a too small sample mostly yields non-conclusive results, implying again that the subjects enrolled were unnecessarily exposed to experimentation. Procedures for sample-size calculations and power estimations as applied in the design of clinical trials are described by Meinert (1986).

Balancing the errors: an ethical decision

The methodology of statistics itself induces ethical problems, and implies compelling ethical choices by the experimenter in close co-operation with the statistician. Sampling necessarily introduces sampling variance, which is the basis for two types of errors which are inherent to statistical inference, and thus to statistical decision-making. When choosing between a null hypothesis (H_0) denoting an equality and a research hypothesis (H_1) indicating a difference or an effect, one is confronted with two possible errors:

- type I error which occurs when a correct null hypothesis is rejected (the so-called α risk)
- type II error in which a null hypothesis is accepted while it is false (the β risk).

These two risks are related in the sense that in order to decrease one of them the other must be increased. In fact, the statistician is confronted with a dilemma which is similar to that of a judge. A judge who wants to avoid the risk that a criminal should remain unpunished has to convict every suspect (set the type II error equal to 0). Of course, in such a situation, many innocent people will go to jail (a very large type I error). On the other hand, acquitting all suspects will eliminate the risk of convicting innocents (a very large type II error makes it possible to eliminate the type I error).

As the null hypothesis (usually) implies that a treatment has no effect (or no different effect from another treatment), the consequence of a type I error is to conclude that a treatment is effective (or different), while in reality it is not. Analogously, a type II error implies that the effectiveness of a treatment is not recognized.

Depending upon the costs (including the ethical impact) of making the two possible wrong decisions, the experimenter and statistician have to determine an optimal combination of both risks. This optimal combination should be completely dependent upon the study under consideration. For instance, the 'ethical cost' of wrongly rejecting a new test to detect HIV infection (while others exist) is lower than that of wrongly rejecting a new effective treatment of AIDS (while no such treatment is available). As decreasing one of the risks while leaving the other unaltered can only be obtained by increasing the sample size, the experimenter and statistician are always confronted with the following ethical problems:

- increasing the sample size, and thus increasing animal and/or human experimentation;
- choosing between a higher probability of rejecting an effective treatment and a higher probability of accepting an ineffective one.

In the latter choice, often the risk of the type I error (α) is emphasized. This results from the fact that, when performing a statistical test, the risk can be determined beforehand while this is not the case with the probability β of the type II error. Indeed, by definition, the β risk depends on the true effect of the treatment (or difference between two treatments), which is unknown. Therefore, the β risk can only be estimated under a number of hypotheses and usually (but unjustifiably) has less attention paid to it.

Furthermore, in most applications, a type I error implies the conclusion that a treatment is effective when it is not. Besides the ethical problem of the consequences of making a wrong result public, the error also confronts the researcher with the 'scientific' cost of having published a wrong conclusion. Indeed, very often only 'positive' results are submitted (or accepted) for publication in the scientific literature, which is not the case for those obtained by the risk of a type II error. This publication bias is a further motivation not to overemphasize the importance of the choice of α.

As it is good research practice in general, and good clinical practice in particular, to repeat experiments, a wrongly published conclusion will usually be detected (rather quickly). Taking into account a 5 per cent risk of making a type I error, the probability that this error would not be discovered after three independent repetitions of the same experiment is 0.000125, which is very small. An unpublished conclusion, being the result of a type II error, has only a small probability of being repeated, and will not soon be detected.

Ethics and statistical analysis

Statistics is an *a priori* science and should be applied as such. Otherwise the frequently heard slogan 'with statistics one can prove anything' has a basis of truth and is difficult to refute. Therefore, the ethical application of statistics implies that any statistical analysis should *a priori* be carefully planned and described in detail. Planning of the statistical analysis in the context of clinical research implies a description of the patients that will be considered in the analysis, the variables that will be analysed, and the tests that will be applied.

Patients to be considered

The protocol of a clinical trial generally describes in much detail the profile of the patients that may be enrolled in the trial. Mostly this concerns general patient characteristics such as age, the patient's disease profile (type, duration, intensity of the disease), restrictions concerning concomitant diseases and treatments (formulated in a set of exclusion criteria), as well as restrictions concerning previous participation in the same trial or other clinical trials and the requirement that the patient has given written or witnessed consent to participate. A discussion of the ethical aspects of consent can be found in Pocock (1984) and elsewhere in this volume (Ch. 4, *Balancing methodological rigour and ethical treatment*; Ch. 18, *Review procedure and review committees for research protocols involving humans*; Ch. 19, *Alzheimers disease: necessary elements in the review of research proposals*; Ch. 21, *Dissent on informed consent*;).

Notwithstanding the efforts made to describe accurately patients who might be included in the trial, inclusion and/or exclusion criteria are frequently violated and patients are enrolled who strictly speaking should not have been. Are these patients to be considered in the analysis or should they be excluded? The general tendency is to perform the analysis of clinical trials according to the 'intention-to-treat' principle, implying that such patients are retained for the evaluation. This type of analysis is based upon the principle that if an investigator judged the patient to be suitable for inclusion, one must respect his clinical opinion, and consider the patient evaluable. Though this principle surely merits application, there may be specific situations where patients violating the protocol requirements should be excluded, especially when protocol violations occur frequently. Besides the intention to treat analysis one might then wish to perform a per protocol analysis in which only patients are considered who strictly fulfil the protocol requirements. Therefore, the statistical analysis plan should unambiguously describe the patients who will be considered in the analysis and list the specific reasons for eventual exclusion of patients from the analysis.

An analogous problem arises when patients are enrolled in the trial, but prematurely withdrawn from the study, either because of study-related factors (for instance inefficacy or intolerance of the study medication) or because of the occurrence of an exclusion criterion during the study (for instance the diagnosis of an intercurrent disease mentioned as the reason for exclusion of a patient from the study) or because of reasons unrelated to the study (the patient withdraws his consent and refuses to continue, or is lost to follow-up, etc.). Such cases not only pose the problem of yielding incomplete data, thus making the analysis more complicated, but usually also introduce bias into the data, posing the question whether such patients should be included in the analysis or not. Suppose that in a trial, with follow-up visits 2 and 4 weeks after onset of treatment, some patients withdraw after 2 weeks. Evaluation of the results after 4 weeks without taking the withdrawals into account might give a biased view on the treatment effect.

Indeed, if the most frequent reason for withdrawing after 2 weeks appears to be drug inefficacy, the evaluation after 4 weeks without precautions will give a too optimistic view. On the other hand, if patients discontinue the treatment after 2 weeks because they feel healed, not taking this fact into account when performing the evaluations after 4 weeks, will lead to the treatment effect being underestimated. The statistical analysis plan should unambiguously describe how the data of patients prematurely discontinuing will be dealt with. Again, in the light of the intention-to-treat principle, it is general practice that the data of patients withdrawing, for whatever reason, are retained for analysis. In order to deal with the abovementioned problem of biasing the analysis, an 'endpoint analysis' can be carried out. In such an analysis, data missing due to non-attendance of one of the trial visits are estimated by the observations made at the previous visit (the last valid observation is carried forward to the following visits). Note that this implies that for patients withdrawing before the first visit under treatment, the baseline observation (made before onset of treatment) will be considered as the last available observation. The exact details on how these situations will be dealt with should also be described in the statistical analysis plan.

Variables to be analysed

Further crucial information to be mentioned in the analysis plan concerns the variables that will be evaluated. Again, sufficient information should be given to calculate or determine the variables to be considered unambiguously. For instance, in a hypertension trial, it is evident that the variables of interest will be defined on the basis of the blood pressure recordings. But even for a simple measurement such as blood pressure there is a multitude of possibilities for evaluation. The variables considered in the evaluation can be the actual recordings of systolic and diastolic blood pressure, but an evaluation can also be made of the mean blood pressure (defined as a weighed average of diastolic and systolic blood pressure). The evaluation can be based upon the actual blood pressure recordings after treatment or upon the change in blood pressure during treatment. One can be interested in the actual magnitude of the change in blood pressure during treatment or merely in the fact of whether patients respond to treatment, response being defined on the basis of the actual blood pressure measurements (e.g. if diastolic blood pressure drops below 95 mmHg). It is an absolute requirement that an exact enumeration of the variables that will be evaluated and the way they have to be calculated must be provided.

As more and more sophisticated instruments are used in clinical trials, the amount of information obtained is sometimes dazzling. Investigators frequently make the mistake of trying to evaluate all possible variables, sometimes without having a clear picture of the relevance of the information that can be obtained from the analyses. However, one should be aware that with an increasing number of evaluations, the risk of finding a false positive result also rapidly increases. In fact, when a statistical test is performed at the 5 per cent level of significance, one accepts a 5 per cent probability to conclude that the test is significant when in reality the null hypothesis (no effect) is true. If two statistical tests are performed, both at the 5 per cent level of significance, the probability of a false positive result in at least one of these tests approaches 10 per cent. Thus, when many tests are performed the probability in finding at least one which is significant when in fact the null hypothesis is true is very large. The risk then exists that too much importance will be attached to the variable found to be significant, and even that only the results of the significant variable will be reported (published) while non-significant results will not be mentioned. Therefore, the relevance of the variables that will be analysed should be indicated by defining the variable or the few variables which are most important for drawing the conclusions of the investigation (the primary variables). The other variables are supportive and their interpretation has to be made in view of the results obtained for the primary variables.

Analysis plan

Finally, the statistical analysis plan has to enumerate all hypotheses that will be tested and the statistical tests that will be applied for that purpose. A schematic overview of statistical tests frequently used for the analysis of clinical data is discussed by Spriet & Simon (1985). The possible variants of particular tests that will be used should be mentioned. For instance, will the chi-square test for two-by-two contingency tables be used with or without continuity correction? It is important to mention this in advance, since the Yates corrected chi-square test is usually somewhat more conservative. Also for chi-square tests, if categories have to be grouped for a valid application of the test, it should be foreseen which categories will be grouped (different groupings might yield different conclusions). A discussion of such issues is given by Fleiss (1981) and Matthews & Farewell (1988).

It is easy to realize that anticipating all possible problems that might arise with either patients or data, when writing the analysis plan, can be difficult, or even impossible. Therefore, the ideal procedure in analysing data from clinical investigations is to organize, after the data management phase but before the analysis phase, a pre-analysis session to discuss eventual problems with the data with all persons involved in the investigation. Then all problems with patients or data can be discussed and, if necessary, adaptations can be made to the analysis plan. It is evident that this meeting should take place without knowledge of the type of treatment patients received, prior to the disclosure of the randomization list.

Drawing conclusions: the research hypothesis *versus* the statistical hypothesis

Research methodology in general, and statistical methodology in particular, ask for a scientific theory to be tested. While the scientific theory would explain the mechanisms by which aspirin interferes with blood coagulation, the research hypothesis which is the object of the statistical test is not the mechanism, but the effect or result of this mechanism. Let us for example, consider the hypothesis that aspirin diminishes the number of platelets in the blood. Accepting this hypothesis does not mean that the underlying theory is true, which we are not able to falsify on the basis of the (testable) results. Too often it is forgotten that different theories may lead to the same results, and there is confusion between the acceptance of the results (the consequences) of a theory and acceptance of the theory itself. The absence of a one-to-one relationship between theory and consequence may lead to misinterpretation.

One well-known problem of the kind mentioned above is that of spurious correlation. Let us suppose that we construct the following scientific theory: the membership of a service club decreases the probability of a particular disease. Suppose that a statistically significant difference is observed between members and non-members. This does not imply that the theory is true, since the consequence is not falsified. It is more probable that the true theory is that higher social classes (which provide a majority of members of service clubs) have access to better medical facilities.

This problem is especially acute in retrospective studies, for which the tendency exists not to test an *a priori* theory against the data but to conceive a theory consistent with the data.

Another well-known problem of this kind is experimental bias. Experimenting on a new drug, the physician is likely to pay more attention to the patient than in normal conditions. In order to prevent confusion between two theories (theory 1, the success rate is higher for the new drug; theory 2, the success rate is higher due to better follow-up by the physician) the experimental plan should blind the physician. Ideally, the experiment should also be blind for the patient to be able to distinguish between theory 1 and a third theory: the placebo effect. The double-blind methodology attempts to discriminate between the research hypothesis and two straightforward alternative theories. But even in this case it is for example not excluded that the drug effect is accompanied by a placebo effect.

Data management

The chain is only as strong as its weakest link: correct statistical conclusions can only be obtained on the basis of correct data. Therefore, good statistical practices go hand in hand with good clinical practices aiming to assure high quality of data obtained from experimentation. This implies that strict procedures should be followed to ensure the correctness, the validity and the completeness of the data used in the statistical analysis of clinical data.

For clinical trials the standard procedure to attain this goal is to have the clinical trial monitor perform data verifications at the investigator's site, to manually check the completeness of the data (to verify whether all data that were to be recorded for the study are indeed mentioned in the case report forms (CRFs)), and to search for eventual contradictions. Obviously these procedures can be, and should be automatically performed by means of computer programs once the data are entered. However, early detection of problems can urge the investigator to be more attentive when subsequent CRFs are filled out and eventual systematic errors resulting from incorrect interpretation of the study protocol can be detected and prevented for future enrollment of patients. More elaborate verification at the investigator's site includes verification of the data transcribed in the CRF with the source documents (e.g. hospital file of the patient, laboratory results, radiographies. See also Ch. 17, *Good clinical practice: burden or blessing?*). This not only allows the correctness of the CRF data to be checked, but also whether all information relevant to the study has been mentioned in the CRF.

Extensive care should also be taken when entering data into the computer. A first precaution to reduce the error rate when performing data entry is to perform double-data entry. Most advisable is to have the data entered by two different persons, and to compare the two resulting data entry files for differences, preferably by a third person. Since the third person takes the decision on the data to be used in the analysis, it should preferably be someone with extensive knowledge of the study and of the information collected. Obviously this procedure may be time consuming, especially for large trials, but it ensures a low error rate. Another possibility, offered by some computer programs especially developed for data entry, is to have the data entered a first time, and to check the correctness of the data entered by setting the system into a so-called 'verify mode'. The data already entered are not displayed on the screen. It is then possible to key in the data a second time, and for each entry it is immediately checked whether the second entry corresponds to the first entry. In case of a difference between the two entries, both the first and second entry are shown on the screen, and the possibility is given of entering the correct value. Also with this procedure at least two persons are involved in entering the data, and since the person performing the second data entry has to take the decision for correcting the data, it should preferably be someone with extensive knowledge of the study and of the information collected. If the choice is made for single data entry then extreme attention should be paid when entering the data, which then again should be performed by someone with extensive knowledge of the study.

Another helpful tool for reducing the error rate when entering the data is to make use of a data entry program, which for each numeric variable only allows the entry of values within a predefined range. In this way typing errors resulting in invalid values of numerical data can already be prevented when entering the data. Also helpful is the possibility of using skip rules for conditional variables (variables that only have to be filled in when a previous variable takes a certain value).

A comparison of single- and double-data entry has been described by Reynolds-Haertle & McBride (1992). Not only is the comparison between the error rates of the two procedures interesting, but also the large between-person variability, and the observation that the error rates were different for different pages of the CRF. It appeared that one third of all errors were due to a single question. This urges the case for careful design of the CRF (well organized, straightforward).

Subsequently, all data entered should be listed on paper in a comprehensive way for a final inspection. A certain percentage (depending on the size of the trial) of the listed data should be compared with the CRFs. This might not only reveal data entry errors but also errors in the development of the data base itself. In cases where only a single entry was performed, the checking of all data can ensure the quality comparable to that of double entry.

After data entry, computerized data verification is warranted. Basically this should consist of the calculation of descriptive statistics for all numerical data (mean, standard deviation, minimum, maximum, extreme values for continuous variables, frequency distribution for discrete variables). Evaluation of the correctness of minimum and maximum values is of course necessary, but the value of the standard deviation in relation to the mean, minimum and maximum may also indicate errors in the data. Even more telling, but unfortunately also more time consuming to prepare and therefore perhaps preferable to restrict to primary variables, are graphical representations such as histograms or box-plots.

The verification procedures should not only be applied to the actual data entered, but also to derived data. If the weight of a patient is recorded on three successive visits at 1 month intervals, the variation 65 kg, 80 kg, 65 kg will not show up to be erroneous when evaluating the data at each visit. It is then necessary to calculate extreme values of the differences between visits in order to draw attention to a possible error. In the same way calculation of periods (numbers of days) between dates might reveal evident errors in the recording of dates.

The previously described procedures should become standard when performing data entry and will ensure a high quality of data used. Nevertheless, alteration or falsification of data, a practice which unfortunately also seems to occur in scientific research, and has been reported in the literature, most probably will not show up even when applying all procedures described above. Detection of deliberate alterations of data, for instance to be able to enroll more patients into a trial, can result from a careful inventory of the data and a verification of the entered data with the source data. An example of data alteration, and its detection, is described by Neaton *et al.* (1991). The detection of fabrication of data might even be more difficult. In general it can be expected that the falsifier of data will avoid drawing attention to problems with the data (e.g. corrections of the data in the CRF, abnormal values of data). It therefore may appear that CRFs containing fabricated data are rather clean as compared to average data, with very few strike-outs, and filled in rather systematically (all in the same handwriting, the same ball-point, only slight variations between evaluations of the same variables performed on several occasions, etc.). Obviously, the person most likely to observe the characteristics of the way CRFs are filled in is the trial monitor in the first place, but also the person performing the data entry. Furthermore, another series of data checks (not necessarily geared to the detection of alteration or fraud), can be performed. A first example is the verification of the day of the week that visits occur or investigations are performed (for most trials it is very unlikely that these occur on Saturday or Sunday). For laboratory data it can be checked whether the frequency of data out of the norm is not too small. Indeed, invented data may tend to have a too small frequency of abnormal data, because the falsifier might fear that data out of the norm might induce questions from the monitor.

However, since laboratory normal ranges generally correspond to 95 per cent tolerance limits, even in a normal population 5 per cent of the patients will have results outside the norms (in a disease population this frequency might even be higher). Also, in real data, correlations will exist between variables. It might be difficult not to disturb the correlation between variables when data are invented. A nice example is described by Bailey (1991). In order to detect patients with data deviating from the normal, not necessarily in the values of individual variables, but especially in the relationship between variables, the calculation of the Mahalanobis distance between the data of an individual and the sample mean might be useful (Evans, 1993).

Conclusions

Statistics is a scientific discipline concerned with formalized techniques allowing conclusions to be drawn, in a scientifically correct way, conclusions from experiments. It is a science that provides objective tools (confidence intervals, *P*-values) to a variety of other disciplines. These tools are used to convince fellow researchers that the conclusions drawn from experiments are correct or at least plausible. Unfortunately, far too often misuse is made of the formalism of statistics. Partly this is possible because still too often the meaning of hypothesis testing, the types of statistical errors, and the feeling of the exact meaning of the *P*-value are only half understood, and also due to the lack of knowledge of the fundamental principals on which specific statistical tests are based. On the other hand, especially for results published in journals, it is sometimes difficult to evaluate the quality of the data on which the tests were applied and to have a clear picture whether the published results are representative for the results obtained from the entire experiment. Therefore, ethical and methodological considerations are intertwined during all phases of data collection and statistical analysis.

References

Bailey, K.R. (1991): Detecting fabrication of data in a multicenter collaborative animal study. *Controlled Clin. Trials*, **12**, 741–752.

Evans, S. (1993): Statistical aspects of the detection of fraud. In: *Fraud and misconduct in medical research*, eds. S. Lock & F. Wells, pp. 61–74. London: BMJ Publishing Group.

Fleiss, J.L. (1981): *Statistical methods for rates and proportions*, 2nd edn. New York: John Wiley & Sons.

Matthews, D.E. & Farewell, V.T. (1988): *Using and understanding medical statistics*, 2nd edn., pp. 20–66. Basel: Karger.

Meinert, C.L. (1986): *Clinical trials – design, conduct, and analysis*, pp. 71–89. New York: Oxford University Press.

Neaton, J.D., Bartsch, G.E., Broste, S.K., Cohen, J.D., & Simon, N.M. (1991): A case of data alteration in the multiple risk factor intervention trial. *Controlled Clin. Trials*, **12**, 731–740.

Pocock, J.S. (1984): *Clinical trials – a practical approach*, pp. 100–109. Chichester: John Wiley & Sons.

Reynolds-Haertle, R.A. & McBride, R. (1992): Single versus double data entry in CAST. *Controlled Clin. Trials*, **13**, 487–494.

Spriet, A. & Simon, P. (1985): *Methodology of clinical drug trials*, pp. 157–197. Paris: Karger.

The ethics of animal and human experimentation, edited by P.P. De Deyn.

4

Balancing methodological rigour and ethical treatment: the necessity of voluntary, informed consent

Holly M. Gorman* and Francis C. Dane†

†*Department of Psychology*, **Department of Internal Medicine, Mercer University, 1400 Coleman Avenue, Macon, GA 31207-0001, USA*

Summary

Since the antivivisectionist movement of the early 19th century, most guidelines for the ethical conduct of research have been proposed in response to perceived harm to subjects. In this chapter, we argue that the inherent conflict between maintaining methodological rigour and preventing harm to research subjects can be resolved by paying particular attention to the social psychological variables that affect the process through which biomedical researchers obtain voluntary, informed consent. The processes underlying conformity and obedience to authority are likely to decrease subjects' abilities to refuse an opportunity to volunteer for research, and researchers must act to reduce such influences whenever such processes are likely to operate. Similarly, subjects' knowledge levels may pose challenges to informed consent. Under such conditions, we argue that it is the researcher's obligation to explain procedures and other necessary information such that prospective subjects are able to understand the information. Consent by proxy should be employed only when the subjects' intellectual ability limits understanding. Lack of knowledge on the part of prospective subjects, however, should be overcome rather than serve as justification for consent by proxy.

Introduction

Virtually all formal guidelines for ethical research have been introduced in response to what was perceived as unnecessary harm to research subjects. The first guidelines, for example, were promulgated by members of the antivivisectionist movement in 1822, at which time a bill that included penalties for inflicting cruelty upon research animals was approved in Great Britain (Dewsbury, 1990). Two years later, the

Society for the Prevention of Cruelty to Animals (later The Royal Society) was founded in London and became the first professional society to establish guidelines for researchers. The American Society for the Prevention of Cruelty to Animals was founded for similar purposes. In one country after another, Descartes's proposition that animals experienced no pain because they had no soul (Jaynes, 1970) was being replaced by guidelines regarding the fact that some harm was inevitable in the conduct of animal research.

Guidelines concerning human research subjects also developed in response to questionable research practices. In the United States, for example, passage of the National Research Act (Final Regulations, 1981) was prompted by the US Public Health Service's failure to treat a control group infected with syphilis, even though its own and others' research results had already established penicillin as a cure (Seiler & Murtha, 1981). The first international guidelines, the Nuremberg Code, were developed in response to atrocities committed by the Nazis in the name of research (Nuremberg Military Tribunal, 1948; Mappes & Zembaty, 1986; Monette *et al.*, 1986). The Nuremberg Code clearly established voluntary consent, including the subject's right to cease participation at will, as an essential element of ethical conduct in research.

Later, the Declaration of Helsinki (World Medical Association, 1964) introduced the notion of consent by proxy as a means by which to satisfy voluntary consent for legally incompetent subjects (Mappes & Zembaty, 1986). Most recently, the World Health Organization (WHO) (Bankowski & Levine, 1992) revised its uniform guidelines as a result of developments in AIDS research in underdeveloped countries (Marwick, 1991). WHO approved consent by proxy, but only as a last resort in situations in which it is clear that the prospective research subjects are not capable of granting informed consent.

Clearly, voluntary, informed consent is at the core of existing ethical guidelines. It is equally clear that those who are capable of conducting research have an ethical obligation to do so (Mindick, 1982; Dane 1990), and that biomedical research inevitably involves harming some subjects. Furthermore, because the questions addressed by biomedical research must lead to some protocol in which humans are subjects (Lavertu & Linares, 1990) for the express purpose of benefiting society (Bankowski & Levine, 1992), there exists an inherent conflict between methodological rigour and avoiding harm to research subjects. Voluntary, informed consent is the means by which we are able to resolve that conflict.

Voluntary participation

Animal research has received considerable attention in recent years partly because it is presumed that animals cannot volunteer to participate in research (Driscoll & Bateson, 1988). The same issue is at the heart of coercion concerning humans, i.e. the extent to which humans freely consent to participate.

Coercion of humans does occur, particularly in countries in which the government exerts considerable control over citizens (Lavertu & Linares, 1990). When such governments require research participation for the 'greater good' of society, researchers must consider whether the participants have played a role in the development of the societal goals. We maintain that government sanction does not free the researcher from the responsibility of avoiding coercion.

Coercion, however, is not limited to behaviour forced through explicit threats of negative consequences for refusal. Peers can exert considerable influence (Asch, 1951, 1952, 1958; Tajfel, 1982; Abrams & Hogg, 1990), and there is no reason to believe that groups of potential research participants are an exception to conformity influence (Lavertu & Linares, 1990). Protecting the confidentiality of one's participants, therefore, becomes part of avoiding coercion through conformity pressure. If members of the group are not aware of who is and who is not participating, they cannot exert influence upon those who prefer not to participate.

Research in the legal arena (Kassin & Wrightsman, 1980, 1981; Wells, 1980) also indicates that offers of reward can create coercive conditions. More important, an individual's decision to engage in an activity in response to a reward is much less likely to be perceived by others as coercive. Thus, excessive monetary inducements or certain offers of relief from symptoms are likely to result in coercion. Judgements concerning what is 'excessive' monetary inducement or 'exaggerated' symptom relief must be made from the viewpoint of the potential participant. What are petty amounts of money to the researcher might be a day's, week's, or month's earnings to the participant. Similarly, delay of death may be sufficient inducement to be considered coercive.

Finally, we note that the authority inherent in the researcher's social position may exert considerable influence upon the prospective participant (Milgram, 1974). If such authority can convince individuals to harm another, as was demonstrated in Milgram's research, it is reasonable to conclude that authority may coerce an individual to risk self-injury at levels greater than what would otherwise be acceptable. The Helsinki Code (World Medical Association, 1964), for example, includes specific advice to avoid situations in which the participant is dependent upon the researcher. We contend dependency may not be completely avoidable insofar as a researcher's authority, in the form of expertise and social position, is not avoidable. Therefore, it is the researcher's responsibility to ensure that voluntary consent includes informed consent.

Informed consent

The key element of informed consent is not the comprehensive nature of the information, but its relevance to the subject's decision to participate (Parsons, 1969). Any risk to the physical or mental health of the participant is necessary information, for one can reasonably expect health risks to alter a decision to participate. Because health risks are an inherent aspect of biomedical research, it is of utmost necessity that researchers exert every means necessary to obtain informed consent (Bankowski & Levine, 1992).

One can and should, however, distinguish between informed consent and educated consent (Ingelfinger, 1972; Beauchamp & Walters, 1978; Childress, 1981; Beauchamp & Childress, 1989). Becoming aware of information is a necessary, but not sufficient, condition for understanding the implications of information with respect to research participation. That is, informing an individual about the risks involved in research is no guarantee that the individual will understand a sufficient amount of the information to make an educated decision.

In some instances, there may exist an *a priori* assumption that the subject is not capable of making an educated decision. In many countries, for example, children are legally prevented from granting informed consent (Barber, 1976). Indeed, most children are incapable of educated consent, primarily because formal operations (Piaget, 1984) – the ability to use abstract reasoning – is not usually achieved until adolescence (Berk, 1991). Without formal operations, children are not able to evaluate potential risks. Presumably because adults have the intellectual ability to grant educated consent, one looks to the child's legal guardian for proxy consent (There is more on this in Ch. 27, *Research involving children: scientific and ethical aspects*)

In other instances, the impetus to employ proxy consent results from a belief that the prospective subjects do not have sufficient knowledge to understand relevant information. Lack of knowledge, however, is considerably different from reduced intellectual capacity, and the researcher is therefore obliged to develop alternatives to standard informed consent procedures (Lavertu & Linares, 1990) without undermining the subject's right to grant consent. The issue here centres on Beauchamp & Childress's (1989) reference to the dual meaning of the phrase 'informed consent.' One meaning refers to the autonomous choice of the subject, and the other meaning refers to the social rules of informed consent as an institutional process. Autonomous choice occurs when the subject authorizes participation with complete understanding of the situation; i.e. the subject grants educated consent. The social rules of informed consent deal with guidelines that have been developed for a particular institution; i.e. one's review board requires presentation of the risks and the subject's signature on the form describing the risks, but does not require any guarantee (other than the subject's signature) that the subject understands the risks. We contend that, in the absence of an *a priori* reason to conclude subjects are incapable of consent, it is the researcher's responsibility to present information in a form that can be understood by prospective participants. One cannot expect prospective subjects to assert their ignorance and ask for clarification (Veatch, 1982). Nor should one decide that ignorance, as opposed to intellectual capacity, is sufficient grounds to deny informed consent.

In contrast, there may exist research protocols in which deception is required for methodological rigour. We do not refer, of course, to deceiving subjects about risks attendant to their participation; such deception is clearly not ethical. Instead, we refer to deception concerning the purpose of the research, the research hypotheses, or similar aspects of the study. Although some argue that deception in a study involving risk is tantamount to preventing informed consent (Monette *et al.*, 1986; Beauchamp & Childress, 1989), we contend that deception may be permissible, provided certain conditions obtain. First, as we noted above, the deception should not reduce the subject's ability to understand the risks associated with participation, including the subject's willingness to terminate participation. Second, the deception must be a necessary aspect of the methodological integrity of the study. Subjects in a placebo group, for example, should be 'warned' about the same side-effects as subjects receiving the experimental drug whenever levels of general anxiety can be expected to affect the medical condition under investigation. Finally, the subjects should be made aware of the deception at the conclusion of the project and be made aware of the importance of the research. Smith's (1981) research indicates that subjects do not object to being deceived when the consequences are not overly unpleasant, when they do not feel coerced into participating, and when the research seems justified by its scientific importance.

To some extent, the power inherent in the research position, in this case expert power (French & Raven, 1959), may be as strong an influence upon informed consent as deception. The prospective participant may be unwilling to admit his or her inability to understand the information provided by the researcher. Conversely, the researcher may not be able to set aside his or her expertise so as to frame the decision in a manner suitable to the prospective participant's knowledge base (Tversky & Kahneman, 1974, 1980). In such instances, a community member should be utilized as a moderator (Lavertu & Linares, 1990). That is, rather than assume that the prospective subjects are incapable of understanding the relevant information, the researcher may have to accept that he or she is incapable of presenting understandable information. Recognizing one needs assistance with communicating information about one's own study, however, is likely to be a difficult process (Nadler & Fischer, 1986).

Conclusions

Since the establishment of the Nuremberg Code, voluntary, informed consent has been an essential component of biomedical research with humans. Recent developments concerning consent by proxy raise several issues that must be addressed. Although conformity pressure, lack of education, and deception are each capable of undermining prospective subjects' capacity, we contend that the authority and power of the researcher may be the greatest challenge to voluntary, informed consent. The importance of biomedical research, coupled with the researcher's status, may make it extremely difficult for prospective subjects to exercise their right to refuse to volunteer and to exercise their right to withdraw from an ongoing study. The educational difference between the researcher and the subjects may reduce the ability of the researcher to present understandable information to the subjects, thereby reducing the subjects' ability to evaluate risk. To compensate for these difficulties, we recommend researchers utilize moderators to explain the research and associated risks whenever status or education discrepancies are large.

References

Abrams, D. & Hogg, M. A. (1990): Social identification, self-categorization and social influence. *Eur. Rev. Soc. Psychol.* **1**, 195–228.

Asch, S. E. (1951): Effects of group pressure upon the modification and distortion of judgments. In: *Groups, leadership, and men*, ed. H. Guetzkow. Pittsburgh: Carnegie Press.

Asch, S. E. (1952): *Social psychology*. New York: Holt, Rinehart & Winston.

Asch, S. E. (1958): Effects of group pressure upon modification and distortion of judgments. In: *Readings in social psychology*, 3rd ed., eds. E. E. Maccoby, T. M. Newcomb & E. L. Hartley, pp. 174–182. New York: Holt, Rinehart & Winston.

Bankowski, Z. & Levine, R. J. (eds.) (1992): *Ethics and research on human subjects: International guidelines* (proceedings of the XXVIth CIOMS conference). Geneva, Switzerland: World Health Organization.

Barber, B. (1976): The ethics of experimentation with human subjects. *Sci. Am.* **234** (2), 25–31.

Berk, L. E. (1991): *Child development*. Boston: Allyn and Bacon.

Beauchamp, T. L. & Childress, J. F. (1989): *Principles of biomedical ethics*. New York: Oxford University Press.

Beauchamp, T. L. & Walters, L. (1978): *Contemporary issues in bioethics*. Encino: Dickinson.

Childress, J. F. (1981): *Priorities in biomedical ethics*. Philadelphia: Westminster Press.

Dane, F. C. (1990): *Research ethics and methods*. Pacific Grove, CA: Brooks/Cole.

Dewsbury, D. A. (1990): Early interactions between animal psychologists and animal activists and the founding of the APA committee on precautions in animal experimentation. *Am. Psychol.* **3**, 315–327.

Driscoll, J. W. & Bateson, P. (1988): Animals in behavioural research. *Anim. Behav.* **6**, 1569–1574.

Federal Register (1981): *Final regulations amending basic HHS policy for the protection of human research subjects.* **46** (16), 8366–8392.

French, J. R. P., Jr. & Raven, B. H. (1959): The bases of social power. In: *Studies of social power*, ed. D. Cartwright, pp. 150–167. Ann Arbor: University of Michigan Press.

Ingelfinger, F. J. (1972): Informed (but uneducated) consent. *N. Engl. J. Med.* **287**, 465–466.

Jaynes, J. (1970): The problem of animate motion in the seventeenth century. *J. Hist. Ideas* **31**, 219–234.

Kassin, S. M. & Wrightsman, L. S. (1980): Prior confessions and mock jury verdicts. *J. Appl. Soc. Psychol.* **10**, 133–146.

Kassin, S. M. & Wrightsman, L. S. (1981): Coerced confessions, judicial instruction, and mock juror verdicts. *J. Appl. Soc. Psychol.* **11**, 489–506.

Lavertu, D. S. & Linares, A. M. (1990): Ethical principles of biomedical research on human subjects: their application and limitations in Latin America and the Caribbean. *Bulletin of PAHO* **24** (4), 469–478.

Mappes, T. A. & Zembaty, J. S. (1986): *Biomedical ethics*. New York: McGraw-Hill.

Marwick, C. (1991): WHO expected to revise international ethical research conduct guidelines. *JAMA* **266**, 187.

Milgram, S. (1974): *Obedience to authority*. New York: Harper & Row.

Mindick, B. (1982): When we practice to deceive: The ethics of metascientific inquiry. *Brain Behav. Sci.* **5**, 226–227.

Monette, D. R., Sullivan, T. S. & Dejong, C. R. (1986): *Applied social research*. New York: Holt, Rinehart & Winston.

Nadler, A. & Fisher, J. D. (1986): The role of threat to self-esteem and perceived control in recipient reaction to help: theory development and empirical validation. *Adv. Exper. Soc. Psychol.* **19**, 81–122.

Nuremberg Military Tribunal (1948): *Trials of war criminals before the Nuremberg military tribunals*. Washington, DC: US Government Printing Office.

Parsons, T. (1969): Research with human subjects and the 'professional complex.' *Daedalus*, Spring, 325–360.

Piaget, J. (1984): Piaget's theory. In: *Handbook of child psychology*, Vol. 1 (4th ed.), ed. P. Mussen. New York: Wiley.

Seiler, L. H. & Murtha, J. M. (1981): Victory at HHS: Final regulations for the protection of human subjects of research provide a balanced compromise. *SASP Newsletter* **7** (2), 6–7.

Smith, C. P. (1981): How (un)acceptable is research involving deception? *IRB: A Review of Human Subjects Research* **3** (8), 1–4.

Tajfel, H. (1982): Social psychology of intergroup relations. *Ann. Rev. Psychol.* **33**, 1–39.

Tversky, A. & Kahneman, D. (1974): Judgment under uncertainty. Heuristics and biases. *Science* **815**, 1124–1131.

Tversky, A. & Kahneman, D. (1980): Causal schemas in judgments under uncertainty. In: *Progress in social psychology*, Vol. 1, ed. M. Fishbein. Hillsdale, NJ: Erlbaum.

Veatch, R. M. (1982): Limits to the right of privacy: reason, not rhetoric. *IRB: A Review of Human Subjects Research* **4**, 5–7.

Wells, G. L. (1980): Asymmetric attributions for compliance: reward vs. punishment. *J. Exp. Soc. Psychol.* **16**, 47–60.

World Medical Association (1964): *Declaration of Helsinki.*

The ethics of animal and human experimentation, edited by P.P. De Deyn.
©1994 John Libbey & Company Ltd., pp. 43–58.

5

Decision making in ethics: a challenge for clinician and researcher alike

Erich H. Loewy

Professor of Medicine, University of Illinois College of Medicine at Peoria and Professor of Humanities (Ethics), University of Illinois at Chicago

Summary

The process of making decisions in ethics, like the process of making decisions in any field, must, if it is to be generally successful, follow a logical process. Because its steps are well understood, a logical process has the advantage not only that it generally results in a more satisfactory outcome but also that it is easier to analyse, criticize or justify such an outcome retrospectively. Any discussion of ethics, especially across various belief systems and cultural contexts, must ultimately rely on rationality and on shared human needs and experience.

Unfortunately, decision making when it comes to dealing with practical ethical issues, is often done in a far more diffuse, undisciplined and basically disorderly manner. Often the source of unresolved conflicts can be traced to such a lack of approach. In this paper I want to offer some thoughts on various ways of approaching such problems and then see if we can apply these thoughts to ethical problems in the therapeutic as well as in the experimental sphere. To do this I shall: (1) briefly discuss the use of traditional ethical theories and approaches, contrast them with newer developments especially as they relate to casuistry, virtue and care ethics and then go on to sketch out a possible resolution; (2) describe the method I have used in dealing with actual cases in my work as an ethics consultant; (3) differentiate between therapeutics and experimentation; and (4) suggest a few ways in which what has been offered might be used in approaching ethical problems both in therapeutics and experimentation. It is obvious that such an undertaking is an ambitious enterprise and one which cannot be finished in a paper, in a volume or, for that matter, in a life-time; not only because contexts change, insights widen and problems adapt, but because, along with John Dewey (1991), I do not believe that problems can ever be solved: the best we can do is to make an 'indeterminate situation more determinate' (or as I, more of a pessimist, would put it: to make an indeterminate situation somewhat less indeterminate).

Theories and approaches

It is fashionable today to claim that humans from diverse cultures and belief systems will have great difficulty in discussing ethical problems because they do not share a common framework of discourse and are, therefore, 'moral strangers': persons who know virtually nothing about each other and are unable to comprehend the little they do know. All that we can know about each other is that all seek to live their own lives according to their own values and that, therefore, our desire to be free from outside interference is the one desire we all share. It follows that we have no means of discussion across the gulf of various belief systems and cultures and are thus left with the one obligation of respecting each others' freedom (and of punctiliously keeping contracts freely entered into) (Engelhardt, 1991). Such a point of view, of course, leads to an ethic in which obligations of beneficence are not ethical obligations at all but are, at best, either required by membership in a particular freely entered enclave or are demoted to being aesthetic and, therefore, not enforceable. In short, such a philosophy (and its libertarian predecessors) undergirds capitalism and ends in the inevitable exploitation of the weak by the strong.

Unfortunately there is not the time or space to dwell here on the fascinating history and theory of collectives and their formation. Suffice it to say that our vision of collectives underpins the way we think about individual as well as communal obligations. The idea of 'moral strangers' would make it virtually impossible to deal with the cultural complexity of ethical decision making in the everyday praxis of medicine or in the working out of ideas of communal justice. The question of being left strictly alone to pursue one's own life plans is hardly the only (and not generally the main) question when it comes to decision making either for individual patients or for questions more broadly dealing with allocation issues. And the notion of 'moral strangers' is flawed. As sharers of a common planet, of a common set of feelings and experiences underpinned by a common biology, we know a lot more about each other than merely that we wish to lead our own lives in our own way. We are perhaps not 'moral friends' but we certainly are 'moral acquaintances' (Loewy, 1983).

In a virtual lexical order (since latter points necessitate the prior fulfilment of those that come before it) all humans (and I would argue, to perhaps a lesser extent, most sentient creatures) share at least the following: (1) an interest in 'being': being alive, being on a habitable planet, existing; (2) distinct biological needs like food, water, shelter and others; (3) social needs (while these may differ starkly they all are social needs and we all need them at one time or another); (4) a common sense of logic which enables us to agree on some very fundamental things: the existence of causality, the fact that p and non-p are mutually exclusive, things without which we would have difficulty getting out of bed in the morning; (5) a desire, as much as possible, to evade suffering; and (6) the drive to lead our lives freely, to pursue our own self-chosen destiny and to make our own choices. Note that our desire to be free, to be 'individuals,' necessarily rides piggy-back on the fulfilment of the prior five. These six conditions, I hasten to add, are not 'principles': rather they are the necessary conditions for the development of all else. Nor does this imply that I base moral principles on biological facts: rather, I maintain that biological facts are the necessary condition for developing such principles. Nothing we do can be done outside of the framework of our inevitable and common biological structure. Discourse, praxis or the development of theories is not possible without communication and negotiation, a thing which 'moral strangers', whose only obligation is to leave each other alone, can only do in a very limited way: in a way so limited that it cannot suffice in a complicated and interdependent world. Since all ethics in dealing with people, relationships and collectives is ultimately social, these conditions are what we must keep in mind when we begin to think about decision making. Obligations which emerge from such a view are far richer than are those which a minimalist ethic would suggest.

Traditionally the approach to ethical problems has been an attempt to develop certain principles, to derive these from traditional ethical theory and then to apply such principles in an almost Newtonian fashion (much as a law is applied to a given case) to the problem at hand. Most of us have been less than satisfied with this method as used in the everyday approach to actual problems encountered in daily life (Toulmin, 1984). On the one hand, we have found that binding us to a rigid set of absolutist principles (with really no acceptable standards of deciding which principle 'trumps' another when they conflict) is unhelpful. An absolutist approach may lead to viewing a problem bereft of context (a process which not only does not help solve but in fact distorts the problem) or to acrobatic attempts to twist the facts of the problem so that they may somehow allow the principle to lead to an outcome we decided would be desirable. Such an acrobatic attempt distorts the problem as well as the principles. And it basically violates what ethics enjoins us to do: use our own rationality (not simply external rules) in dealing with the problem at hand. Doing otherwise, simply and legalistically 'applying' preset principles can, in fact, be framed as failing to act autonomously: something not even the most confirmed deontologist would embrace!

The attempt to escape from the all too rigid clutches of absolutist principles, on the other hand, has led to fleeing into the embrace of formlessness, and likewise leaves one little better off. While one may initially feel more satisfied with what one has done (after all, by allegedly not having a yardstick one has apparently acted on some more visceral urging) one is soon left in the unpleasant position of being unable to defend (to oneself or to others) a course of action which perforce is composed of emotion, past experience and internalized beliefs. Even if it were possible to act without a guiding principle (and I would argue that one cannot, in the human condition, act without principles for even doing so entails the use of at least the principle of acting that way) it would be a course of action which one could defend only by an appeal to one's own peculiar emotions, past experiences and internalized beliefs.

In response to the insight that principles often are of little help in bringing practical problems to a satisfactory conclusion (that they often increase determinacy only in so far as one 'knows what to do' but not insofar as producing a real, albeit a perforce tentative, resolution) several schools of thought ranging from situationalism through virtue ethics to, most recently, a so-called 'care ethic' have been developed. Here is not the place to detail the strengths and weaknesses of each. Suffice it to say that situationalism or 'agapism' as it has been termed, is really a form of act utilitarianism in which the aim is to use 'love' (undefined) as a measure of the good (Fletcher, 1966, 1982; Frankena, 1973). Virtue ethics seeks to use a basically Aristotelian notion of virtue in the sense of skill in bringing about solutions to ethical problems. Moral persons will make ethically acceptable decisions in grappling with such problems and will become increasingly skilful (or 'virtuous') in dealing with such problems. To get an idea of how to deal with problems, we must look to people who are skilled in making ethically good judgements ('virtuous' judgements): virtuous judgements are judgements made by persons skilled in this activity. To get an idea of what constitutes a good judgements, we must examine the judgements such 'virtuous' people make (MacIntyre, 1966, 1983; Frankena, 1982). Casuistry, in many ways similar to virtue ethics and certainly very much related to it, is really a method more than it is an ethical theory: in fact, all of these alternatives have that about them. By studying index cases which have found resolution in the past and by using a system of reasoning at least as old as the Jesuits (and some would argue going back to the Talmud) we can deal with our problems (Jonsen & Toulmin, 1988). These three visions of ethics or, at least and hardly the same thing, of ethical problem solving share a reliance on precedence (other similar cases) which allow us to formulate 'rules of thumb' so as to get on with the task at hand. Such rules of thumb and such general insights are, I think, an important lesson: not only is it not surprising that such a methodology was developed in the Anglo-American world with its heavy emphasis on 'case law' instead of on statute in its legal structure, but such a methodology is, in fact, one we very often use successfully in solving all sorts of problems. However, such a method in itself can become a strait-jacket almost as tight as a reference to 'principles': unless used with discernment, rigid reliance on prior cases in dealing with current problems simply exchange one form of rigid pattern following for another. Such methods lack a framework for adjudication, lack standards which allow us to determine whether the solution brought about with such skill (or the index case or rule of thumb referred to) is in itself a 'good' solution. One cannot allow the circle of 'a virtuous person makes good decisions and a good decision is what virtuous persons make' to complete our ethical vision or pre-empt our ethical judgement. We can, lacking such a framework, become very skilled indeed in making ghastly decisions, decisions whose ghastliness we have no way of determining.

Some have suggested that an ethic of caring, or the 'care ethic' as it has come to be called, represents a step forward: away from a coldly analytical attempt to examine and resolve ethical problems and best suited to dealing with concrete ethical problems (Gilligan, 1982; Nodding, 1984; Loewy, 1994a). Although it has been suggested as especially useful in health-care ethics, its ramifications and application extend far beyond this field. Care ethics, as I understand it, is basically an a- or truly an anti-intellectual kind of ethic in that it tries not only to value feeling over thought in dealing with problems of ethics but that, indeed, it would almost entirely substitute feeling for thought.

'Care based' has been opposed to 'justice based' reasoning: the one, it is suggested, a typically female, the other a typically male activity (Gilligan, 1982). There is, incidentally, some evidence that maleness or femaleness have little to do with the approach used: female attorneys or physicians tend to use the same method of reasoning as their male counterparts and male nurses reason like their female colleagues. Justice-based reasoning reasons along rule-based lines and finds resolution for problems by an appeal to rules which in turn are based on some ethical theory. It is 'cold', analytic and, somehow, not quite human. Care-based reasoning evades this sterility: it looks at each situation with concern and caring and finds resolution by examining its own inclinations and instincts. Therefore, it lends itself far better to dealing with what are, after all, uniquely human, uniquely existential and uniquely situational and contextual problems. Care-based ethics is doing what one's innermost instincts counsel one to do in a situation in which one is deeply involved instead of in a situation from which one stays remote.

It is unclear, when one reads writings in this field, if the 'care ethic' is a theory, a method, a way of thinking or feeling, or whether it is all or none of these. Writings in the field fail to make clear or convincing distinctions, and claim all of these (and, indeed, suggest more) at various times. It cannot be the case that an ethic based on 'caring' alone is a theory unless that theory, pure and simple, were to be 'act as your feelings (or instincts or "guts") tell you'; but it is rather a direction of how to apply something than it is a theory. Is it a method then? But if a method, a method for what? For applying itself? It is difficult to see how a concept like 'caring' can be more than a concept: an important concept, one which can make an ethic alive and breathing but neither in itself a theory or a method. At best, and not insignificantly, it would seem that what has been sketched is a tool to implement the making of choices and the carrying out of actions in human and often difficult situations. Searching for a resolution to an ethical quandary or problem without much caring about it or applying such a solution carelessly is surely not what we would want to see done: that makes caring an awfully important part of seeking or applying a good solution to a troubling problem but that does not make 'caring' central to the resolution or to its application (Loewy, 1994a).

Care ethic takes a path quite opposite to 'principle based' ethics: do away with a formal framework and do what your inclination commands. The background assumption (a patently false one, I think) is that one's 'natural' inclination will be to do 'the right and good thing'. Whereas Kantian ethics (Kant, 1989), for example, look on human inclinations with a rather jaundiced eye, care ethics sees inclinations through rose-coloured glasses. The idea that one's inclinations (those things we care about doing) will lead one to do right is not by any means a version of Rousseau's pre-social and amoral being endowed, however, with a primitive 'sense of pity' (Rousseau, 1965, 1972). Since following one's gut feelings (the way 'caring' plays itself out) rather than attending to (mere) formal principles takes place in a very distinct society which has already conditioned the way our gut will feel (take the 'gut feelings' of a youthful member of a Nazi youth organization, that of a Christian fundamentalist or that of a member of a Buddhist or Quaker group) it is a quite different thing. Rousseau's a 'primitive sense of pity' which pre-exists social organization is a starting point for ethics: in my view it is, as Schopenhauer (1986) remarked, the *'Triebfeder'* or 'driving force' of ethics; but Rousseau's 'sense of pity' is not an 'ethic' but a feeling which stimulates and perhaps even enables ethical discourse and action (Engelhardt, 1991). It can, just as can other feelings, be suppressed, distorted or fostered depending upon the kind of community we belong to. The way care ethics as I understand it plays itself out is the opposite of Kant's: being praiseworthy is following your inclination and ignoring formal conditions; being blameworthy is doing the opposite. Feelings cannot be verified or judged: I can never know how another really feels and to say that one 'ought to feel that way' or that one ought to like or dislike Mozart, jazz or peanut butter may be predictive (since I know your liking for Haydn and Beethoven I conjecture that you would like Mozart) but it cannot be judgmental; feeling a given way cannot, in itself, be praise- or blameworthy. Caring, as a guide to action, in that sense escapes any possible verification or moral judgement.

Feeling, when underwriting undisciplined and intuitive action without theory, has no head and, therefore, no plan and no direction; theory eventuating in sterile rules and resulting in action heedlessly based on such rules lacks humanity and heart. Neither one nor the other is complete in itself. There is no reason why we should necessarily be limited to choosing between these two extremes (Loewy, in press).

Theoretical ethics, what has been called 'justice-based reasoning' and what has been called 'care-based reasoning' when properly linked can form a useful model. Theoretical ethics develops theories of the good life, of what it is that constitutes an ethically proper framework and seeks to give convincing reasons for its recommendations. Examples of this are legion and the search, even though the solutions are hardly common ranges from Plato and Aristotle, through Bentham, Mill, Kant, Moore, Dewey, McIntyre and Nozick, to name just a very few among hundreds. Indeed, there are few philosophers who have not at least had a few things to say about basic theories of morality. Our principles and rules are derived from such considerations. What has been called 'justice-based reasoning' derives its rules of justice from some moral theory or way of looking at things. These rules, however, are not simply 'derived' in a mathematical or linear sense: it is a to-and-fro adjustment in which rules and theory inform and correct each other. Analysing an individual problem means laying it out in detail, drawing relevant distinctions, and examining various options in light of these considerations, in light of our rules and in light of the ethical theory to which they conform. Often this is a quite unconscious process and often such theory and principles are not consciously invoked until ideas clash and conflict occurs. Once possible options have been evolved and examined, the individual case (which has always explicitly or tacitly been part of the process) moves into centre stage. Attempting to use the options in a fashion which is unmindful of context or individual peculiarity is to apply it uncaringly and it is here that 'care-based reasoning' finds its usefulness. Care, it is hoped, has been exerted all along: we have, one hopes, cared about what we are doing and we have undoubtedly hardly been free from examining our 'gut feelings' about the case. *But*, and this is the major 'but,' we have not leapt from feeling to adjudication: rather we have used our feelings as a starting point to help guide us, to modulate but not to control our thinking. Applying what we have learned and fitting it to the individual case again is not a linearly derived activity. It comes to us neither from looking to the options we have found nor from the feeling in our guts as to what we should do. Such individualization in turn relates to justice-based reasoning and theory in a critically interdependent fashion. As we deal with the individual case, we may call into doubt the options derived by 'justice-based reasoning' and modulated by the way we feel about the case: we may correct, as it were, our justice-based reasoning just as our justice-based reasoning may correct our gut feelings. In the real world with real problems, justice as well as caring (both, as Nelson (1992) has pointed out, virtues but quite different ones) are necessary elements in almost all ethical decisions: it is not that they are juxtaposed or somehow antagonistic but rather that they have to be meshed and jointly brought to bear on the problem at hand. This, since they are quite different virtues, is not altogether impossible: after all, virtues can be seen as reinforcing rather than as competing with one another.

The relationship, it seems to me, is a homoeostatic balance between these various forces all of which properly come into play not only in dealing with particular problems but likewise in thinking about 'theory-' and 'justice-' or 'care-based' reasoning. Even the most abstract reasoning is informed by experience with or at least knowledge of concrete problems. To say that theory, justice and caring are related in a linear fashion is to oversimplify a complicated and necessarily involved process. They are inevitably intertwined, interrelated and mutually reinforcing and corrective. In dealing with real problems, in real situations or, for that matter, in speculating purely on ethical theory one cannot, in truth, say where one begins and the other ends. Moreover, once a 'solution' has been found or a rule or theory corrected, it is not conceived as a fixed solution, rule or theory valid in all such future cases but as a step in our future learning and growth. Having made an indeterminate situation more determinate (or perhaps merely made a quite indeterminate situation somewhat less indeterminate), we do not accept it as 'fixed' or 'certain' but rather as having been settled for the time being. Rather than a fixed conclusion which *ends* discussion, it provides a new starting point for our never ending quest (Dewey, 1988, 1991).

Dealing with actual cases

It may be fruitful here to sketch my approach to actual clinical problems as an ethics consultant. Later on, I hope to show that such a method can be adapted to grappling with ethical problems in the realm of experimentation. In American hospitals, ethics consultants are finding an increasing role. They act in difficult ethical problems in many ways similar to the way consultants from other fields act when it comes to complex problems in their fields. Ethics consultants try to help physicians and other care-givers as well as patients and families to think through difficult ethical problems. Properly they are not in competition with functioning ethics committees (which are quite a different thing, by the way, from *'Ethik Komitee's'* in Germany or Austria where the term means what in the Anglo-Saxon context are called Institutional Review Boards (IRBs) but rather can supplement and assist each other (Loewy, 1990).

Problem solving, whether the problem is one in ethics, technical medicine or auto-mechanics follows similar rules. The method of inquiry is the same; the material it is applied to, and therefore some of the details of application, may differ (Dewey, 1983, 1991). What one does, is to pose testable hypotheses and by tests appropriate to the material at hand affirm or refute them: the 'solution' thus found is one which is not ultimate but is one which allows us to proceed with the job at hand: that is, the proof of the pudding is in the eating. As time goes on the solution itself calls up other problems which are dealt with in a similar manner. Thus problem solving is a process of learning, growth and adaptation. In the hope of making things even more workable, we use our (temporary) 'solution' as a springboard for further inquiry (Dewey, 1991).

My work as a consultant uses what I have come to call a 'travel agent' model. I set out to find answers to three questions, questions which must be sequentially posed and sequentially grappled with. These questions are like those a travel agent must ask: (1) where are we?; (2) where are we going? (the *quo vadis* question); and (3) how do we get from where we think we are to where we think we want to go? The attempt to deal with the second before the first or the third before the second question leads to chaos, frustration and confusion. And yet when problems in ethics are discussed on the ward that, in my experience, is exactly what is often done. No self-respecting scientist or travel agent would attempt to grapple with the second question before the first had been at least tentatively answered!

The first question is largely a technical one: it depends upon 'medical facts', things like diagnosis and prognosis which only physicians expert in the particular field in question can supply. And since rather critical decisions must be made, one is well advised to insist that the 'medical facts' are supplied by those well qualified to deal with such particular problems: the 'medical fact' that someone is permanently vegetative or permanently ventilator bound must be affirmed by a specialist in the respective field. It is important here to realize that technical 'facts' are no more absolute than are moral ones: 'facts' are discriminated and understood in the embrace of 'values' and cannot be entirely separated from them. But since, in order to get on with the problem at hand, we must rely on such information and cannot do without it, such medical information must be well understood and accepted by all actors. When there is dispute, it may be because some 'fact' is not believed (the patient's wife may not believe the diagnosis or physicians may differ in their assessment) or because the certainty of such 'facts' is unclear to all. In the first instance, ethics consultants cannot help: only more expert opinion can help provide a solution. The second instance (the one dealing in one way or another with certainty) may present itself in two ways: the first is exemplified by the question: 'what if a miracle should happen?'; the second by the question: 'are you sure?' The first of these is easy to answer: 'if God wishes to bring about a miracle, no human can stand in God's way.'

The second is more difficult to deal with. No one can, in the human condition, ever be absolutely certain; all we ever can ask is a degree of certainty appropriate to the importance of the action. No matter how important, however, absolute certainty cannot be had and since we must act (failing to act is, after all, likewise acting) we must act on what seems most and not what seems to be the least probable. Probability should be as high as we can obtain – with prudence and by the use of the best experts available; but high probability, not certainty, is what we will ultimately have to act upon. Ambiguity is inevitably an unavoidable part of the human condition.

It is important not only to be aware of what we know but, likewise, to be aware of what we cannot know or what would be most difficult or hazardous to know. And our knowledge, as well as what we do not know, cannot know or can know only at a price perhaps not worth paying, must be shared with all concerned and must be clearly understood. The role of the ethicist in the first question is one of informing him or herself and then being sure that all actors not only are fully informed but also have a reasonable understanding of what the information means in the context of the case at hand. Knowing medical 'facts,' knowing what cannot be known and understanding probabilities can serve as a firm foundation so as to proceed to the second question.

The *quo vadis* question is the question ethicists can be most useful in helping to sort out. One part still relies on additional medical information. Physicians must sketch the 'realm of the possible' to us. We must know the best-case scenario as well as what is most likely to happen. Will the patient (should everything 'go right') end up semi-conscious in a nursing home or is there a fair possibility of some (how much?) functional recovery? Knowing where we want to go must first be predicated on where it is possible to go: it is futile to want the impossible just as it is foolish to pursue the unwanted. But knowing what is possible does not suffice to sort out what is desired. The question 'where could I go?' precedes but does not answer the question 'where do I want to go?'. Such a question can be answered only with reference to a patient's own values and life story: preferably it is a question a patient answers for him or herself but all too often it becomes one relatives, friends and health-care givers must grapple with. Such a question is a biographical one that requires an intimate understanding of a given patient's life story, cultural setting and personality. It may be answered in quite contradictory ways by persons whose life story, cultural setting and personality are different: both continued aggressive treatment and abandoning such treatment may, depending upon the person who acts or for whom one must act, be an appropriate course of action. The course of action must fit.

Eric Cassell (1984) speaks of life as a work of art: a work of art which from cradle to grave we are in the process of creating and which only we can best create ourselves. Imagine Mahler finishing Schubert's 'Unfinished' or Van Gogh finishing a Rembrandt self-portrait! While one could not paint without knowing the 'facts' of paint make-up or compose without understanding the 'facts' of harmonic theory, the 'facts' alone would not help in bringing such a work of art to fruition. Dealing with decisions involving individual patients is quite similar: while we must know 'the facts of the case,' and while we must understand what it is possible to do, this alone is unhelpful in making such a decision. It is best when patients are able to make such decisions themselves: ethicists here can help patients explore values and think through problems; when that is not possible, only 'getting inside the patient's skin' by understanding their past and their values can help to approximate their work of art. It is essential to understand what patients hold dear: would considerable physical impairment with no intellectual impairment be acceptable or would it not? Would the converse? Would a patient be reasonably content if intellectual function were to be somewhat dimmed but physical function would remain well enough to go for walks, play with grandchildren or enjoy dinner? What kind of a patient is this patient: one who would gladly take great risks, one who still has expectations (a book to be written or a daughter to graduate) or one who felt that life had been good and was now completed, the symphony written, the portrait's last stroke done? Ultimately in answering these questions, definite goals and priorities are set. Is the prime goal cure, relief of suffering, prolongation of life? And, if there is more than one goal (say preventing suffering and curing), which should take precedence over the other.

The last question (one of means: how do we get from here to there?) is, once the ground has been thoroughly laid, not a difficult one to answer. It is here that, just like a travel agent, the ethicist must explain the scenery or the difficulties to be encountered along the particular ways chosen. It is the ethicist's task to help affirm the patient's (and not their own!) values: choices made are not in themselves 'right or 'wrong' but appropriate or inappropriate to a given person and a particular context. It is not at all rare that in a given problem aggressive treatment may be a not inappropriate course of action while in a similar problem concerning another patient 'comfort only' measures would not be inappropriate: the choice made depends on the patient's (and not the consultants' or the physicians') vision of their work of art. As far as that is possible, it should be authentic. This, of course, does not deny that some choices are ethically quite inappropriate and cannot be supported: of course, that can be the case. It does imply that in reconciling world views and life stories, many ways of proceeding could be ethically acceptable.

It is in grappling with the second and third question that theory, principles and values play their role and it is here that these have to be individually applied. Understanding 'what makes the patient tick' is, in part at least, understanding what principles, values and ways of thinking and acting he or she would have chosen for themselves. The task of the ethicist is to guide patients in an affirmation of their own values in the context of communal ones and to coordinate them with the principles, values and beliefs of the health-care givers and the institution.

Dealing with such questions often involves negotiation. Physicians may feel that it is too soon to give up or that not sufficient was known to have reasonable certainty while patients or families may want to quit. Patients as well as health-care givers have world views and life stories which make certain courses of action impossible for them to pursue: the moral agency of physician, nurse, institution and patient are equivalent insofar as they must all be respected. Negotiating a framework of toleration ('although it is not what I really would like to do, I can go along this far but no further') is one of the important tasks consultants can help perform: physicians who feel that they are still obliged to treat while relatives or patients themselves wish to stop, may be willing to set a time when they would be willing to stop; would patients or families be willing to go along? Almost invariably when 'facts' are understood, values sorted and consequently goals chosen and prioritized, negotiation will be successful. In the very rare cases that it is not, suggesting a change of health-care givers (after referring the problem to the full ethics committee) may be necessary.

Therapeutics and experimentation

In popular language, the term 'experiment' is used to refer to anything whose outcome seems rather uncertain. Beyond this, certain innovations (for example, in art or music) are often termed 'experimental.' Thus, experiment has the sense of 'trying something new' or of innovation. Although that meaning is part of the whole concept, it does not satisfy what we mean by 'experiment.' The difference is not trivial: trying to do something that one does not have reasonable assurance that one can do is, in a sense, 'an experiment.' Trying to use a particular antibiotic for an as-yet undiagnosed infection or trying a surgical instrument in a somewhat different way or under somewhat different circumstances is, however, not what 'experiment' implies in the way it is used in medicine. In the way the word is used in science, experiments are conducted to establish systematic and significant connections between objects and processes in nature, society or thinking (Dingler, 1928). In their simplest forms as mere unorganized observations they are nothing new – having undoubtedly been performed since the dawn of man or of higher animals and they are described in antiquity and in the Middle Ages (Röseberg, 1990). But methodical experimentation is a rather recent development not really utilized until, among others, Newton and Bacon's introduction of the scientific method in the 17th century.

Methodical investigation seeks to bring about new or to revise old knowledge. The outcome is not known: it has no 'track record'. As such it is a 'logically distinct' activity from therapeutics which is interested in bringing about the patient's good (Thomasma, 1988). Therapeutics has a track record: patients are treated in one way rather than another precisely because of this. If a patient profits from an experiment, that is well and good; it may even be hoped for but it is neither predictable nor the main mission of experimentation. Bringing about a 'good act of healing in the face of illness' is not the main task of the experimenter. Therapeutics, on the other hand, while it may create new information does so by happenstance: the primary task of the physician treating a patient is 'to bring about a good act of healing in the face of illness' not to bring about a better understanding of the disease process (Pellegrino, 1979).

Of course, experimentation can be done in a variety of different ways. It can be done: (1) on healthy persons (a) for the sake of gaining physiological, pharmacological or other knowledge, or (b) under controlled circumstances to produce an illness; (2) on ill persons (a) which could possibly help them deal with the illness, or (b) under circumstances which may not benefit them but would help gather new knowledge about their illness (Loewy, 1994b). Furthermore, experimentation may be performed on adults capable of giving consent or on others whose ability to consent is far more questionable (the critically ill, the demented, children, mentally impaired or senile persons, prisoners or medical students). And that is only human experimentation: animal experimentation, in which consent is out of the question, presents quite different and equally troublesome problems. The question of the propriety of using sentient life forms who can suffer but who cannot consent for experimentation is a most troublesome one but one which will not be dealt with in this chapter.

Experiments, since the horrors of Nazi Germany in Europe and of Tuskeegee in the United States have become known, have rightly been under considerable scrutiny (Mitscherlich, 1978; Jones, 1981). Stimulated by these horrors, international codes have emerged and have found their application. In most countries committees which evaluate experiments and experimental process from an ethics point of view have emerged: in the Anglo-Saxon context these are called IRBs; in German-speaking countries they are what is usually referred to as *'Ethik Komitee.'* Such boards or committees are constituted to judge the ethical propriety of the experiment and of the experimental process. Beyond this, regrettably not within the scope of this discussion, such boards have begun to look into the propriety of animal experiments and experimentation.

There are several problems with judging the ethical propriety of a given experiment. When it comes to seeking subjects it is, of course, best to use persons most capable of consenting: that is, uncoerced persons who are capable of understanding what is at stake and who make a free decision to participate. Indeed, Hans Jonas (1974) argued long ago that consenting to an experiment falls well beyond the bounds of social obligations, that it is supererogatory, and should be based on a strong sense of personal commitment. Furthermore, he suggests that rather than allow persons of lesser training to participate, subjects should ideally come from among experimenters and others intellectually most capable of full understanding. There is a large bit of at least theoretical truth in such a view. Nevertheless, this fails to exhaust or even satisfactorily answer most of the problems: putting oneself at risk (especially at significant risk) cannot, unless one has a special role obligation, be morally obligatory; but what about if there is virtually no risk or if doing so is merely inconvenient but the information to be gained is of critical importance? What about if I am asked to take a small risk to help save my wife's or my best friend's life? Furthermore, as has been argued recently, personal commitment alone may be the result of a distorted psychic process (Fethe, 1993). Is it, furthermore, really true or practically possible that those best educated are the experimental subjects of choice? What about experiments which necessitate the use of children or of demented or retarded persons? Should such experiments be stopped? Space does not allow us to discuss these vexing and ever-recurring problems: what we are after is not so much an answer (tentative as it may be) to such problems but a methodology of approach.

The physician-investigator has a major ethical problem: he or she simultaneously has to pursue two logically distinct ends. Seeking new knowledge and benefiting individual patients is sometimes difficult, if not impossible, to reconcile. The suggestions heard from time to time that there might well be two different individuals involved with the same patient (one to look after the patient's good – an 'ombudsman' of the experiment – and one to conduct the experiment itself) has merit. Furthermore, it has precedence: in organ donation the team harvesting and the team transplanting are and ought to be distinct. In discussing consent, a method much like that described can be useful at the bedside. The 'facts of the matter' (what will be done) must be sketched by the investigator and clearly communicated to the patient and those advising on process. When it comes to the *quo vadis* question, investigators must clearly inform patients of their expectations and, most importantly since this is an experiment, must share with them their vision of the foreseeable and the range of the unforeseeable outcomes. It is here that patients and investigators need to examine their principles, beliefs and values in the context of the individual social situation.

Grey zones are frequent: not all work done with patients is done in exactly the same way as before nor does it (or can it) follow a pre-set algorithm. Innovation, trying out new ways of diagnosing, treating or operating, is a daily event and one which falls between the cracks. On the one hand it is motivated by a genuine desire to help a patient; on the other, it is motivated by the sort of curiosity which has allowed medicine to progress. It is not really an experiment: it is not systematic, there is some, even if not a substantial or disciplined, track record with similar procedures in not quite the same but similar circumstances, and its main purpose is to help a given patient rather than to generate new information; but neither is it therapeutics based on a solid track record. Often it is the forerunner of later formal experimentation: seeming to have 'worked', it stimulates disciplined investigation. Since it is usually done *ad hoc* – a particular and usually unforeseen situation comes up which the physician decides to handle in a somewhat different way – it does not fall under the purview of an IRB nor under the strict canons of experimental process. As such, it falls between the cracks and is not without danger. Once again, it is well to share what one knows and what one does not know with patient and family, to make them partners in the undertaking and to allow them to integrate what is done or what is proposed into the totality of their lives.

This is not a perfect world. Institutions like IRBs (or '*Ethik-Komitees*' in German-speaking countries) have certainly helped scrutinize and regularize experimental procedures: even though they are hardly foolproof (a review of any given medical journal for any length of time will show not a few questionable experiments), they are better than nothing. The danger, of course, is that by the very nature of peer review, investigators judge each others' proposals and may easily fall prey to the very human temptation to allow another investigator's work to pass unchallenged in the hope that theirs also will be: a clear instance of 'you scratch my back and I will scratch yours' (Loewy, in press).

Review Boards of IRBs have several tasks which are not quite the same as those of ethics consultants or (in the Anglo-Saxon sense of the word) ethics committees. While some ethics consultants see themselves as investigating and judging technical medical facts, most ethics consultants or committees do not consider investigating or judging such facts to be their mission: they rely on experts to inform them. In point of fact, consultants and committees are ill equipped to make such judgements: being trained to help think through ethical problems, keeping up with the literature in the field, focusing on the ethical in contrast to the technical question, perforce reduces the time one can devote to technical questions even if (and this is not generally or necessarily even desirably the case) ethics consultants happen to be trained as physicians. Assuming that one, as an ethics consultant, understands the technical aspects of medicine well enough to judge those who practice it every day is a form of hubris. On the other hand, the first task for IRBs is to judge whether an experiment is designed to provide the information sought: putting people at risk in a poorly designed experiment whose results would not be useful is not ethically defensible. Thus at least some members of IRBs must know a good deal about experimental process and statistical questions. They – perhaps with help in difficult situations but nevertheless – must judge the validity of the experiment: by virtue of having no track record, by virtue of being an experiment and not a proven way of proceeding, this is difficult and demands a focus on process. Only after that is done must IRBs grapple with the nature of the experimental subject and with questions of informed consent. The task of IRBs is thus much less one of individual focus (the life story of the particular subject is not the question) and much more one of adhering to more general canons of experimental procedure and process. It is logically distinct from that of ethics committees or consultants just as therapeutics is logically distinct from experimentation. IRBs are concerned with the protection of unidentified lives and while they are constituted to protect individual lives they must do so by general rules rather than by individual judgements.

Closing comments

In this chapter, I have been concerned with a methodological approach, one which, mindful of the differences, is applicable at the bed-side as well as experimentally. An idea of ethical theory and the rules of such theory is helpful in going about one's task: it is helpful in providing guidelines and prima facie rules but destructive when applied in a cookie-cutter fashion to the problem at hand. Ethical theories differ, often differ greatly, but in the final analysis tend to eventuate in similar courses of action (Toulmin, 1984). I believe that this, as well as the fact that quite dissimilar religions tend to have very similar basic moral rules, can be traced to our common human condition and our common human experience. If we were to fall into the trap of looking at others as moral strangers, instead of at least as moral acquaintances, it would be difficult to deal with the complex multicultural ethical problems on the ward or to deal with what is and what is not ultimately allowable experimental process. Here is not the place to deal with these problems in detail, merely to show that the method described and the ethical considerations previously considered can be applied to ethical problems in experimental as well as in clinical medicine. Again, it is a hypothesis-forming approach in which various possibilities and options are examined. The ethical problems in setting up experiments can be likewise examined under the three rubrics mentioned before. To know where we are, we need to examine the tentative proposal and the alternative ways of grappling with it. Here IRB members (at times helped by particular 'experts' in the particular question at hand as well as by 'experts' in statistics and design) must decide if the experiment merits performance: a poorly designed experiment, since it cannot yield the information sought, is a priori ethically not admissible. Once this hurdle has been cleared, we must ask where we are going: a most difficult question in experimentation. The outcome of an experiment (by the very nature of 'experiment') is unknown: perhaps the best and easiest definition is that it has no scientifically acceptable 'track record.' Just because something does not have a track record and just because we have no very clear idea of what exactly it will lead to, does not mean it is necessarily entirely unpredictable: we have some, even if only a tentative, idea of what we wish to investigate and what the alternative outcomes might be. But our level of probability is far less and our uncertainty far greater. Unforeseen outcomes are far more possible in experimentation than they are likely in therapeutics. For that very reason, persons who participate or their surrogates must be well informed not only about what we know (which beyond the purpose and experimental design is, by the nature of the task, preciously little) but must be fully informed of the fact of its unpredictability. They may benefit, if they are already ill; on the other hand, they may lose heavily. When patients are willing to take such a risk, they do so in view of their life, their life's story, their values, their hopes and their fears. But these individual life stories and values cannot be known to the members of the IRB: their decisions perforce affect lives they cannot know about. It is, therefore, important that members are mindful of our common human heritage of needs and experience: what one might call the existential a prioris of ethics.

Experimental method has to be best suited to produce knowledge, not best suited (should there be a conflict) to help an individual patient. And patients must, if we are to conduct experiments in an ethically acceptable manner, be quite aware of that. And yet things are not that easy, for even the strictest scientific experiment done purely to gather knowledge by a remote scientist must ultimately positively or negatively affect society and individual lives. The outcome may open a variety of possibilities heretofore precluded and as such play a significant role in bettering (or, unfortunately, in making worse) individual and communal lives.

The suggestion of having an ombudsman who would be familiar with the individual patient and with their individual lives, values and hopes (especially when experiments entail the active treatment of severe illness) has distinct merit. Too often individuals, their needs, fears and lives, get lost when only one person is 'in charge' and when that person's main interest, and one could argue moral obligation, is the gathering of knowledge. The addition of such an ombudsman could serve much as does the ethics consultant explaining, negotiating and analysing. I have tried to sketch a method of making decisions in ethics which is woven together from an understanding of ethical theory, personal involvement and an explicit process which attempts to pose and answer questions in a sequential manner. Such a method has the advantage of allowing us to separate the problem into component parts while remaining mindful of the need to view the whole problem with compassion. There is a critical and often ignored logical difference between the activity of experimentation and that of therapeutics. Nevertheless, whether we deal with the identified and identifiable lives in the clinic or with the necessarily unidentified lives when it comes to judging experimental protocol, the final common denominator is that our decisions ultimately affect individual lives and destinies and that these individual lives and destinies are subjects of their lives and destinies. Using a disciplined method which yet has space for individualization (easier in clinical than in experimental work but not impossible in either) may go a long way in dealing with problems which ultimately affect individuals who must act out of their particular cultural context and life experiences.

References

Cassell, E.J. (1984): Life as a work of art. *Hastings Center Report* **14(5)**, 35–37.

Dewey, J. (1983): Logical conditions of a scientific treatment of morality. In: *The middle works of John Dewey*, Vol. 3, ed. J.A. Boydston, pp. 3–39. Carbondale, IL: Southern IL University Press.

Dewey, J. (1988): The quest for certainty. In: *The later works of John Dewey*, Vol. 4. ed. J.A. Boydston Carbondale, IL: Southern IL University Press.

Dewey, J. (1991): Logic, the theory of inquiry. In: *The later works of John Dewey*, Vol. 12, ed. J.A. Boydston. Carbondale, IL: Southern IL University Press.

Dingler, H. (1928): *Das Experiment: Sein Wesen und Seine Geschichte*. München: Reinhardt.

Engelhardt, H.T. (1991): *Bioethics and secular humanism*. Philadelphia, PA: Trinity Press.

Fethe, C. (1993): Beyond voluntary consent: Hans Jonas on the moral requirements of human experimentation. *J. Med. Ethics* **19**, 99–103.

Fletcher, J. (1966): *Situation ethics*. Philadelphia, PA: Westminster Press.

Fletcher, J. (1982): Situation ethics revisited. *Rel. Humanism* **16**, 9–12.

Frankena, W.J. (1973): *Ethics*. Englewood Cliffs, NJ: Prentice Hall.

Frankena, W.F. (1982): Beneficence in an ethics of virtue. In: *Beneficence and health care*, ed. E.E. Shelp, pp. 63–82. The Netherlands: Dordrecht.

Gilligan, C. (1982): *In a different voice: psychological theory and women's development*. Cambridge, MA: Harvard University Press.

Jonas, H. (1974): Philosophical reflections on experimenting with human subjects. In: *Philosophical essays: from ancient creed to technological man*, pp. 105–131. Chicago, IL: University of Chicago Press.

Jones, J.H. (1981): *Bad blood: the Tuskeegee syphillis experiment*. p.11. New York, NY: Free Press.

Jonsen, A.R. & Toulmin, S. (1988): *The abuse of casuistry*. Berkeley, CA: University of California Press.

Kant, I. (1989): *Grundlegung zur Metaphysik der Sitten*, ed. W. Weiscvhedl. Frankfurt: Suhrkamp Verlag.

Loewy, E.H. (1983): *Freedom and community: the ethics of interdependence*. Albany, NY: SUNY Publishers.

Loewy, E.H. (1990): Ethics consultation and ethics committees: a functioning model for reaching consensus. *Hospital Ethics Committee Forum* **2(6)**, 351–359.

Loewy, E.H. (1994a) Care ethics: a concept in search of a framework. *Cambridge Quarterly of HC ethics* **3(4)**.

Loewy, E.H. (1994b): *Ethische Frayen in der Medizin.* Vienna: Springer Verlag (in press).

MacIntyre, A. (1966): *A short history of ethics.* New York, NY: Macmillan.

MacIntyre, A. (1983): *After virtue.* Notre Dame, IN: University of Notre Dame Press.

Mitscherlich, A. (1978): *Medizin ohne Menschlichkeit: Dokumente des Nürnberger Ärzteprozesses.* Frankfurt: Fischer Taschenbuch.

Nelson, L. (1992): Against caring. *J. Clin. Ethics* **3(1)**, 8–15.

Nodding, N. (1984): *Caring: a feminine approach to ethics and moral education.* Berkeley, CA: University of California Press.

Pellegrino, E.D. (1979): Toward a reconstruction of medical morality: the primacy of the act of profession and the fact of illness. *J. Med. Philos.* **4(1)**, 32–55.

Rousseau, J.J. (1965): *Discours sur l'origine et les fondements de l'ingalite' parmi les hommes.* Paris, France: Gallimard.

Rousseau, J.J. (1972): *Du contrat social,* ed. R. Grimsley. Oxford: Oxford University Press.

Röseberg, U. (1990): Experiment. In: *Europnische Enzyklopdie zu Philosophie und Wissenschaft.* Band I. (Hgb: Sandkühler HJ). **1**, 977–980. Hamburg: Felix Meiner Verlag.

Schopenhauer, A. (1986): *Preisschrift über die Grundlage der Moral.* In: *Arthur Schopenhauer, Sämtliche Werke, Band III.* Frankfurt: Suhrkamp.

Thomasma, D.C. (1988): Applying general medical knowledge to individuals: a philosophical analysis. *Theoretical Med.* **9**, 187–200.

Toulmin, S. (1984): The tyrrany of principles. *Hastings Center Report* **14(5)**, 31–39.

Section II: European legislation. Two examples: The Netherlands and Belgium

The ethics of animal and human experimentation, edited by P.P. De Deyn.

6

Legislation in Belgium concerning animal and human experimentation

Herman Nys

Department of Medical Law, Center for Biomedical Ethics and Law, University of Leuven, Kapucijnenvoer 35, B–3000 Leuven, Belgium

Summary

Belgium, like most other member states of the European Community (EC), has no legal regulation of research on human beings. This gap is in a limited way covered by provisions in the Criminal Code (such as voluntary injury) and the medicines' law. Moreover self-regulation plays an important role in the regulation of research on human subjects in Belgium. The Belgian Order of Physicians requires researchers to supply every experimental protocol to an ethics committee licensed by the Order. The licensing criteria mainly deal with the composition of the committee and some formal aspects. Substantial rules are lacking. Presumably most committees refer to the Declaration of Helsinki and the Good Clinical Practice for Trials on Medicinal Products in the EC.

From the point of view of the protection of the rights of the subject, the situation is far from satisfactory. While in neighbouring countries such as France, Germany and, in the near future, The Netherlands, legislative measures exist aiming at the protection of research subjects against abuses, Belgium tends to become an island in a sea of restrictive and limiting legislation. The fact that more than 100 ethics committees have been approved by the national council of the Order of Physicians is not reassuring. The danger of 'forum shopping' is not imaginary.

Unlike human experimentation, animal experimentation has been the object of legislation, which is discussed briefly.

I: Human experimentation

Current legal situation

In Belgium, there has never been any statute specifically regulating the conduct of research on human beings. In the absence of any specific statutory framework we must look to the common law. Also some provisions in the law on the practice of medicine and the medicines' law of 1964 are of relevance (Nys, 1993).

In particular, so-called non-therapeutic research or 'non-therapeutic biomedical research involving human subjects (non-clinical biomedical research)' (see Declaration of Helsinki of the World Medical Association) is considered with great distrust, especially by criminal lawyers. Any intervention that infringes the physical integrity of the patient can be qualified in legal terms as voluntary injury (Article 392, Criminal Code). The consent of the research subject cannot justify this infringement. Neither is it justified by a therapeutic purpose, which lacks by definition in non-therapeutic research. Following this reasoning, non-therapeutic research is illegal in Belgium. Nonetheless, there are no examples of prosecutions against researchers, physicians or manufacturers for undertaking this kind of research. The least one can say is that at the moment much legal uncertainty surrounds non-therapeutic research.

Article 6bis §1 of the law of 25 March 1964 concerning pharmaceutical preparations or medicines' law (*Moniteur belge*, 17 April 1964) empowers the Crown to determine the general conditions under which manufacturers, importers and wholesale dealers in pharmaceutical products may allow clinical trials with pharmaceutical products or may encourage them. This article has been incorporated in the Law of 25 March 1964 by the Law of 21 June 1983 (*Moniteur belge*, 15 July 1983). It is of fundamental significance in the sense that it may be considered as a principal recognition of the lawfulness of clinical trials with pharmaceutical products. The Crown may indeed not be deemed to regulate activities that are illegal. The exact meaning of 'clinical trial' in article 6bis, however, remains uncertain. In the Declaration of Helsinki, clinical research ('medical research combined with professional care') is treated differently from non-clinical biomedical research. In this sense, the meaning of clinical trial would be limited to therapeutic research, so that article 6bis does not offer a solid legal basis to non-therapeutic research.

It is furthermore questionable whether article 6bis §1 of the medicines' law offers the possibility of regulating medical research with human beings in a satisfactory way. First, it enables the Crown only to determine 'general' conditions, not detailed prescriptions. Second, these general rules cannot be directed towards physicians and researchers but only to manufacturers, importers and wholesale dealers. Third, this article only regards (therapeutic?) experiments with (new) pharmaceutical products, not with procedures, techniques, other products and so on. Finally, article 6bis §1 has not been implemented, although some efforts have been made between 1983 and 1988 by different state secretaries of health.

A final provision that has to be mentioned here is article 7 of the International Covenant on Civil and Political Rights of the United Nations (New York, 19 December 1966). According to article 7 no one shall be subjected to torture or to cruel, inhuman or degrading treatment. In particular, no one shall be subjected without his free consent to medical or scientific experimentation. This Covenant was approved in Belgium by the law of 15 May 1981 (*Moniteur belge*, 6 July 1983) and thus has the force of law in Belgium.

Not formally binding regulation

The lack of legislation on human experimentation in Belgium is far from unique. When considered in a European context, it is rather the common situation. Only Denmark (1992) and France (1988) have comprehensive legislation in this field. Other member states of the EC, such as Germany, have enacted legislation limited to clinical trials with pharmaceuticals. In the Netherlands, a comprehensive law is under preparation (Ch. 7, *Dutch legislation on human and animal human experimentation*).

The lack of legislation however does not mean that rules governing human experiments do not exist. In Belgium, as in most other European countries, self-regulation plays a more important role than statutory enactments in research on human subjects (Leenen *et al.*, 1993).

Self-regulation

Guidelines of the Order of Physicians. To a certain extent, the lack of specific legal rules regarding research with human beings is compensated by self-regulatory mechanisms. The code of professional ethics of the National Council of the Order of Physicians contains some requirements as to medical research (Arts. 89 to 94). They have been supplemented by rules laid down in an advice of the same National Council of 14 April 1984. This advice has been replaced by an advice of 15 February 1992 containing new rules on so-called experiments with human beings (National Council, Order of Physicians, 1992).

Biomedical research with human beings requires that an experimental protocol should be transmitted to an ethics committee. Physicians and researchers are obliged to answer the questions asked by that committee. They have to submit the full text of the advice of the committee to the research subjects. Any change of the experimental protocol has to be transmitted to the ethics committee. This committee has to be informed of the course and results of the experiment (first rule of the advice of 15 February 1992).

The composition of an ethics committee has to be such that its members are capable of understanding biomedical as well as ethical problems. An ethics committee may consult experts. Persons who are directly responsible for managing or financing a health care institution cannot be a member of the ethics committee of this institution (second rule).

An ethics committee is composed of at least eight members. The majority of them have to be physicians. Some members should come from outside the health care institution; at least one of these has to be a physician. Both sexes are to be represented (third rule).

A member of an ethics committee who is directly or indirectly involved in a research project has to abstain from taking part in the decision-making process (fourth rule).

A favourable advice about an experimental protocol requires the approval of at least two-thirds of all the members of the ethics committee. All members and all persons consulted are bound to a duty of secrecy (fifth rule).

A physician who participates in biomedical research with human beings has to ascertain whether the experimental protocol has been transmitted to an ethics committee approved by the National Council of the Order of Physicians, and whether its advice was favourable.

The experimental protocol describes the purpose, object and risks of the project, the information to be given to the subjects and the way these subjects will give their consent (oral or written). The protocol also has to mention whether an insurance policy covers the risks inherent in the project (sixth rule).

When publishing or lecturing on the results of the experiment, the researcher has to mention the ethics committee to which the experimental protocol has been submitted and its advice (seventh rule).

A physician who participates in biomedical research with human beings that has not previously been submitted to an ethics committee is liable to disciplinary prosecution and sanctions (tenth rule).

It is obvious that these rules are more of a formal nature and do not contain substantial requirements. The code of professional ethics of the Order of Physicians however, contains some substantial rules. For example, Article 90 permits 'experiments on a healthy subject' only insofar as the subject has reached the age of majority (18 years of age) and is capable of giving free consent, which is not the case for prisoners.

The foregoing has made it clear that medical research with human beings is, from a legal point of view, far from satisfactory. While in neighbouring countries such as France, Germany and, in the near future, the Netherlands, legislative measures exist aiming at the protection of potential research subjects from abuse, Belgium is becoming more and more an island in a sea of restrictive and limiting legislation. The fact that more than 100 ethics committees have been approved by the National Council of the Order of Physicians is not reassuring. Doubts have been expressed as to the expertise of many of these committees. What makes things worse is that a researcher is free to select the ethics committee to which the experimental project will be submitted. Therefore, the danger of 'forum shopping' is not imaginary.

Declaration of Helsinki. The requirement of the advice of an independent review committee (ethics committee) has been inspired by the Tokyo version (1975) of the Declaration of Helsinki of the World Medical Association.

This declaration is in itself also an example of self-regulation. As Annas rightly remarked: 'the Helsinki Declaration was simply this: recommendations to physicians by physicians' (Annas, 1992). The Declaration of Helsinki is just a set of ethical principles and has no legally binding authority (Fluss *et al.*, 1992).

This statement should be nuanced however, with respect to Belgium and the other EC member states. A royal decree of 22 September 1992 (*Moniteur belge*, 5 december 1992) has taken the appropriate measures necessary to comply with Commission Directive 91/507/EEC, O.J. L 270/32. This Directive modifies the Annex to Council Directive 75/318/EEC on the approximation of the laws of Member States relating to analytical, pharmacotoxicological and clinical standards and protocols with respect to the testing of medicinal products. Part 4 of this Annex relates to the clinical documentation accompanying applications for marketing authorizations. Evaluation of these applications shall be based on clinical trials. Part 4 of the Annex contains general requirements (A) and rules regarding the conduct of trials (B). Of great importance are the rules under the heading '1. Good Clinical Practice' and more specifically 1.2. It states that all clinical trials shall be carried out in accordance with the ethical principles laid down in the current revision of the Declaration of Helsinki. One can argue that through royal decree the current revision of the Declaration of Helsinki has become part of the Belgian law and is formally binding.

The consequences of this conclusion may however not be exaggerated. The Declaration of Helsinki is recognized by most as providing the fundamental guiding principles for conduct in biomedical research involving human subjects (Fluss *et al.*, 1992). One did not need a reference in a formally binding text for this. Further, the obligation to conform to the Declaration of Helsinki is only directed to the applicant of a marketing authorization. This implies a double limitation: one in a personal sense (the researchers themselves do not fall under the legally binding obligation to adhere to the Declaration of Helsinki; for them it remains an ethical obligation) and one in a material sense (research on human beings other than clinical trials is outside the scope of this legal obligation). Most important to me is that the reference to the Declaration of Helsinki in the royal decree of 22 September 1992 has left one of the main deficiencies of the Declaration of Helsinki unchanged, namely the lack of a statutory mechanism to control its application and to interpret its dispositions. Eminent authors have criticized the Declaration in this respect. 'The rules (of the Declaration of Helsinki) are tenuous, unaccompanied by any real controls, traditional sanctions, or other means of enforcement' (Fluss *et al.* 1992, p. 160). 'The Declaration of Helsinki, analogous to a legal statute, requires opportunities for interpretation; only then could it become a viable document' (Annas, 1992, pp. 205–206; idem Bergkamp, 1988, p. 74). Admittedly, permission to market a pharmaceutical may not be agreed when a clinical trial did not respond to the principles of the Declaration of Helsinki. This kind of post factum control is however not satisfying from the point of view of the protection of the rights and interests of the trial's subjects.

Good Clinical Practice in the European Community

The Declaration of Helsinki is also referred to in 'Good Clinical Practice for Trials on Medicinal Products in the European Community', in a way that remembers the wording in the annex to the royal decree of 22 September 1992 and the directive 91/507. 'The current revision of the Declaration of Helsinki is the accepted basis for clinical trial ethics, which must be fully known and followed by all engaged in research on human beings' (1.1) and 'The principles of informed consent in the current revision of the Helsinki Declaration should be implemented in each clinical trial' (1.8). A question difficult to answer is whether the 'good clinical practices' mentioned in part 4 of the annex to the royal decree and the directive (2.1.2) are really 'Good Clinical Practice for Trials on Medicinal Products'. If the answer is positive, this would enforce the formal binding value of the latter.

Whatever the answer is, 'Good Clinical Practice' demonstrates the same deficiencies as the Declaration of Helsinki, namely its lack of control mechanism (Dillmann, 1992).

Non-binding regulation and the protection of the rights of the subject

From a substantial point of view, 'Good Clinical Practice' offers a stronger protection to the subject than the Declaration of Helsinki. Whereas the 'Good Clinical Practice' requires a 'favourable opinion on the procedures and documentation' of the ethics committee (1.5), the Declaration of Helsinki requires only that the experimental protocol should be transmitted to 'consideration, comment and guidance' of the committee (1.2). 'Good Clinical Practice' is also more specific than the Declaration of Helsinki as to the task of the ethics committee in protecting the subject of the trial, . The Glossary preceding Chapter 1 of 'Good Clinical Practice' defines an ethics committee as 'an independent body, constituted by medical professionals and non-medical members, whose responsibility is to verify that the safety, integrity and *human rights of the subjects* participating in a particular trial are protected'. This formulation leaves different questions open: is it appropriate to label such a review board as an 'ethics committee', given this task? What are the consequences for the composition of the committee? What are the consequences of a favourable opinion as to the liability of the members of the committee when, e.g., the right to informed consent has not been fully respected during the performance of the trial? Nonetheless, if this task is taken seriously, the protection of the rights of the subjects is guaranteed more strongly than in the vague wordings of the Declaration of Helsinki.

The privacy of the subjects is another example of stronger protection from 'Good Clinical Practice'. Whereas the Declaration of Helsinki requires that 'every precaution should be taken to respect the privacy of the subject', Chapter 3 of the 'Good Clinical Practice' contains a detailed regulation for data handling. And although these regulations are not free from criticism (Roscam Abbing, 1990), it is an important step forward in the protection of the subjects of experiments.

With regard to the informed consent of the subject, 'Good Clinical Practice' may be criticized for offering sometimes less, sometimes scarcely more protection than the Declaration of Helsinki. In Helsinki I (1964) informed consent was not even listed as one of the basic principles (Fluss *et al.*, 1992). Helsinki II (1975) however places greater emphasis on the notion of informed consent. Principle 1.9 of the basic principles (rather than just those applying to clinical and non-clinical biomedical research) requires that the researcher obtains the 'freely given informed consent' of the research subject (after he has been informed of the aims of the research, the methods to be employed and any potential risks). Principle 1.10 cautions that great care should be taken if the subject is in either a dependent relationship to the researcher or may consent under duress. Although the 1975 revision has introduced the requirement for informed consent, Katz (1992) suggests that in subsequent revisions the requirement of respect for persons will become more pre-eminent in language and in its position among the basic principles.

As to the principles of informed consent, 'Good Clinical Practice' refers to the Declaration of Helsinki (1.8). Thus, both documents do not differ in principle. There are however some differences in the way the principles have to be applied.

With regard to therapeutic research (or in the wording of the Declaration of Helsinki: medical research combined with professional care) the Declaration implicitly allows it without the informed consent of the subject: 'if the physician considers it essential not to obtain informed consent, the specific reasons for this proposal should be stated in the experimental protocol for transmission to the independent committee' (II. 5) (Bergkamp, 1988, p. 74). According to Katz: 'In clinical research the emphasis (in the Declaration of Helsinki) is not on consent but on the imperative of physicians' freedom' (Katz, 1992, p. 232).

Also 'Good Clinical Practice' leaves room for therapeutic research on incompetent persons without informed consent (Roscam Abbing, 1990). This may be concluded from 1.13: 'If the subject is incapable of giving personal consent (e.g. unconsciousness or severe mental illness or disability), the inclusion of such patients may be acceptable if the ethics committee is, in principle, in agreement and if the investigator is of the opinion that participation will promote the welfare and interest of the subject. The agreement of a legally valid representative that participation will promote the welfare and interest of the subject should also be recorded by a dated signature. *If neither signed informed consent nor witnessed signed verbal consent are possible this fact must be documented with reasons by the investigator.*' Admittedly, 'Good Clinical Practice' may offer somewhat more protection in the sense that the ethics committee has to give its approval, while the Declaration only requires notification of the motives to this committee (although the formula in 'Good Clinical Practice' 'in principle, in agreement' could lead some researchers to think that *in practice* no agreement is required). Another difference is that principle II. 5 of the Declaration is as such not limited to incompetent persons, while principle 1.13 of 'Good Clinical Practice' is indeed so.

Both the Declaration of Helsinki and 'Good Clinical Practice' allow non-therapeutic experiments on patients. The Declaration of Helsinki is explicit at this point: 'The subjects (of non-therapeutic biomedical research involving human subjects) should be volunteers – either healthy persons *or patients* for whom the experimental design is not related to the patient's illness' (III.1). Again, information and consent are not highlighted for non-therapeutic biomedical research (Katz, 1992), thus one has to apply the basic principles. Principle 9 of these requires the subject's freely given informed consent, preferably in writing.

Principle 1.14 of 'Good Clinical Practice' requires that consent should *always* be given by the signature of the subject in a non-therapeutic study. Although principle 1.14 does not mention patients as subjects of non-therapeutic studies, it neither excludes them explicitly (Roscam Abbing, 1990). Whether patients may be subjected to non-therapeutic research even with their express consent is however a highly debated item. Even more questionable is whether a legal representative may consent to a non-therapeutic experiment when the subject, a patient or healthy person, is incompetent to do so. 'Good Clinical Practice' does not allow for this. The Declaration of Helsinki however could be understood otherwise. While the principles under III do not refer to informed consent, principle 11 of the basic principles that does apply to both II and III provides for the informed consent of the legal guardian in case of legal incompetence. This is clearly at variance with article 7 of the International Covenant on Civil and Political Rights (see above). According to De Blois (1990, p. 30): 'The objective of article 7, namely the protection of the personal integrity of the person subjected to experiments [. . .] can only be served in a proper way if the experiments which are permitted without the free consent of the person concerned are of a purely therapeutic character.'

Towards legally binding rules

The main question that arises here is whether the Declaration of Helsinki and 'Good Clinical Practice' offer satisfactory protection to the subjects of medical experiments in Belgium.

I am convinced that this question has to be answered negatively. Both the Declaration of Helsinki and 'Good Clinical Practice' focus on biomedical research and the researcher, not on the subject. Their main purpose is to enable the performance of biomedical research in ideal circumstances which requires a sufficient number of subjects. Only if minimal protective measures are respected by all engaged in biomedical research, are people prepared to participate either as volunteers or as patients in research projects. In its Introduction, the Declaration of Helsinki states: 'Medical progress is based on research which ultimately must rest in part on experimentation involving human subjects [. . .]. Because it is essential that the results of laboratory experiments be applied to human beings to further scientific knowledge and to help suffering humanity, the World Medical Association has prepared the following recommendations as a guide to every physician in biomedical research involving human subjects.' Only in principle 1 of part III (non-therapeutic biomedical research) a reference can be found to 'the duty of the physician to remain the protector of the life and health of that person on whom biomedical research is being carried out.' But it is not only the life and health of the subject that need protection, but also his rights as a person. Admittedly, the approach of 'Good Clinical Practice' is different with regard to the protection of human rights. The foreword to 'Good Clinical Practice' states: 'Pre-established, systematic written procedures for the organization, conduct, data collection, documentation, and verification of clinical trials are necessary to ensure that the rights and integrity of the trial subjects are thoroughly protected.' But the sentence goes on '[. . .] and to establish the credibility of data and to improve the ethical, scientific and technical quality of trials.' The interests of biomedical research seem equally important as the rights of the subjects.

Besides this utilitarian approach, another point of criticism is the substantial differences between the Declaration of Helsinki and the 'Good Clinical Practice' (e.g. informed consent). These differences cause uncertainty among European, *in casu* Belgian, researchers but especially for the subjects. Finally, the lack of a control mechanism and real sanctions (see above) mean that the Declaration of Helsinki and 'Good Clinical Practice' cannot be considered as an effective tool for the protection of the rights of the subjects.

As Leenen *et al.* (1993) have shown, legislation on the protection of human subjects of research and experimentation is increasing, though slowly. Different 'models' of legislation (France, Denmark, The Netherlands, Germany) are at the disposal of the Belgian legislator. This is not the appropriate place to go into details as to the contents of this legislation. The Recommendation No R(90)3 of the Committee of Ministers of the Council of Europe to Member States concerning medical research on human beings, adopted on 6 February 1990, recommends the governments of the Member States (Belgium is one of them) to adopt legislation in conformity with the principles appended to the recommendation. According to Fluss *et al.* (1992, 167), the emphasis in this Recommendation on the notion of informed consent is 'quite significant'. 'It marks a definitive turn away from the Declaration of Helsinki and it underlines that it is absolutely necessary to obtain the informed consent of the person undergoing medical research.

II: Animal experimentation

Unlike human experimentation, animal experimentation has been the subject of legislation. An act of 14 August 1986 on the protection and welfare of animals (*Moniteur belge*, 3 December 1986) contains in its chapter III rules on the conduct of animal experiments.

Substantial requirements

Article 20 §1 prohibits any animal experiment that does not comply with article 3, 15. The latter defines animal experiments and enumerates the lawful purposes of such experiments. An animal experiment is every intervention or observation on a living animal with a view to verify a scientific hypothesis, to collect information, to harvest or to test products, to preserve micro-organisms or tumours, to check reactions of animals, to teach with visual aids or to assure the education of people.

Article 24 of the act on the protection and welfare of animals contains the following substantial rules.

(a) Animal experiments should be limited to what is strictly necessary;

(b) Animal experiments may only be conducted if the envisaged result cannot be achieved by other means;

(c) Animal experiments may only cause pain, suffering or harm insofar as it is inevitable for the intended purpose;

(d) Animal experiments that cause pain, suffering or harm may only be conducted under sufficient anaesthesia, unless the pain, suffering or harm caused by the intervention is smaller than that caused by the anaesthesia.

This requirement is not applicable if anaesthesia is excluded for scientific reasons. In that case, the animal should not be used anymore for a similar experiment, unless a repetition is necessary to achieve the ultimate purpose of the experiment.

If an animal can only survive an experiment in pain and suffering, it should be killed painlessly. If the completion of the experiment requires the animal to stay alive, it should receive any treatment required.

Procedural requirements

The act on the protection and welfare of animals contains a system of mandatory notification of laboratories using or keeping vertebrates in order to perform animal experiments (article 21 §1). The act also provides for a system of mandatory licensing of laboratories performing animal experiments that may cause pain, suffering or harm (article 21 §2). Also, enterprises that rear or trade animals for experimental uses have to be licensed (article 22).

Ethical aspects

Article 28 empowers the Crown to establish a committee of experts to study the ethical aspects of animal experiments. At the time of writing this article (October 1993), this committee has not been established.

Animal experiments and higher education

According to article 30 §1 of the act on the protection and welfare of animals, animal experiments with didactic purposes are only permitted in a university, provided they are indispensable for the education of the students and that no equivalent didactic methods exist. They have to be conducted under the responsibility of competent teaching personnel.

Also the French and Flemish communities have enacted rules to stimulate alternatives to the use of animals for didactic purposes.

References

Annas, G.J. (1992): The Nuremberg Code in U.S. Courts: ethics versus expediency. In: *The Nazi doctors and the Nuremberg Code. Human rights in human experimentation*, eds. G.J. Annas & M.A. Grodin, pp. 201–219. New York: Oxford University Press.

Bergkamp, L. (1988): *Het proefdier mens. De normering en regulering van medische experimenten met mensen*, p. 385. Alphen aan den Rijn: Samsom.

De Blois, M. (1990): Experiments on human beings and international law. *Leiden J. Int. Law*, **1990**, 18–34.

Dillmann, R.J.M. (1992): De E.G. en geneesmiddelenonderzoek. *Medisch Contact* **47**, 502–505.

Fluss, S. *et al.* (1992): The Nuremberg Code: an international overview. In: *The Nazi doctors and the Nuremberg Code. Human rights in human experimentation*, eds. G.J. Annas & M.A. Grodin, pp. 149–173. New York: Oxford University Press.

Katz, J. (1992): The Consent principle of the Nuremberg Code: its significance then and now. In: *The Nazi doctors and the Nuremberg Code. Human rights in human experimentation*, eds. G.J. Annas & M.A. Grodin, pp. 228–238. New York: Oxford University Press.

Leenen, H., Gevers, S. & Pinet, G. (1993): *The rights of patients in Europe*, p. 189. Deventer-Boston: Kluwer.

National Council of the Order of Physicians (1992): *Official Bulletin* **55**, 35–38.

Roscam Abbing, H.D.C. (1990): EG aanbevelingen inzake experimenten met geneesmiddelen met mensen. *Ned. Tijdschr. Geneeskd* **134**, 2124–2125.

Nys, H. (1993): Belgium. In: *International encyclopaedia of laws. Medical law*, ed. H. Nys, vol. 1. p. 146. Deventer-Boston: Kluwer Law and Taxation Publishers (loose-leaf).

The ethics of animal and human experimentation, edited by P.P. De Deyn.

7

Dutch legislation on human and animal experimentation

Frans C.B. van Wijmen

University of Limburg, PO Box 616, NL-6200 MD Maastricht, The Netherlands

Summary

Medical experiments on both humans and animals are important to the development of new drugs and medical techniques in the field of health care. Test persons and laboratory animals run a certain amount of risk when they are involved in medical experiments. To minimize the risks legal protection of both human and animal test-subjects will be necessary. To this end two bills were submitted to the Dutch Parliament in 1992. In this contribution the main objectives of both the bill on human experiments and the bill on animal experiments will be described.

Introduction

When medical experiments on humans or animals are carried out, test-subjects run a certain amount of risk, while they will not benefit themselves from the experiment. Besides the test-subjects, several other parties with different interests are involved with medical experiments (e.g. society, researchers, universities, academic hospitals, research organizations and the pharmaceutical industry). To find a balance between the interests of all the parties involved and to minimize the risks for test-subjects, a system of preceding medical, ethical and legal verification of experiments on humans and animals has been developed.

In the Netherlands, legislation on animal experiments exists for quite some time. Currently a legislative proposal has been put to the Dutch Parliament to add a new paragraph to the existing law, in which the mandatory review of animal experiments by a committee has been laid down.

Until now no legislation existed on experiments on humans. In 1992 a bill has been tabled in which regulations for the protection of human test-subjects – patients as well as healthy test-subjects – has been laid down.

Outline

In the previous chapter, Professor Nys already pointed out the features of juridical parameters and the contours of professional codes with regard to medical experiments which have been developed by both official and private organizations world-wide. This chapter focuses firstly on the explanation of the content of the Dutch bills. Secondly a comparison between the two bills will be made to show that the result of the legislative process leaves room for self regulation to the field of health care and research.

Thirdly a brief discussion on the way the bills contribute to the protectionof human and animal test-subjects will be described.

Some historical remarks

More than a century ago considerations were made to regulate the use of animals by law in the Netherlands. During the parliamentary discussion on the Dutch Penal Code of 1881 substantial attention was given to the protection of animals and legislative review of animal experiments was recommended. In the Netherlands the discussion concerning the moral acceptability of the 'use' of animals dates further back than the exchange of ideas over patients' rights, which only started in the 1970s. The regulation of animal experiments has been in the lead, which has also been reflected in terms of legislation: the Animal Experiment Act is already more than 15 years old. In the field of animal experimentation, activities have been developed on European level in order to attune the policy and measures for the protection of animals in Europe: both the European Council (1985) and the European Community (1986) issued guidelines for the protection of animals, on which the Dutch bill of January 1992 was based. Hoever, initiatives fromthe field resulted in self regulation: review committees have already been dealing with animal experiments for more than 10 years in the Netherlands.

The protection of human rights in general began after the Second World War. As far as experiments with humans were concerned, the Dutch Health Council drew attention to its legal regulation in 1955. More than 15 years later the predecessor of our current National Council for Public Health published an advice in which legislation was recommended. The review of medical experiments in hospitals then became mandatory by means of accreditation norms for hospitals. In 1987 a draft for the legislation of medical experiments was published and finally in April 1992 a bill was put before Parliament. However, as in the case of animal experiments, initiatives from the field – especially the TNO (a Netherlands organization for applied scientific research) and Professor Noach (who established the first medical-ethical committee in the Leiden Academic Hospital) – resulted in self regulation: medical-ethical committees have already been dealing with experiments on humans for more than 15 years.

Headlines Bill on animal experiments

Pursuant to the current Animal Experiments Act the bill requires a licence to carry out animal experiments. Conditions to obtain a licence relate in particular to:

– responsible limitation of the number of animals;
– the discomfort caused to the animals;
– the limiting of multiple use of laboratory animals. The use of alternatives, if available,

is mandatory;
– the expertise of the researchers; and
– the care and treatment of the laboratory animals.

The concept of animal experiments and the objectives for which they are permissible are amply formulated.

In 1977, only section 18 of the Animal Experiments Act was applicable, which brought into existence a national Advisory Committee concerning Animal Experiments (hereafter also called the 'Section 18 – Committee'). Further introduction took place in January 1986, after the Animal Experiments Decree when a number of Legislative stipulations were issued and became operational. The licence holder must appoint a veterinary doctor or another expert for the supervision of the animals; the Decree further defines the duties and authority of this so called 'Section 14 – Functionary'. Demands are further formulated for those who actually carry out experiments and for those responsible for the care of the animals. The Decree also contains directions for legal registration.

Some important provisions laid down in the European convention of the Council of Europe of 1985 and the European Community Guidelines of 1986 include the promoting of research for alternatives, the explicit choice of animals and their numbers and the single use of laboratory animals for experiments where intense pain, great discomfort and associated equivalent suffering are involved. The Dutch Bill intends to comply with the European Community Guidelines.

The central standard for comparison

Experiments on animals are not allowed to be carried out if general interests are not in balance with the suffering and discomfort of the laboratory animals. This is the central standard for comparison of interests which is formulated in the bill. Violation of this prohibition is a punishable offence. In an earlier proposal it was stated that general interests of the experiment must be 'relatively proportional' to the suffering and discomfort of the laboratory animals. This terminology could cause problems because, according to arbitrary criteria, a major interest could justify serious damage. Quite rightly this has been replaced in the Amendment by 'weighed against'. The explanatory memorandum clarifies that the interest must always be greater than the discomfort. However, it remains difficult to measure the level of discomfort.

Extremely serious discomfort

In case of extremely serious discomfort the experiment must be of interest to essential needs of mankind or animals. 'Discomfort', which in plain Dutch stands for 'inconvenience' does not cover the meaning correctly. It would be better to use 'harm' or 'harm to health' (including pain and injury) in combination with (serious) discomfort. A definition in section 1 of the Animal Experiments Act makes it possible to prevent continuous repetition of formulations.

Another question is whether review of an intended animal experiment is not required if there is no 'discomfort' for the animals. This would not be correct because without discomfort an infringement of the laboratory animal's health or well-being is also very well imaginable, for example with biotechnological (genetic) research. Preceding ethical review of this type of experiments is also recommendable.

With regard to experiments that may cause extremely serious discomfort to an animal an extra 'severe' standard of comparison has been introduced: the experiment must be of importance for the essential needs of mankind or animals. This provision originates from European regulations. Earlier classification defined slight, moderate and serious discomfort. The limits between serious and extremely serious as well as the interpretation of the exact meaning of 'essential' is unclear. Clarification and objectivity are necessary.

The norms to be reviewed

No animal testing may be carried out without advice having been issued by the review-committee for animal experiments, which carefully relates the research protocol with a view to the aforementioned comparison of interests to norms laid down in the Animal Experiments Act. An earlier proposal introduced the system which, in the case of negative advice form the review-committee ('with the advice meaning the research would not be carried out or not be carried out in accordance with the protocol'), would mean that the protocol's licence holder – accompanied by his written point of view – would have had to make a submission to the committee for further advice. The licence holder has to wait up to a maximum of three months for this further advice. Once this had been issued he could, regardless of its contents, still decide to carry out the animal experiment or have it carried out. This invoked widespread objections. The Secretary of State for public health has still backed down. He draws a parallel with the Bill concerning medical experiments wih humans, where initially also the freedom of the researcher existed, also after negative advice, to go his own way, but where, partly upon the instigation of the Council of State, in the second instance a choice is made for a mandatory ositive advice. Quoted from the Memorandum in Reply this is explained as follows: 'If the licence holder has received a negative advice from the committee for animal experiments, he requests, if he still wishes to carry out the experiment, the judgement of the committee. He is not allowed to carry out the experiment if that judgement is also negative. If the committee fails to issue its judgement within three months, then the judgement is deemed to be negative; the license holder can submit an appeal to the Court of Appeal in respect of every negative judgement (fictitious or otherwise).'

The system of approval

The minister of Health can issue an approval, based upon the advice of the committee hearing, provided the requirements stated hereafter regarding the composition of the committee have been complied with. The Minister can withdraw the approval under two circumstances:

* if the committee for animal experiments no longer meets the necessary requirements;
* if the committee fails to exercise or impropelry exercises its controlling duties.

In addition the Minister has the authority to withdraw the approval of the committee if 'within the space of one year, the number of times advice is requested is less than determined in a General Governmental Decree'.

Establishing a network of committees for animal experiments fits within the concept of self regulation. It is not clear why a system has been chosen in the Bill that requires the

Minister of Health to accredit review-committees for animal experiments. With the proposed legislation concerning medical experiments involving humans this incurs substantial (constitutional) objections and furthermore this runs seriously against deregulation endeavours.

Composition of committees for animal experiments

In order to get an approval participation is required, based upon stipulated conditions, of experts in the field of animal experiments, of the laboratory animals and their protection and of the ethical review: in addition one member of the committee must be someone who is not involved in carrying out animal experiments; finally it is not permitted that any person involved in the experiment participates in the deliberations of the committee concerning his own protocol. The Bill gives no ruling on the proportion of members originating from the three areas of expertise, nor is it determined whether any of the categories may have a majority. At least the latter is desirable.

Sanctions

The Animal Experiments Act knows qua system a number of prohibitions and obligations with which the proposed amendments will be extended. Violation of the prohibitions and failure to meet the obligations will be punishable. The surveillance is in the hands of the Veterinary Inspection Organization which have investigational authority.

Headlines Bill concerning medical experiments

The basis for the legislation concerning medical experiments with humans is that for the execution of scientific research in the field of medicine, whereby people are involved in experiments, certain norms and regulations must be complied with. A positive aspect of this Bill is that the norms, upon which the acceptability of a medical experiment must be reviewed, are reproduced clearly and in an orderly manner. On the one hand, it concerns norms related to the scientific merits of the experiment, and on the other hand, norms which have in mind the protection of the people being tested, such as informed consent as a condition for voluntary participation, protection of privacy and stipulations concerning insurance against possible damage.

More and more it needs to be explicitly declared that a proposed experiment conforms with the intended norms and regulations. To this end the researcher must present the research protocol to a committee, by tradition popularly named the medical-ethical committee. These committees are not introduced by the government but upon the initiative of the interested parties. In order to guarantee the quality of the committee's functioning, requirements are made regarding their composition and there is a system of accreditation by a Central Committee which is going to be brought to existence by law. Therefore an experiment may only be carried out if an accredited local committee has issued a positive judgement regarding the research protocol. Should the committee's decision amount to a rejection then reappraisal is possible by way of the Central Committee. For experiments in certain categories the protocols may be assessed directly by the Central Committee for the sake of uniformity.

Tasks and authority of the Central Committee and the local committees

One of the aims of the future legislation is the improvement of the existing review organization. The most important problem is the heterogeneity of committees and accordingly the quality of the review. A Central Committee which accredits local committees also has the authority to withdraw the accreditation. Other tasks of the Central Committee include the reappraisal of a protocol, initially negatively judged, and in certain cases issuing a primary judgement. It is explicitly determined that the Central Commitee ought to supervise the local committees: the latter must send (summaries of) protocols and subsequently the judgement issued. Based upon this, the Central Committee can obtain insight into the quality of the committee's work. According to the explanation in cases of poor quality the Central Committee can act individually in the communicative area; if structural differences between committees are involved, for example in relation to judgement, then the Central Committee can exercise its authority by issuing guidelines. Local committees can also request support from the Central Committee and can even 'provoke' guidelines. Coordination in multi-centre trials is a task described expressly for the Central Committee. All in all the review organization is more clearly outlined than in the preliminary draft.

Composition of the Central committee and local committees

The basic components for the composition of the central and local committees in terms of their disciplines are established by legislation. The first noticeable thing is that – contrary to the preliminary draft – there is no longer mention of 'one or more persons who are thought to be able to represent the interests of people involved in experiments in the Netherlands'. The explanation now states for example that those concerned with ethics will be particularly concerned with the protection of the person to be tested and (an argument which in connection with the foregoing is not very logical) that the people involved in the experiments do not form a demarcated group whose interests could be represented. Indeed, it is not about representing interests, but about the (experience) expertise of the test-subjects. It is true that in practice it is not easy to find people with this point of view, but where that has succeeded these committee members add an essential element to the expertise already present in the committee. A "layman's opinion" has its own meaning, in addition to the opinion of other members, who are all professional in one way or another, from whom the lawyer and the nurse sometimes choose the perspective of the patient's protection.

The 'basic composition' of the local committee is 'lighter' than that of the Central Committee: not named are persons who are expert in the field of pharmacology, nursing and the behavioural sciences. The explanation offers no clarification. Also for the local committees it is required to have the names of the three disciplines added. Medicinal experiments form in total an important share of patient-related research; nurses – often professionally involved in experiments themselves – judge the participation of patients from their own point of view; behavioural sciences expertise brings its own methodological knowledge, whilst many experiments partly encompass non-biomedical aspects. Another solution is to leave the control of the composition to the Central Committee, which furthermore could affect the desired uniformity by issuing sector associated guidelines.

Recognition requirements for local committees

Apart from the composition the Bill also names the following requirements for the recognition of a local committee:

- regulations must be sufficiently equipped for the cooperation of external experts;
- it must be apparent from the regulations for which 'wide circle' the committee is destined;
- within reasonably acceptable limits the committee must receive a minimum number of protocols for judgement as determined by the Central Committee (art. 14, second section)

The Central Committee withdraws recognition when:

- the committee no longer conforms with the above-mentioned requirements;
- the committee's compliance with its legal responsibilities is insufficient;
- the committee amends its regulations to an extent that a proper execution of its task is no longer reasonably assured (section 20, first paragraph).

Comparison between the Bills for animal and human experimentation

It is obvious that animal and human experimentation is important for the development of health care in general and medicine in particular. In Western society many experiments in which animals and human beings are involved take place daily. Examples in the past show that sometimes researchers do not make the right estimate of the balance between social (and their own) interest and the pain and discomfort of persons and animals.

The pleas for legal protection of humans and animals involved in scientific research are unanimous. The Dutch legislator happens to discuss proposals to regulate previous review of human and animal experiments on the same time: bills are submitted to Parliament in January and April 1992.

Having sketched the headlines of the proposals for the regulation of both kinds of experiments there is the opportunity now to make a comparison. We have seen there is a great difference in development: more than one hundred years ago legislators cared about the well-being of animals and there had been stipulations for the use of animals in the Dutch Penal Code of 1881. The attention for human rights in general and the legal protection of humans involved in medical experiments dates from the period after World War II. In the last decades international documents – public (Universal Declaration of Human Rights, European Convention of Human Rights) as well as private documents (Declaration of Helsinki) – have been published in favour of dignity and self determination of individual human beings.

In 1977 the Animal Experiments Act appeared with regulations to reduce animal experiments, to safeguard a proper use of laboratory animals and to benefit the quality and responsibility of those who are charged with the performance of animal experiments and with the care of animals. A system of previous reviewing protocols for research projects both for human and animal experiments was introduced privately in the 1970s.

The incentive to regulate protection of animals by the way of review-committees came from European Conventions (1985, 1986). As to the human medical experiments a revision of the Constitution in 1983 inspired preparation of legislation.

There are resemblances in both bills:

- starting point is a prohibition to carry out an experiment with any human or animal without a positive advice of a review-committee
- such experiments are only acceptable when there is a good benefit–risk ratio, a balance between common interest (such as advancement in health care, amelioration of drugs and methods) at the one hand and the well-being (in terms of risks, potential injury or damage, discomforts and inconveniences) of test subjects involved on the other hand;
- in order to make a proper comparison there are norms and criteria concerning the quality of the research protocol and the protection of humans and animals;
- there will be a Central Committee which has to accredit local committees and which have the task to assess and ameliorate the quality of the functioning of the local committees;
- in total there are controlled systems to check the quantity and quality of the use of animals and humans for scientific research.

Besides corresponding elements there are also differences between the Bills for regulation of human and animal experiments:

- the Animal Experiments Act is a product of legislation from the 1970s which is characterized by a jungle of rules and the necessity to work out more rules by means of decrees and orders; the future Human Experiments Act is more tight and sober qua design in accordance with the modern philosophy of legislation (government steps back and leaves more responsibility to private partners);
- in the Animal Experiments Act norms and criteria for the acceptability of experiments are diffused whilst in the future Human Experiments Act they will be concentrated in two specific sections;
- The Animal Experiments Act requires the concept of centralism (e.g. the Minister of Welfare, Health and Cultural Affairs accredits the review-committees) whilst the starting point in the Human Experiments Act is so called 'conditioned self-regulation': as much as possible private parties have to regulate their affairs on their own or together;
- thus the Animal Experiments Act leaves the impression of tight and detailed regulations whilst on the contrary, the future Human Experiments Act symbolizes a new approach of legislation.

Conclusion

If we consider it in its entirety once more, we must come to the conclusion that one hand of the legislator does not know what the other is doing: for the review of animal experiments an organizationally greedy system is proposed, whilst the regulations concerning experiments with humans fulfil a contemporary concept of balance between legislation and conditioned self regulation much better. Legislative processes are long winded. Inner monologues are unknown to the legislator, just as flexibility is not one of his most noticeable characteristics. A concept, which was in blueprint more than three or four years ago often still carries with it the legislative technique of the preceding decade: the 1970s, expectant in finely meshed detail, and the 1980s, searching for a new style of dealing with the government in the field of health care. It is regrettable that the practice of animal experiments will not be able to pluck the fruits of a completely new style of dealing with the legislative government and with its citizens. We may hope that this does not negatively influence the quality of legal protection of both humans and animals.

References

Bergkamp, L. (1992): Regels voor medische experimenten (Rules for medical experiments). Beschouwingen over het wetsvoorstel. *Tijdschrift voor Gezondheidsrecht* **16**, 372–388.

Duijnstee-Bijvoet, W.E.M. (1993): Regulering van experimenten (Regulation of experiments). *Kwaliteit en Zorg* **1**, 125–130.

van Wijmen, F.C.B. & den Uyl, A. (1987): Toetsing van dierproeven (Review of animal experiments). Verslag van een onderzoek betreffende een wenselijke regeling van dierproeven, Vakgroep Gezondheidsrecht Rijksuniversiteit Limburg. Ed. Samenwerkingsverband van de Nederlandse Vereniging tot Bescherming van Dieren en de Nederlandse Bond tot Bestrijding van de Vivisectie.

van Wijmen, F.C.B. & den Uyl, A. (1989): Wettelijke regeling voor toetsing van dierproeven (Legal regulation for the review of animal experiments). *Tijdschrift voor Diergeneeskunde* **114**, 269–279.

van Wijmen, F.C.B. (1987): *Experimenten met mens en dier (Human and animal experimentation).* In: Terugblik en vooruitzien. Serie onderzoeksrapporten vakgroep Gezondheidsrecht Rijksuniversiteit Limburg. Maastricht, Sept 1987, 19–40.

van Wijmen, F.C.B. (1992): Het Nederlandse wetsvoorstel inzake medische experimenten (The Dutch bill concerning medical experiments). *Vlaams Tijdschrift voor Gezondheidsrecht* **13**, 86–95.

The ethics of animal and human experimentation, edited by P.P. De Deyn.

8

Animal research: some legal aspects

Laurens van Veenendaal

Rudolf Magnus Institute for Neurosciences, Universiteitsweg 100, NL-3584 CG Utrecht, The Netherlands

Summary

An animal experiment cannot be performed, in contrast to the old legislation, when negative advice is given by the Animal Experimentation Commission, and the (central) Advisory Commission of animal experimentation. If the experiment is performed regardless, the licensee risks the criminal Court calling his actions 'without a reasonable objective' or 'needless', due to this negative advice. Unreasonable or needless abuse could be seen as a violation of the Dutch Criminal Code (regarding animal abuse), and could be convicted. Although the new Dutch legislation regarding animal experimentation prefers to hold the licensee legally responsible, the person performing the experiment, the experimenter, will not go free entirely upon violation of the Law on animal experiments. They all have a so-called *Garantenstellung*, which means that in the evaluation of certain actions, the liability is determined in accordance with the social role or function the person in question has accepted. The liable person has a certain 'quality', and a corresponding responsibility.

It would be a mistake to assume that under certain circumstances they might be deemed to be criminal offences and that grounds for justification would therefore need to resorted to. Another reason to reject this approach is that it fails to cohere with reality as this is experienced by the persons conducting the experiments. People who conduct experiments with animals do not view these experimental acts as ones which are, in principle, criminal offences. But this is precisely what approaches to grounds of justification do. Instead of using this legal fallacy we would be better off looking for a construction which fits better with the interests of the animal experiments that are conducted in real life.

I want to make clear that responsible animal experimentation according to professional standards, and being socially adequate, is not the kind of behaviour that should be the province of the Criminal Code. Such actions are controlled by professional codes, rules for right conduct and morality. Violation of these rules should be judged by the Veterinary Inspector General, and in some instances the Disciplinary Judge. Only when flagrant violation appears to have occurred, can it be assumed that the animal experimentation falls outside the boundaries of admissibility, and that the Criminal Code should intervene.

From past to present

Ever since Antiquity, (medical) scientists have performed human and animal experiments in order to learn more about the human body and about the problems of health and disease, and to discover (better) treatment modalities and drugs for patients (for a history, see Chalkly (1974) and Clendeling (1960)). Many centuries later, whilst rediscovering Antiquity during the Renaissance (in the 16th century) man renewed his interest in the study of nature (Withington, 1964). Experimentation on animals became more common, and it was realized that, especially in the case of mammals, there are no essential differences between humans and animals. Until the 20th century, ethical and legal guidelines hardly existed for researchers. Apparently, trust in scientists was such that it was not doubted that they would comply with current morality. Unfortunately, this trust was sometimes abused. After World War I (1914–1918), where 'trial-and-error methods' still prevailed (Macdonald, 1989a, b), a change in social reaction occurred, largely due to the crimes against humanity during World War II (1940–1945) (Redlich, 1978). During the first half of the 20th century, social resistance against abuses in (medical) research emerged. During the 1947 criminal action at Nuremberg, the Military Tribunal formulated the Nuremberg Code, the first international document with regard to the regulation of medical experiments. In the Netherlands, government regulation, although not established before the 1960s, became increasingly strict (Derksen *et al.*, 1989). Thus, a 1958 Law on Provision of Medicines was modified several times during the 1960s and the 1970s, and during the process, implementing orders with regard to pharmacy, preparation and delivery of pharmaceutical products, and registration of medicines were enacted and changed. The two latter orders deal with clinical experimentation on human subjects. In 1977, an act on animal experimentation was entered onto the Dutch Statute book. This Law and the Order on Animal Experimentation was not fully enacted before 1986. One year later, on 21 December, 1987, following a long period of preparation, a Concept Bill on medical experiments was published.

In the meanwhile, public emancipation has proceeded. People have become more mature and more aware of their right to self-determination. The need has been growing to reflect on the ethical aspect of medical practice in general, and in particular on human and animal experimentation in science. A certain amount of control of experimentation is deemed appropriate to secure the quality of current medical practice on the one hand, and to make sure, on the other, by checking research projects that medical progress does not entail undue suffering. It goes without saying that the increase in the medical–technical possibilities has given rise to many new ethical and legal questions. In the Netherlands, the foundation of this discussion is provided by articles of the Constitution: *the Government takes measures for the promotion of public health (art. 22, para. 1), and subject to and under legal restriction, everybody has a right to bodily integrity (art. 11).*

In article 22 paragraph 1, the legislator has deliberately chosen the term 'promotion of public health' instead of 'protection'. The reason is that 'protection' suggested protection against imminent danger, and infers the preservation of any already existing or obtained condition. Promotion, moreover, includes measures to increase public health (*Explanatory Memorandum of the Constitution, 1975–1976*). As such, this article is the foundation of the Dutch Law on Animal Experiments. The article is directed towards legislator and government, and it has a scope such as to leave plenty of room for government policy; it supposes an active government (Akkermans, 1992). The Government is obligated to take action. It concerns the instruction to take action on behalf of certain interests within the bounds of financial and economical possibilities. This instruction cannot, in principle, be legally enforced. When government action is demanded, it will be manifested in legislation or prescriptions for implementation. All this might also mean that promotion of public health as in the Constitution article 22 paragraph 1 may require the progress of medical science. Accordingly, human and animal experimentation might be necessary. By its policy on subsidies, the Government can support certain scientific projects, and can thus also declare its partiality towards specific projects. The Government can, moreover, become responsible for the realization of the research, and it can direct the course of scientific research by means of legislation.

A subject that is inseparably connected to the act of experimentation itself is animal research. Dutch law with regard to medical experiments maintains that: *it must be evident from the research protocol that sufficient amounts of research has been performed an animal subjects and/or tissue cultures to justify research on human subjects.* Also: *it is acknowledged that part of the experiments termed medical is performed on animals, and is regulated, therefore, by the Law on Animal Experiments.* The Tokyo–Helsinki Agreements, for that matter, prescribe animal experiments to be performed before the application of novel medical techniques or therapies to human beings. From the explanatory memorandum it is clear, moreover, that the Council for International Organizations of Medical Sciences, in collaboration with the World Health Organization (WHO), has issued the 1982 *Proposed International Guidelines for Biomedical Research* based on the Tokyo-Helsinki Agreements. In the Netherlands, the guidelines of the Foundation for Basic Medical Research (FUNGO) and the Health Organization for Applied Natural Science Research (TNO) are based on the Tokyo–Helsinki Agreements also. The policy of the Dutch Government is thus that animal experimentation is allowed only with respect to certain interests, that the number of experiments should be as small as possible, and that the experiments should be performed with extreme care. This is achieved through a legal system of licensing of institutes that perform animal experiments, and the conditions thus imposed. These conditions mainly comprise the responsible limitation of the number of animals used as well as the amount of animal discomfort, and the limitation of repeated use of experimental animals. An important part of the regulations refers to yearly obligatory registration and reporting to the Veterinary Inspector General of all issues with regard to animal experimentation and experimental animals. Licensees are further obligated by law to leave the care and handling of the animals to persons who meet the professional standards and who took the obligatory courses. The licensee is also obligated to put the welfare of the experimental animals in the institution under the surveillance of a professionally trained individual. The Governmental Advisory Commission on animal experimentation issues plays an important role in all this. The members of this commission are specialists in the field of animal experimentation, experimental animals, and animal welfare. Last but not least, the promotion of so called alternatives to animal experiments is of the utmost importance. We mention the Platform for alternatives to animal experimentation which ensures cooperation between government, industry, and animal welfare organizations.

The Dutch Law on Animal Experiments dates from 12 January, 1977. Article 18, which regulates the installation of an Advisory Commission, was enacted immediately. Articles 1, 10, 13, 16, 17, 20, 25, and 29 were enacted on 2 September, 1980; all other articles with the exception of article 19, on 1 January, 1986. Further based upon this Law, rules have been implemented in the Act on Animal Experiments of 10 December, 1985. Recently, a change of and a supplement to the Law and related Act on Animal Experiments came about. This was necessary, in the first place, to comply with Guideline 86/609/EG, (Pb-EG L358) of the European Convention, as well as the European Agreement with regard to the protection of vertebrate animals used for experimentation and other scientific purposes, which was realized at Strasbourg on 17 March, 1986. An important new part of the Law consists of regulations regarding Animal Experimentations Commissions (DEC). These commissions, which have been operational for some years, now get a legal basis. It is established that animal experiments have to be submitted to ethical review before they can be performed. The construction is thus that every licensee should ensure evaluation of the ethical aspects of all animal experiments to be performed under his licence. This evaluation is the task of the so-called Animal Experimentation Commission, which offers advice about the (un)acceptability of the experiment considered, after balancing the benefit of the animal experiment against the harm inflicted on the experimental animals. The licencee has to determine a rule for this which takes the prevailing law into account. New also is the licence requirement for breeding and selling animals for research purposes; this requirement is outlined in the Guideline and the Agreement. The institutions in question are obligated to comply with care and registration requirements also. The change further contains an increased strictness by the Guideline and the Agreement of the criteria which should be applied while balancing the benefit of the experiment against the discomfort (*Explanatory Memorandum of the Law on Animal Experiments, 1991–1992*).

As I have shown, an animal experiment cannot be performed, in contrast to the old legislation, when negative advice is given by the Animal Experimentation Commission, and the (central) Advisory Commission of animal experimentation. If the experiment is performed regardless, the licensee risks the criminal Court calling his actions 'without a reasonable objective' or 'needless'. Unreasonable or needless abuse could be seen as a violation of Article 254 and 455 of the Dutch Criminal Code (regarding animal abuse), and could be convicted as such. In view of all this, the one who performs the experiment should make sure that the licensee, or the person leading or ordering the experiment, acts in keeping with the law. Although the new Dutch legislation regarding animal experimentation prefers to hold the licensee legally responsible, the person performing the experiment, the experimenter will not go free entirely upon violation of article 25. Liability of the corporation is part of the Criminal Code (article 51). The question remains however: is it this person who performed the challenged action? More so, because at present the experimenter, as well as the supervising authorities, must be properly qualified. This applies to, e.g. the article 9 and article 14 officials, but also to the person performing the experiment. They all have a so-called *Garantenstellung*, which means that in the evaluation of certain actions, the liability is determined in accordance with the social role or function the person in question has accepted. The liable person has a certain 'quality', and a corresponding responsibility. This applies to the action, as well as to refraining from action where action was necessary.

A critical remark would be in place here. The entire professional community, in collaboration with animal welfare groups, has succeeded not only in reducing the use of experimental animals during the last few years, but also in establishing self-regulating ethical frameworks by which responsible action becomes an *internal aspect* of the experimenter. Jurisprudence cannot be found which deals with irresponsible action or deliberately ignoring the relevant legislation. Why then has the frightening aspect of the Criminal Code been employed? It is even more oppressive because the role of government supervision has been drastically changed. Besides the supervising task outlined in article 20, the government supervision officials presently also have, on the basis of article 26, the authority to trace the offences outlined in article 25. This general authority has been assigned to the supervising officials on the basis of Criminal Code article 141. Thus, the practical consensus that has been reached with the supervising officials has come under increased pressure. They no longer have the function of advising supervisors, interlocutors, etc., but they also have become criminal prosecutors. This might lead to legal problems; the Criminal Code is, moreover, unsuitable to judge animal experimentation-related actions. The problem is that judges will have to use criteria that are relatively vague (i.e. difficult to interprete for outsiders). There is more similarity with disciplinary jurisdiction of the sort used in veterinary medicine, which would be a much more appropriate tool than the Criminal Code with regard to the nature of the animal experimentation issue. The role of government supervision would also come out better.

Social adequacy

A criminal act is understood to be human behaviour within the parameters of a criminal offence, which is unlawful and to which blame may be ascribed. I am aware that penal codes and scholarly writings about that body of law recognize a distinction between justification and excuse. However, no very precise theory is advanced to make this distinction, and most scholars and reformers evince little concern in connection with this sloppy state of affairs. Greenawalt (1984) for example, argued that Anglo-American criminal law should not attempt to distinguish between justification and excuse in a fully systematic way. However, a few possibly prophetic voices are crying in the wilderness, among whom is George P. Fletcher (1985) whose voice is the loudest and the most eloquent. He tells us that in distinguishing justification from excuse, our own practices and level of understanding compare unfavourably with those of legal systems in the civil law tradition, and that this failing correlates with deeper and more pervasive attitudes, such as 'flat' thinking and legal positivism. He proposes techniques for common law jurisdictions to remedy present inadequacies in dealing with justification and excuse. Aside from the impressions outlined above, Eser and Fletcher (1987) offer an excellent view of these problems in Anglo-American law, Russia, Germany, Poland and Scandinavia.

However, in all cases, it is the description of a criminal act which retains a dominant position. The circumstances which prevail under which the unlawfulness and culpability of an act are carried out are deemed to be included in the description of that act. But determining that a description of an act meets the criteria of its being unlawful and the perpetrator culpable only indicates unlawfulness and culpability, it does not demonstrate that the act itself meets these criteria, only the description thereof. Criminal law assumes that whoever meets the terms laid down by the criminal code is guilty of a criminal offence and in that sense acts unlawfully, with the exception of those cases in which this assumption is inapplicable. Rules are given which form exceptions to the main rule, which take the shape of a counter-norm or grounds for justification. Grounds for justification may only be deployed to make an exception to the norm, as a generally applicable rule, in certain situations, so that – exceptionally – the conclusion may be drawn that no punishment shall be meted out, all this under cover of a textual penalty provision for the act in question. Grounds for justification hence appear incidentally, that is, in cases where, on the grounds of exceptional circumstances prevailing, it is judged that punishments shall be refrained from for an act which does meet the textual demands made in the description of an unlawful act. However, animal experiments may not be tested by this criterion.

Animal experiments fail to meet the legal description of an unlawful act. A reason to reject this approach is that it fails to cohere with reality as it is experienced by the persons conducting the experiments. People who conduct experiments with animals do not view these experimental acts as acts which are, in principle, criminal offences. But this is precisely what the approaches to grounds of justification do. Instead of using this legal fallacy we would be better off looking for a construction which fits better the interests of animal experiments which are conducted in real life.

The solution may be found if the assumption is made of 'acceptable risk', as this is done, for example, in connection with driving on the roads. Simply participating in this entails the possibility of damage being sustained by others. However, because this is a socially acceptable risk, 'participating' as such is not covered by criminal law. The theme of 'acceptable risk' does however manifest itself in a substantially different case where grounds for justification are present. In the case of 'acceptable risk' acts are retained, due to interpretation, outside the bounds of the textual scope of the description of the unlawful act.

In the case of 'acceptable risk' the act is, in concrete, of the type indicated by the description of the unlawful act but remains one to which no criminal conviction accrues, as an exception, and, in connection with 'acceptable risk', the reasoning must be that the acts are of another type than that covered by the descriptions of unlawful acts. The theme of 'acceptable risk' is a completely different matter viewed in terms of criminal law dogma. It is covered by the broader denominator of the 'Theory of Social Adequacy'. Applying the theory of social adequacy as shall be set forth below, leads to certain professional groups in society falling outside the scope of a given norm, and as a result, also falling outside the scope of the punitive provisions attached to it.

Socially adequate behaviour is typified by human relations in a social context. A doctor, a docker, a train-driver, a nurse, in brief anyone and everyone, occupies a certain position in society as well as having a function. This requires certain (specific) knowledge, insights or skills. When these are correctly exercised and deployed, bearing in mind the applicable rules, each individual will take his or her rightful place and function in society and in relation to one another and one may speak of adequate behaviour. In many cases this behaviour will be professional. Aside from this, everyone is part of society by dint of being human. People are socially committed.

In brief, people can not be conceived of outside the historical and social context which congrues with their function. Should acts be in balance with the social position occupied, then this behaviour is socially adequate. This certainly applies to the professional group presently under scrutiny. In other words: socially adequate behaviour is that which is played out in its entirety within the frame of reference of the 'normal' ordering of life which has historical roots. In Hart's terms: socially adequate behaviour is that which congrues with the social rules of a group (Hart, 1961). For professional groups these norms are partly formulated by professional standards and an ethical system, the points of departure of responsible animal experiments. These acts are not those intended to be covered in a description of an unlawful act as set forth in the Criminal Code. The subject conducting such an act, for example, in conducting professional activities, is not part of the circle of persons covered by the Criminal Code. The theory of social adequacy leads to the conclusion that certain groups in society fall outside the scope of certain prohibitions and as a result also fall outside the scope of the punitive provisions attached to them.

To summarize: socially adequate behaviour is that which plays itself out within the historically rooted social ordering of life, without any positive or negative connotation being attached to this. Such behaviour is, in a certain sense 'normal'; socially adequate behaviour comprises the freedom of action. It amounts to this behaviour falling outside the terms of criminal justice. 'When behaviour is assessed as being socially adequate, the terms set forth in a description of an unlawful act are not met.' (Jörg & Kelk, 1990). For the professional group presently under scrutiny, this means that criminal law shall firstly come into play when someone deliberately acts in contravention of the norms used by this group. Acts are then no longer deemed to be socially adequate. Only then, and only if there is due cause, may criminal law be deployed an unlawful act, irrespective of the perpetrator's profession. In these cases the criminal justice system shall decide if there are other grounds which justify this behaviour.

An example of social adequacy

A veterinarian was prosecuted for infringing an article of the Livestock Act, 1920, in which 'deliberately herding (having herded) livestock into inadmissible conditions' is scheduled as an unlawful act.

The veterinarian had deliberately had healthy cows brought into a stable infected with foot-and-mouth disease. This was done with the intention of having the animals, which would probably become infected anyway, exposed to and contract it at a favourable period, that is, when dry. This would exactly conform in terms of goal and effect with a prophylactic treatment, lawfully inoculating the livestock against the disease. Moreover, the well-being of the livestock was ensured in a scientifically responsible manner. In the first instance, the Supreme Court, in a decree dated 27 June, 1932, NJ 1933, 60, considered and ruled, that if, in fact, the correctness of the contentions made by the veterinarian were to be ratified then 'no conviction may take place either on the grounds of the punishability of the suspect being excluded, or, on the grounds that it may not be assumed that the Livestock Act, which scheduled that deliberately herding (having herded) livestock into inadmissible conditions covered those acts which were committed by the respondent with the prescribed intent'. The Supreme Court referred the case to the Court in Amsterdam. This Court ruled that the appeal submitted by the suspect on the grounds of his having acted in his capacity as a veterinarian, thereafter by analogy, appealing to the right of appeal retained by the medical profession, did not hold water.

The Court stated that 'inasmuch as medical treatment falls under the textual scope of punishment provisions, revoking the punishability of the medical practitioner may be grounded in the exceptional nature of the protective right retained: that is the right to 'retain, for a given person a healthy body'. The interest which the veterinarian wished to establish: 'the retention for a certain owner of healthy livestock' lacks in the judgement of the Court the character of being an exception.

When the Supreme Court once again reviewed this case in 1933, the ruling of the Court of Amsterdam was quashed. Summarizing, the Supreme Court stated that from the fact 'that according to law only someone licenced to act as a veterinarian may do so already indicates the correctness of the contention that – unless the law expressly determines to the contrary – a veterinarian who acts in accordance with correct scientific insight in the best interest of livestock, is not guilty of unlawful behaviour'.

If this ruling is taken into account in reviewing animal experiments, then, paraphrasing the ruling of Supreme Court, it may be stated that: from the fact that according to the law only someone with a licence may conduct animal experiments then it is already indicated that for the correctness of the statement – unless the law expressly determines to the contrary – an experimenter who acts in accordance with professional standards and correct scientific insight in the best interest of science for the well-being of mankind and animals, is not guilty of unlawful acts. What the veterinarian did was to protect this interest. This is congruent with the definition of socially adequate behaviour. In this ruling, one is able to recognize an interpretation of the assessment of unlawfulness which precedes the description of the unlawful act. It shows the position, which in my opinion, is legally speaking presently occupied by social adequacy. To summarize: would social adequacy consequently be legal as an interpretation of unlawfulness which precedes the description of the unlawful act? In other words; should acts be assessed as being socially adequate, then the question of unlawfulness would not be addressed, neither would be the question of criminal liability.

Summa summarum: more than ever before, our society demands that people continually evaluate what they do, or refrain from doing, in certain situations taking the risks and consequences of their behaviour into account. Technological and economic developments in all fields, changing patterns in society, and the diminution of sharply delineated norms are responsible for this. The life and health of others but also the proper functioning of social institutions depend to a significant extent on the alertness and care taken by each and every one of us. The proper fulfilment of obligations which arise out of the nature of our work or activities remains imperative.

References

Akkermans, P.W.C. (1992): Article 22. In: *Akkermans/Koekkoek, De Grondwet*, p. 348. Zwolle: W.E.J. Tjeenk Willink.

Chalkly, D.T. (1974): Considerations in the protection of humans as subject of research. *Bull. PanAm Health Organ.* **1974**, 289–292.

Clendeling, L. (1960): *Source book of medical history*, p. xiv. New York: Dover Publications.

Derksen, W., Drupsteen, Th.G. & Witteveen, W.J. (1989): *De terugtred van regelgevers: Meer regels, minder sturing?* Zwolle: Tjeenk Willink.

Eser, A. & Fletcher, G.P. (1987): *Rechtfertigung und Entschuldigung (Justification and Excuse): Rechtsvergleichende Perspektiven (Comparative Perspectives).* Freiburg (Germany): Max Planck Institut für auslandisches und internationales Strafrecht, and New York: Columbia University, School of Law. Vol. I, 1987; Volume II, 1988).

Explanatory Memorandum of the Constitution (1975–1976): 13 872, No. 3.

Fletcher, G.P. (1985): The right and the reasonable. *Harvard Law Rev. Assoc.* **98**, 949.

Greenawalt, K. (1984): *The perplexing borders of justification and excuse.* New York: The Columbia Law Review Association, Inc. rev. 1897.

Hart, H.L.A. (1961): *The concept of law.* Oxford: Oxford University Press (Clarendon Law Series).

Jörg, N. & Kelk, C. (1990): *Strafrecht met mate.* Alphen aan de Rijn: Samsom H.D. Tjeenk Willink (zesde druk).

Macdonald, L. (1989a): *Roses on no man's land.* London: Macmillan.

Macdonald, L. (1989b): *Some, they called it Passchendaele.* London: Macmillan.

Redlich, F.C. (1978): Medical ethics under national socialism. In: *Encyclopedia of bioethics*, ed. Warren T. Reich. Georgetown University, New York: The Free Press.

Withington, E.T. (1964): *Medical history from the earliest times*, p. 424. London: Holland Press.

Section III: Animal research: long-standing controversy

The ethics of animal and human experimentation, edited by P.P. De Deyn.

9

Understanding (and misunderstanding) the animal rights movement in the United States

Adrian R. Morrison

Director, Program for Animal Research Issues, National Institute of Mental Health, National Institutes of Health, Room 17C–26, 5600 Fishers Lane, Rockville, MD 20857, USA; and Department of Anatomy, School of Veterinary Medicine, Department of Animal Biology, Laboratories of Anatomy, University of Pennsylvania, 3800 Spruce Street Philadelphia, PA 19104–6045, USA

Summary

The animal rights movement in the United States focused primarily on attacking biomedical research until fairly recently and gained considerable financial support from an uninformed public. Some organizations have misrepresented the value of animal research to attract sympathizers and have targeted various researchers for public vilification and harassment, while underground terrorists have destroyed laboratories. Some health professionals engage in another reprehensible activity: misquoting the scientific literature to cast doubt on the value of animal-based research. There are those who believe in the animal rights philosophy and seek to live it peacefully. Their views can be respected, but they must consider the implications of their beliefs for humanity and denounce those who sully their cause. Scientists must: (1) assure people that their animals are used by necessity and are treated humanely; (2) correct the distortions that the public hears; and (3) educate non-scientists about the process of science.

Introduction

Humans have battled for good health for as long as one can see back into history. Their enemy, Disease, was cloaked in disguises unwittingly provided by humans themselves through their ignorance: the will of the gods or miasmas. The recognition at last in the 19th century that many health problems stemmed from invasion of the body by microbes provided a point of attack leading eventually to the development of preventive health measures and antitoxins, vaccines and antibiotics. As Lewis Thomas (1974), the noted medical scientist and essayist, reminds us:

> 'Everyone forgets how long and hard the work must be before the really important applications become applicable. The great contemporary achievement of modern medicine is the technology for controlling and preventing bacterial infection, but this did not fall into our laps with the appearance of penicillin and the sulfonamides. It had its beginnings in the final quarter of the last century, and decades of the most painstaking and demanding research were required before the etiology of pneumonia, scarlet fever, meningitis and the rest could be worked out. Generations of energetic and imaginative investigators exhausted their whole lives on the problem. It overlooks a staggering amount of basic research to say that modern medicine began with the era of antibiotics.'

Basic biological and behavioural research, much of it depending on studies using animals, has done much more, of course: anatomists, physiologists, biochemists, psychologists, parasitologists, geneticists, zoologists (the list could go on) have all contributed the bits of information underlying modern medical and surgical practice that have resulted in the healthiest generation in history. Just how healthy we are is brought home by Paton's (1993) description of medical practice little more than a half century ago:

> 'One no longer sees infants with ears streaming pus, schoolboys with facial impetigo, beards growing from heavily infected skin, faces pocked by smallpox or eroded by lupus, or heads and necks scarred from boils or suppurating glands. Drugs and a better diet have transformed haggard patients with peptic ulcers. The languid, characteristically brown-skinned case of Addison's disease of the adrenals; the pale, listless patients of chronic iron deficiency or pernicious anaemia; and the cretin or, conversely, the young woman with 'pop eyes' and overactive emotional behaviour – due respectively to thyroid deficiency or excess – are all being treated. The soggy hulk of a patient in the oedematous stage of chronic kidney disease is relieved by diuretics. As a result of polio vaccine and control of tuberculosis, we see few crippled children; as one walks behind a group of youngsters today, varied as ever in shape and size, the marvel is how straight their limbs and backs are. The chronic arthritics with their sticks are being replaced by septuagenarians swinging along on their plastic hips. The patients now are rare that once one saw dying from an infected mastoid, struggling for breath in the last stages of heart failure, or dying from appendicitis, leukaemia, pneumonia, or bacterial endocarditis.'

The success of the animal rights movement

Unfortunately, too many of the general public do not understand how advances from these conditions and how practical applications in medicine in general depend upon basic research. Because of their training and experience, biomedical professionals can readily accept and understand Comroe's & Dripps' finding (1976) that 41 per cent of the papers reporting work judged to be fundamentally important to the 10 most important advances in cardiology were concerned with studies that sought knowledge for the sake of knowledge itself. Non-scientists, however, have no way of evaluating this important study. And this lack of understanding provides fertile ground for the animal rights movement to sow their seeds of discontent about the use of animals in basic biomedical research.

Furthermore, fewer and fewer people have contact with the animal world, at least as active users of animals other than keeping them as pets. The United States is probably an extreme example. At the present only 2 per cent of the citizenry live on a farm compared with 50 per cent in 1880 (Strand & Strand, 1993, p. 5). Having little understanding of how the living and dying of various animals contribute to their own existence in so many ways, too many are susceptible to the fanciful view of animal life that animal rightists promote.

The leaders of this movement have taken advantage of another aspect of the public's character: the willingness of most people to accept that others are at least trying to act honourably most of the time, however imperfectly. Even though we are, at the same time, sceptics to varying degrees, confidence ('con') men still do remarkably well in our society. And so, through clever misrepresentation of biomedical research and its value to society, animal rights leaders (con men really) have been able to attract quite a few intelligent people to their cause.

The animal rights movement in the United States has had continuing success in spite of the many well-publicized atrocities committed by some of its adherents. The movement has thrived on the phenomena I have already noted: relative ignorance of the nature of science amongst the public (science illiteracy, in other words), naivety concerning the natural world, and the seemingly limitless capacity for distorting the truth revealed by the leadership of the animal rights movement. Other factors have also contributed to animal rightists' success: clever selection of targets in the form of laboratories doing very invasive studies on animals for purposes not well-understood by people – head injury and behavioral research rather than cancer research, for example – to maximize contributions from a compassionate public not wishing to see animals harmed; timidity and ineptitude of institutional administrators in responding to attacks; and indifference and fear among scientists.

These factors together have translated into a considerable amount of money coming into the hands of activists from contributors. The 1992 budgets displayed on Internal Revenue Service forms of the 26 most visible and active animal rights, protection and welfare groups totalled $577 million (Strand and Strand, 1993, p. 55). Because of takeovers of traditional welfare organizations by radical followers of the animal rights philosophy (Strand & Strand, 1993, p. 71) and a melding of the two concepts into 'animal protection' (see below), contributors may be fooled into supporting something in which they really do not believe. Individuals willing to engage in terrorist acts under the aegis of the Animal Liberation Front have also created a negative balance of millions of dollars by destroying research facilities, and stealing animals and data, which stimulates others to spend more on added security (United States Department of Justice and Agriculture, 1993).

Even as overseeing of animal use in the laboratory has resulted in a level of housing and care that outdistances that afforded any other animals in the United States, the terrorist attacks and attempts at introducing more burdensome legislation continue. Because of the tremendous human good done by medical researchers, the continuing relentless attacks on various researchers investigating serious problems, such as head injury, are clear evidence of the misanthropy that drives the most forceful and radical segment of the animal rights movement. Also, as Nicoll (1991) has noted, activists continue to press for local and state legislation blocking the release of animals from pounds for research even though those animals will eventually be killed anyway. This drives up costs as the supply diminishes, forces purchase of costly purpose-bred animals and, of course, impedes research.

Although misanthropy may explain part of the drive for more legislation, at least on the part of radical activists, a genuine concern for animals and ignorance of the nature of scientific inquiry among many of our citizens are significant elements as well. A variety of organizations supported by such individuals are currently grouped under the banner of the 'animal protection community.' However, those organizations with conventional animal welfare concerns are finding even the most radical animal rightists crowding under that honourable banner, and some are finding that their organization and its assets have been taken over by radical animal rightists (Strand & Strand, 1993, p. 71). It would seem that reference to animal protection, rather than animal welfare, had to emerge in the literature of organizations uncomfortable with research on animals and of groups overtly hostile to it once biomedical researchers (and other animal-user groups for that matter) demonstrated that they, too, had animal *welfare* concerns, contrary to what the animal rights movement had been saying about them. Of course, emphasizing a common cause, 'animal protection,' leads to a usefully confusing blending of the belief shared by most of us that animals have a 'right' to good care when in our hands, with the extreme view that rats are our moral equals.

Do not interpret this analysis to mean that I am belittling those who believe that one has no right to use animals in any fashion, however impractical I think that essentially religious philosophy to be. Herzog (1993a), a behavioural researcher who works with animals, performed a very interesting qualitative survey of 23 rank-and-file animal rights activists; and it is clear that they have strongly held beliefs and struggle to live their convictions consistently. He points out that they are essentially 'religious' fundamentalists, believing firmly in their cause. Herzog reported an antagonism toward science, not surprisingly; but there was no discussion of whether these individuals would refuse medical treatment for the rest of their lives as do some religious sects nor whether they had concerns that their activities might lead to unnecessary suffering of their fellow humans if medical research were impeded by activist activity. Because those who lead the movement continue to misrepresent the benefits that have come to us and how that research is conducted, I think those who follow have an obligation to investigate the matter and, at the very least, reject lies as a foundation for sincere concerns.

Having read the results of Herzog's survey, I am convinced that some *followers* in the animal rights movement could be persuaded that they should not prevent others from benefiting from medical research. If educated in the *process* of science – I shall return to this theme at the end of this essay – how could they, for example, deny children with cystic fibrosis the chance to enjoy a longer, more comfortable life as a result of the gene therapy becoming available thanks to animal research conducted during the past few years in particular? Could the philosopher Tom Regan (1983)?

Coming from the animal protection community, undoubtedly due to a variety of motives and insights with differing levels of scientific (and political) sophistication, are calls for support of only that research that will obviously benefit human health. Some have 'the illusion that anyone is qualified to make scientific judgements on the value of research, thereby successfully moving the issue from the scientific realm to an arena where moral judgements and personal opinions (however uneducated) determine public policy' (Morrison, 1993). For example, Rollin (1991) – a professor of philosophy, not a scientist – sees the need for permitting only 'patently beneficial research' (Rollin, 1991, p. 154). He continues: 'Obviously, this criterion would exclude a great deal of current invasive animal research, ranging from much, if not most, product testing to military research, to a great deal of 'knowledge-for-its-own sake research' (Rollin, 1991, p. 154–155). Rollin would require a cost (to animals)–benefit (to humans) analysis leading to funding decisions that would be made, not by scientific experts but by 'panels – grand juries as it were – of intelligent interested citizens who would look at research proposals and decide if the benefits exceeded the costs, or if the question being asked was the sort that truly needed to be answered' (Rollin, 1991, p. 156). He does say he would provide them with expert technical advice. Rollin claims that this scheme would 'integrate science and concern for science far more closely into the fabric of society and help accelerate scientific literacy' (Rollin, 1991, p. 156). This incredibly naive proposal indicates to me that a priority concern of scientists should be raising the level of science literacy of our society, but not as Rollin would do it. Practical mechanisms for educating people about biomedical research will be proposed later.

The use of animals and the concept of speciesism

Productive discussions can be held with those who genuinely care about animals and agree to their use but have a limited understanding of science and a concern (fuelled by the animal rights movement) for what *might* be going on in laboratories. On the other hand, Horton (1989) has noted that calls for reaching agreement between animal rights activists and scientists imply that each group is at an extreme when, in fact, scientists are doing society's work. As Goodwin & Morrison (1993) have put it:

> 'No consensus can be reached between those who accept the use of animals for important human needs and those who categorically reject animal use based on a philosophy that views all forms of sentient life as morally equivalent. If the question fundamentally is *whether* to use animals, no middle ground exists. Use cannot be partly ethical, it is either ethical or unethical.
>
> People who genuinely want to discuss the matter with researchers must first disavow the animal rights position. To engage in middle-ground discussions with true believers in animal rights is, at best, fruitless; at worst, it provides animal rights activists with a tactic to shift the uninformed a little closer to the ultimate goal of total abolition of animal use. Only if one starts from the principle that the use of animals is acceptable does the issue of *how* animals are used address the spectrum of legitimate issues.

One end of this spectrum holds that we should spare no expense to provide absolute comfort and procedural safeguards for experimental animals; a corollary of this extreme animal welfare position is that research goals have to be secondary to the absolute commitment to animal comfort. The other end of the spectrum holds that humane treatment should not be a consideration if it involves any extra expense or inconvenience – that animals can be treated essentially like lab equipment. Between these two extremes, the biomedical research community occupies the middle ground. We are engaged in legitimate, important debates about regulations *vs.* costs and about animal welfare vs. human needs ... ' (Goodwin & Morrison, 1993).

Without question, though, a disdain for humanity coupled with an elevation of animals to equal status motivates the most radical and, unfortunately, the most successful animal rights organizations in the United States (and elsewhere for that matter). Repeating a couple of the statements made by a couple of these organizations' leaders will make my point: 'If animal research resulted in a cure for AIDS, we'd be against it,' is a famous utterance of Ingrid Newkirk (1989), National Director of People for the Ethical Treatment of Animals (PETA), the most virulent and dominant of the many radical, 'above-ground' US groups. Chris DeRose (1989) of Last Chance for Animals admits: 'A life is a life. If the death of one rat cured all diseases, it wouldn't make any difference to me'.

Presently, the movement is attacking all uses of animals: biomedical research, toxicity testing, education, food, fur coats, hunting (Marquardt *et al.*, 1993). The extension of attacks to include all uses of animals is a relatively recent development, though; for the most publicized attacks were against researchers and research and testing establishments beginning in the early 1980s. Nicoll & Russell (1990) analysed the animal rights literature and found that, relative to the actual numbers of animals used, an inordinate amount of space was devoted to concerns about the use of animals in research and testing. There is a likely reason for this: few people engage in or understand the value of biomedical research; whereas many enjoy eating meat. If one wishes to obtain funds to fuel a social movement, it would not make sense to attack something most do – eat meat for example – and expect those consumers to contribute to the demise of a favourite activity. Singer (1990) revealed that, in fact, there were political considerations:

> 'American animal researchers are a smaller and politically less powerful group than American farmers, and they are based in regions where animal liberationists live. They therefore made a more accessible, and slightly less formidable opponent . . . '

Now that the movement is well-funded, though, we are seeing attacks on every conceivable use of animals in the United States.

Claims against biomedical research by the animal rights movement

Goodwin (1992) has noted that the attack on animal use in biomedical and behavioral research focused on several secondary 'stop research' arguments when the true agenda was something else, promotion of an ideology that is really anti-societal in that it effectively equates animals with humans:

Research is inherently cruel

For those who value humans above animals, the idea that working to alleviate human suffering is a cruel activity has no merit. It is an idea based on a misconception, that scientists are cold and calculating, caring little about the animals on which they work. Granted, even the most caring scientist can make mistakes or lack veterinary knowledge – no human activity is perfect. These failings are countered, though, by the presence, by law, of Institutional Animal Care and Use Committees (IACUC) and laboratory animal veterinarians that oversee animal experiments (Morrison, 1993). Finally, the United States Department of Agriculture (USDA) reported in 1990 that more than half (58 per cent) of the experiments actually involved no pain or distress at all, 36 per cent required analgesics or anaesthetics and only 6 per cent involved study of pain mechanisms so that chemical pain relief was not possible (USDA). Experiments on pain are very carefully scrutinized by institutional committees, granting agencies and journals; and they can often be designed to permit the animal to escape intolerable pain.

Research is wasteful and duplicative

This argument reveals a lack of common sense and understanding of the process of science. What highly trained individual seeking recognition from his peers would pursue trivial or redundant research? At the same time, replication of findings by other scientists establishes the generality of one's own. With funding levels for *approved* grants from the National Institutes of Health now well below 20 per cent, uselessly redundant research has little chance of survival.

Research diverts funds that could go into prevention or treatment

For those who receive complaints from the public about animal research, this is a frequently heard refrain. Actually, for every $100 spent on health care in the United States, only 40 cents is spent on animal research (Goodwin, 1992). Furthermore, more than half of the grants awarded by the National Institutes of Health are given for studies on people or for those using methodologies not requiring animals (Personal communication, L. Sibal, Office of Laboratory Animal Research, National Institutes of Health).

Alternative methods are now available, making animal research unnecessary

Another suggestion reflecting a profound lack of understanding of science – perhaps leaders of the movement are just being deceitful – is that modern science has passed animal research by, because other technologies have rendered animal use unnecessary. It is often stated that use of tissue cultures, computers and human clinical cases are sufficient to unravel the mysteries of disease. This claim, of course, does not take into account the complexities of the functioning organism. Also, one should not forget that scientists are the individuals who have devised the various alternative methods used in order to address scientific questions in the most appropriate way; they are not wedded to the idea of using animals.

The movement has also argued that biomedical research endangers pets. Of course, 90 per cent of the approximately 20 million animals (United States Congress Office of Technology Assessment, 1986) used in the United States are purpose-bred rats and mice and cannot possibly be stolen pets. The USDA licenses dealers who buy dogs and cats from those who raise them, or from pounds and shelters, where, in fact, several million abandoned or feral animals are killed in the latter each year. Although it is possible that some *wanted* but unclaimed pets could slip through this 'safety net,' the number would have to be small. There is also the possibility of false charges from the animal rights community: In the spring of 1993, a known activist charged a major university with having her pet dog in their animal quarters. In the presence of a USDA veterinarian, she pointed out the dog; however, it did not respond to her loving embrace. After comparing the dog and her pet's medical papers, the veterinarian pointed out that the dog in the facility was an intact male and that the medical records of her pet indicated it had been castrated! (Public announcement, Johns Hopkins University.)

The over-riding principle guiding animal rights activists is that use or 'exploitation' of animals for human benefit is nothing less than 'speciesism,' an idea generally identified with the Australian philosopher, Peter Singer, because of the popularity of his book *Animal Liberation* (1990). Speciesism is 'a prejudice or attitude of bias in favour of the interests of members of one's own species and against those of members of other species' (Singer, 1989). This notion makes no sense to a biologist.

I look at the problem in a practical way: animals use other animal (and plant) species in the over-all scheme of things, and we are animals. Thus, in my opinion, we are also permitted to use other species. This doing-what-comes-naturally argument might appear to be weakened because we recognize right from wrong, and other animals do not operate in this framework. The argument seems to be that consequently we are obligated to act more nobly. In fact, we do. We are the ones who pass anti-cruelty laws. Yet, through our intelligence we can project our lives well into the future so that taking many rats' or dogs' lives because we can foresee a benefit to ourselves or our young seems no different from or less supportable than a cat's killing several animals to give herself energy to feed her young. Both activities meet the needs of survival. Viewed this way, our intelligence makes us no more culpable. One must ignore the realities of Nature and the power of natural impulses to conclude otherwise.

Cohen (1986) turned the concept of 'speciesism' on its head in a way with which I clearly agree:

> 'I am a speciesist. Speciesism is not merely plausible; it is essential for right conduct, because those who will not make the morally relevant distinctions among species are almost certain, in consequence, to misapprehend their true obligations. The analogy between speciesism and racism is insidious. Every sensitive moral judgement requires that the differing natures of the beings to whom obligations are owed be considered. If all forms of animate life – or vertebrate animal life? – must be treated equally, and if therefore in evaluating a research program the pains of a rodent count equally with the pains of a human, we are forced to conclude (1) that neither humans nor rodents possess rights, or (2) that rodents possess all the rights that humans possess. Both alternatives are absurd. Yet one or the other must be swallowed if the moral equality of all species is to be defended.

Vance (1992) cautions that Singer and the other major philosopher of the animal rights movement, Tom Regan, cannot be brushed aside as promoting emotional arguments in favour of animals. Both present the rational arguments typical of analytical ethics although their arguments differ radically. Singer is a utilitarian arguing that animals should be accorded equal consideration because they equally feel pain and that one should act to bring about the best balance of good and bad consequences; while Regan holds that animals have inherent value and ultimately reaches the conclusion that they have moral rights, which affords them protection from experimentation. In addition to presenting quite different philosophical reasons for objecting to harming animals for human benefit, Regan and Singer presented their theses in quite different books. Except for a few sentences explicitly stating the usual distorted descriptions of medical research obtained from the animal rights literature, Regan's book, *The Case for Animal Rights* (1983), is a purely philosophical treatise. Singer, however, devotes more than half of *Animal Liberation* to proselytizing for animal liberation (not animal rights) and describing the evils of research, toxicity testing and agriculture – often out of context, even inaccurately, or ignoring new developments in animal care, as Katz (1993), Nicoll *et al.* (1992), Russell and Nicoll (1994) and Verhetsel (1986) have reported.

Vance (1992) notes that additional work is under way in the philosophical community to shore up weaknesses in Regan's and Singer's thinking and that we should prepare ourselves for more carefully reasoned arguments. I am certain, however, that the most scholarly defense of the proposition that humans should, in general, not be afforded any more consideration than any other animal will not sway the vast majority of people. I am confident that the common man has more common sense.

Educating people about biomedical research

We need to focus our efforts on three things: (1) assuring the public that we are caring for animals as well as we can while doing well-conceived research; (2) revealing the distortions of our literature by the more radical in the movement; and (3) educating the public, particularly young students, in the process of science. The remainder of this essay will address these items.

(1) The care of laboratory animals in the United States has improved over the years as researchers (and society in general) became more sensitive to animal needs and the specialty of laboratory animal medicine (and veterinary medicine itself) matured. Conditions were uneven, though, until a set of standards was mandated by law in 1985. Now, institutions receiving federal funds must have an attending veterinarian and a committee, the IACUC mentioned above, which approves all proposals for experiments using animals before they can begin, and oversees that use via semi-annual inspections. Public Health Service policy (United States Department of Health and Human Services, 1986) states that the IACUC must have five members, including a veterinarian experienced in laboratory animal medicine, a practising scientist experienced in animal research, a person whose primary interest is non-scientific, and an individual with no ties to the institution. The USDA has similar requirements, and using their own inspectorate periodically inspects any facility using animals (excluding rats and mice), not just those receiving federal funds (Morrison, 1993).

Animal activists have made much of the fact that the USDA does not inspect rodent facilities even though rats and mice comprise 90 per cent of the 20 million animals used in research, but these animals are covered under Public Health Service policy (United States Public Health Service, 1992). Both the Office of Protection from Research Risks of the Public Health Service and the Regulatory Enforcement and Animal Care division of the Animal and Plant Health Service of the USDA have the power to investigate complaints against laboratories, demand corrective actions and invoke sanctions – and they use it. The system is working well, and researchers should tell the public so while striving to handle their animals as humanely as possible.

Researchers should also reveal their own ambivalence about working with animals. Herzog (1988, 1991, 1993b) has written a series of thoughtful articles that address this issue and the paradoxes that inevitably arise when putting animals to any human use. All the researchers I know are uncomfortable with having to harm animals, particularly when one has to kill an animal that one has studied over an extended period or when large numbers must be killed for a biochemical analysis. I have described my own feelings, which have been printed in newsletters of organizations concerned with protecting biomedical research and researchers: the incurably ill For Animal Research (iiFAR), National Animal Interest Alliance and Putting People First. Many scientists probably share my thinking:

> I believe animal use by humans is natural and no less appropriate in the scheme of things than animal use by other animals. Therefore, I reject as nonsense the notion of speciesism that the animal rights movement promotes. It is a perversion of biology, not a principle. Vivisection fits into the category of appropriate uses; for it is a function of a legitimate aspect of our nature, which is to explore and increase knowledge. Indeed, increasing knowledge in all spheres, even if it requires the deaths of some animals, is our obligation; for we are the only species capable of undoing 'harm' to the planet caused by us.
>
> This is not to say that the invasiveness of vivisection is something I prefer or participate in without reflection. Because I do experimental surgery, I go through a soul-searching every few months, asking myself whether I really want to continue working on cats – my family has had up to four of them at a time as pets over the years – or other animals for that matter. The answer is always 'yes' because I know that there is no other way for medicine to progress but through animal experimentation and that basic research leads ultimately to unforeseen benefits.
>
> My passion is to alleviate human misery; it takes precedence over everything. The animal rights movement, on the other hand, focuses on pain/suffering in 'sentient beings' in the immediate present. Certainly pain should not be inflicted wantonly or left unalleviated if at all possible. Yet, we humans suffer the same and much more; there lies the difference. What animal can match in suffering the heartbreak of parents, who lose a child to illness or who have given birth to a child with severe birth defects, or the despair of a teenager who learns that life in the future will be incomplete as a result of the car accident that severed his spinal cord? Even chimpanzees cannot participate in the grief of others (Cheney & Seyfarth, 1990). We can, even when learning of a tragedy in the newspaper. This makes us 'special'.

(2) The weakest point the animal rights movement has from an ethical standpoint is their willingness to lie and to misquote the scientific literature. The worst offenders in my eyes are medical professionals, who appear to have no compunction about engaging in this practice, fudging the data as it were.

Students gasp when I show a slide from a book by Brandon Reines (1985), a veterinarian, claiming that a scientist who developed a heart–lung machine for open-heart surgery did so using only human patients and then follow it with a slide revealing the full quotation (Wertenbaker, 1980) in which the scientists describe their use of dogs in a paragraph omitted from the centre of Reines's quotation and replaced by ellipses. Thus, Reines quotes the researcher as follows:

> 'Lillihei himself says, "We were feeling our way along as far as flow was concerned ... Then we got more experience with our heart–lung machine and it worked for all sizes of people"' (Reiner, 1985).

Reines then continues: 'Thus, Dr. Lillihei and his associates made the heart–lung machine safe and effective during the course of practice on actual patients – not from studies on healthy laboratory animals.'

Audacious examples like this abound. Verhetsel (1986) has reported many more misquotations from Reines's books and others often used to support animal rightists' claims, such as Ruesch's *Slaughter of the innocent* (1985) and Ryder's *Victims of science: the use of animals in research* (1983) that try to present a negative image of medical research. Articles by Nicoll & Russell (1992) have exposed the questionable practices of Neal Barnard, a psychiatrist who is President of the Physicians Committee for Responsible Medicine, an affiliate of PETA, as well as those of Singer (Nicoll *et al.*, 1992; Russell & Nicoll, 1994), noted above. Miller (1991) has revealed additional misrepresentations of the literature by a psychologist (Ulrich, 1991) who has turned away from animal research, and by members of the Medical Research Modernization Committee, another group containing health professionals who reject the idea that animal research has been necessary for medical progress and twist the facts to promote their cause.

A useful exercise for students would be to have them read the original writings of scientists and then compare their conclusions with the quotations and interpretations found in the animal rights literature.

(3) Even though most of the public accepts that continued animal research and testing is necessary to ensure the medical progress from which they want to benefit, they are naturally uncomfortable with the idea that harm does come to other creatures, as are we scientists. They want that harm minimized. Again, so do we. Lacking a sophisticated understanding of the *process* of science, however, the public is prone to accept the idea that tighter and tighter control on animal use can only be a good thing. Rollin (1991) predicts this as the wave of the future.

We need to help people learn how science is really done. Any experienced scientist knows that new knowledge comes with difficulty and that luck and insights obtained from unexpected sources play important roles. Of course, a project should start with an hypothesis formulated by a well-trained, well-read individual. It should be pursued, though, with a mind open to the very real possibility that the hypothesis will have to be modified or even abandoned along the way. Observations from a myriad of studies conducted in this manner eventually merge in unexpected ways that lead to a real medical advance. Thomas (1974) sketched out this process in describing the development of antibiotics, and Comroe & Dripps (1976) proved the value of basic research in their analysis of the cardiology literature. One wonders what advances Rollin's 'citizen panels' would have blocked by stopping 'knowledge-for-its-own-sake research'.

More of us should undertake exercises like that of Comroe and Dripps, but in a way that would make them accessible to students. Miller (1985) has called for this and has written as a prologue to a textbook a review based on the excellent book by science historian Judith Swazey (1974) on the development of chlorpromazine as a relief for schizophrenia. He compares the research to the assembling of a complex puzzle from many parts, involving study of the chemical structure of dyes and investigation of the fungus, ergot, and one of its components, histamine, and then antihistamines. Further study of a blue dye effective against malaria led to the development of new antihistamines, all producing drowsiness. A medical treatment for schizophrenia eventually resulted – but not without the additional help of developments in animal learning theory and behavioural tests useful for examining drug effects.

Those of us who have spent years in research have a story to tell even if we are not professional historians like Swazey. Thinking back on a career in sleep research, I marvel at how inspiration from a book outside my field, discussion of a reading with an undergraduate student, an accidental observation by another student, and even the experience of being attacked by the Animal Liberation Front eventually led me to investigate the pathophysiology of post-traumatic stress disorder. It is an interesting story and one I pledge to tell. I hope some of the readers of this chapter will consider doing the same.

References

Cheney, D.L. & Seyfarth, R.M. (1990): *How monkeys see the world.* Chicago: University of Chicago Press.

Cohen, C. (1986): The case for the use of animals in biomedical research. *N. Engl. J. Med.* **315**, 865–870.

Comroe, J.H., Jr. & Dripps, R.D. (1976): Scientific basis for the support of biomedical science. *Science* **192**, 105–111.

DeRose, C. (1989): as quoted in *Biting back* by E. Venant & D. Treadwell. *Los Angeles Times*, April 12: E12.

Goodwin, F.K. (1992): Animal rights: medical research and product testing: is this a 'hang together or together we hang' issue? *Contemp. Top. in Lab. Animal Sci.* **31**, 6–11.

Goodwin, F.K. & Morrison, A.R. (1993): In animal rights debate, the only valid moderates are researchers.*The Scientist* **17** (Sept. 6), 12.

Herzog, H.A., Jr. (1988): The moral status of mice. *Am. Psychol.* **43**, 473–474.

Herzog, H.A., Jr. (1991): Conflicts of interest: kittens and boa constrictors, pets and research. *Am. Psychol.* **46**, 246–248.

Herzog, H.A., Jr. (1993a): 'The movement is my life': the psychology of animal rights activism. *J. Social Issues* **49**, 103–119.

Herzog, H. (1993b): Human morality and animal research: confessions and quandaries. *Am. Scholar.* **62**, 337–349.

Horton, L. (1989): The enduring animal issue. *J. Natl. Cancer Inst.* **81**, 736–743.

Katz, L.S. (1993): How to attack animal agriculture with a pinch of fact and a pound of hyperbole. Coalition for Animals and Animal Research (CFAAR) Newsletter, PO Box 8060, Berkeley, CA 94707–8060 USA, 5/1, 30–31.

Marquardt, K., Levine, H.M. & LaRochelle, M. (1993): *Animalscam: the beastly abuse of human rights.* Washington, DC: Regnery Gateway.

Miller, N.E. (1985): Prologue. In: *Psychology and life,* 11th edn., ed. P.G. Zimbardo, pp. i–vii, Glenview, IL: Scott Foresman.

Miller, N.E. (1991): Commentary on Ulrich: need to check truthfulness of statements by opponents of animal research. *Psychol. Sci.* **2**, 422–424.

Morrison, A.R. (1993): Biomedical research and the animal rights movement: a contrast in values. *Am. Biol. Teacher* **55**, 204–208.

Newkirk, I. (1989): as quoted in *Politics* by F. Barnes, *Vogue*, Sept. p.542.

Nicoll, C.S. (1991): A physiologist's views on the animal rights/liberation movement. *The Physiologist* **34**, 303–315.

Nicoll, C.S. & Russell, S.M. (1990): Editorial: Analysis of animal rights literature reveals the underlying motives of the movement: ammunition for counter offensive by scientists. *Endocrinology* **127**, 985–989.

Nicoll, C.S. & Russell, S.M. (1992): Commentary: animal rights, animal research, and human obligations. *Mol. Cell Neurosci.* **3**, 271–277.

Nicoll, C.S., Russell, S.M. & Lau, A. (1992): Letter to the editor. *New York Review of Books*, Nov. 5, 59–60.

Paton, W. (1993): *Man and mouse: animals in medical research*, 2nd edn., p. 93. Oxford: Oxford University Press.

Regan, T. (1983): *The case for animal rights*. Berkeley: University of California Press.

Reines, B. (1985): *Heart research on animals: a critique of animal models of cardiovascular disease*, p. 52, Jenkintown, PA: The American Anti-Vivisection Society.

Rollin, B.E. (1991): Some ethical concerns in animal research: where do we go next? In: *Animal experimentation: the moral issues*, eds. R.M. Band & S.E. Rosenbaum, pp. 151–158. Buffalo, NY: Prometheus Books.

Ruesch, H. (1985): *Slaughter of the innocent*. Klosters, Switzerland: Civitas Publ.

Russell, S.M. & Nicoll, C.S. (1994): A dissection of the chapter 'Tools for research' in Peter Singer's *Animal liberation. Proc. Soc. Exp. Biol. & Med.* **Oct.** (in press).

Ryder, R.D. (1983): *Victims of science: the use of animals in research*. London: National Anti-Vivisection Society.

Singer, P. (1990): *Animal liberation*, 2nd edn., p. 6. New York: Random House.

Singer, P. (1989): Unkind to animals. *New York Review of Books*, Feb. 2, p. 37.

Strand, R. & Strand, P. (1993): *The hijacking of the humane movement*, Doral Publ.: Wilsonville, OR.

Swazey, J.P. (1974): *Chlorpromazine in psychiatry: a study of therapeutic innovation*. Cambridge, MA: MIT Press.

Thomas, L. (1974): *The lives of a cell*, p. 117. New York: Viking Press.

Ulrich, R.E. (1991); Commentary: animal rights, animal wrongs and the question of balance. *Psychol. Sci.* **2**, 197–201.

United States Congress Office of Technology Assessment (1986): *Alternatives to animal use in research, testing and education.* Washington, DC: US Government Printing Office, OTA-BA–73, Feb, p. 5.

United States Department of Agriculture (1990): *Animal welfare enforcement, Fiscal Year 1990.* Washington, DC: US Department of Agriculture.

United States Department of Health and Human Services. (1986): *Public health service policy on humane care and use of laboratory animals.* Bethesda, MD: National Institutes of Health, Office of Protection from Research Risks.

United States Departments of Justice and Agriculture (1993): *Report to Congress on the extent and effect of domestic and international terrorism on animal enterprises.* Washington DC 20530: US Dept of Justice.

United States Public Health Service (1992): *Protecting laboratory animals (USPHS policy statement).* Obtainable from author.

Vance, R.P. (1992): An introduction to the philosophical presuppositions of the animal liberation/rights movement. *JAMA* **268**, 1715–1719.

Verhetsel, E. (1986): *They threaten your health: a critique of the antivivisection/animal rights (AV-AR) movement.* Tucson, AZ: Nutrition Information Centre.

Wertenbaker, L. (1980): *To mend the heart,* p. 155. New York: Viking Press.

The ethics of animal and human experimentation, edited by P.P. De Deyn.
©1994 John Libbey & Company Ltd., pp. 107–113.

10

Education and training in laboratory animal science

Lambertus F.M. van Zutphen

Department of Laboratory Animal Science, Faculty of Veterinary Science, Utrecht University, PO Box 80 166, 3805 TD Utrecht, The Netherlands

Summary

In several countries, regulations have been issued with the aim of protecting animals which are used for scientific purposes. For European Community (EC) Member States, these regulations are largely based upon the 1986 EC Council Directive on the protection of animals used for experiments and other scientific purposes. Appropriate education and training of persons who are involved in animal experimentation is an important issue in the EC Council Directive and several Member States have already implemented the sections on competence.

In the Netherlands, training in the field of laboratory animal science has been made compulsory by law for animal caretakers (persons responsible for the day to day care of the animals), animal technicians (persons responsible for the performance of methods and procedures), scientists (persons responsible for the design of experiments) and laboratory animal specialists (persons responsible for management and animal quality control or for the welfare of animals used in research). Formal training programmes have been developed for each of these categories.

For animal caretakers and technicians the training programmes take 1.5 and 3 years, respectively. In these programmes practical training is a major component. Scientists are allowed to design and perform animal experiments only after graduating in one of the biomedical sciences (e.g. biology, medicine, veterinary medicine, pharmacology) and having, in addition to that, successfully completed a 3-week course on laboratory animal science. For the animal welfare officer a 1-year postgraduate training programme is compulsory. The contents of these training programmes should contribute to the humane use and care of animals and to the quality of experiments.

Introduction

The use of animals as model for man has a long history and runs parallel to the development of Western medicine. The number of animals increased with the growth of biomedical research. A substantial increase occurred after World War II.

However, in most Western countries animal use is now decreasing, whereas biomedical research is still growing. Several developments have contributed to this decrease, including legislation, ethical evaluation of protocols, and education. Although education in the field of laboratory animal science is also important for the quality of research, until recently the need for this type of training for persons responsible for the design of animal experiments was not widely recognized. During the last decade, education and training in this field has been made compulsory by law in several countries (De Greeve *et al.*, 1993). For European countries two documents controlling the use of animals for scientific purposes are most important. The Convention for the Protection of Vertebrate Animals used for Experimental and other Scientific Purposes was issued by the Council of Europe in Strasburg in 1985 (Council of Europe), whereas the EC Directive for the Protection of Vertebrate Animals used for Experimental and other Scientific Purposes was adopted by the Council of the European Communities in 1986 (EC Council Directive). This latter document is based upon the Convention but its requirements are more stringent. All EC Member States must implement the provisions of the EC Directive via their national laws.

There are several sections in the EC Directive dealing with competence. Article 7 states that animal experiments should be performed solely by a person who is considered to be competent or under the direct responsibility of such a person. In article 14 it is stated that persons who carry out experiments or participate in them, and persons who take care of animals used for experiments, including duties of a supervisory nature, shall have appropriate education and training.

Also, in the USA, specific training of scientists and technicians involved in animal experimentation is no longer optional. Since 1985 the Animal Welfare Act includes provisions as to the training on relevant aspects of laboratory animal science to all personnel using animals in research (USA Animal Welfare Act, 1985).

The provisions on competence aim to contribute to the humane use and care of animals, and to the quality of experimental results. Education and training should also provide the opportunity for obtaining the proper attitude and the notion of including ethical aspects into animal experimentation.

There are several categories of persons involved in animal experimentation: animal caretakers (persons responsible for the day to day care of the animals), animal technicians (persons responsible for the proper performance of methods and procedures), scientists (persons responsible for the proper design and conduct of experiments) and laboratory animal specialists (persons responsible for management and animal quality control, or for the welfare of the animals used in research).

Each of these categories need to be specifically educated in the field of laboratory animal science. Formal training courses have been developed in several countries (Dennis & Van Hoosier, 1989; Olfert & Flowers, 1983; Report of the Working Party on Courses for Animal Licences, 1984; Sarboudy, 1987; Van Hoosier & Dahm, 1983; Van Hoosier *et al.*, 1993; van Zutphen, 1988; van Zutphen 1989). In this contribution a short overview is presented on the requirements on education and training in the Netherlands, with some emphasis on the training programme for the scientist.

Animal caretaker/animal technicians

In the Netherlands, as in most other countries, training in the field of laboratory animal science started with persons who are in charge of the day-to-day care of laboratory animals and those who are performing the experimental techniques. These persons are closely involved in animal experimentation. The training of these categories started more than 40 years ago, mainly as institutional initiatives. It soon became clear that collaboration could improve the quality of the courses, so in 1962 a national working committee on laboratory animal issues (LWL) was established. A main objective of this committee was the coordination of training courses for employees of institutions that use laboratory animals. In 1972, the first textbook on laboratory animal science for animal caretakers and technicians was published (Van der Gulden *et al.*, 1972). This book has been used ever since for all vocational training courses for these two categories of persons.

Legal requirements on competence for these categories were issued in 1985, but it was not before 1993 that the regulations with minimum requirements for the training courses came into effect. The minimum requirements for the animal caretaker are a course of 1.5 year with at least 500 hours laboratory animal science, 150 hours general (basic) education and 800 hours practical training. The minimum requirements for the animal technician are a course of 3 years with at least 1000 hours laboratory animal science, 300 hours general (basic) education and 1600 hours practical training. These courses are presently organized at a limited number of locations. Practical training (on-the-job training) is performed at institutions where laboratory animals are used for research, education or testing.

Scientists

The scientist who is responsible for the design and conduct of animal experiments is the first responsible person for the humane use and care of animals. According to the Federation of European Laboratory Animal Science Associations (FELASA) priority should be given to the education and training of this category. The training in laboratory animal science should preferably be taken before participating in animal experiments. This training should not only contribute to the understanding of the technical aspects of animal use but also to an understanding of the moral and ethical implications. The students should become sensitized to their responsibility for the animals used in their research, and should become alert to the need for searching for alternatives. They should be motivated so that, if animals must be used, they will seek for procedures and techniques which will eliminate or minimize pain and distress whenever possible.

In 1991, FELASA formulated the requirements for the training and education of scientist. According to FELASA, scientists who are responsible for the design of animal experiments can be considered as competent after having completed a full university degree course, graduating with a bachelor's or master's degree in a biomedical discipline (such as biology, medicine, or veterinary medicine) and having taken an introductory course on laboratory animal science. This course should be no less than 80 hours and must provide the tools for a responsible use of animals and high scientific standards.

The introductory course on laboratory animal science must be completed before a scientist is considered fully competent to undertake animal experiments on his/her own full responsibility.

Additional specialized training, e.g. required for surgery or particular techniques, should be obtained through close collaboration with experienced investigators and animal technicians, or by attending specialized courses.

In a recent report of the EC and the European Federation of Pharmaceutical Industries' Associations (EFPIA) on the harmonization of training in laboratory animal science within Europe (1993) the conclusion was reached that international guidelines on education should be established and that the current FELASA proposals are useful as a starting point. It was stated that special attention should be paid to ethics and the use of alternative methods.

In the Netherlands, legal provisions on competence for persons who are responsible for the design of animal experiments were issued in 1985. The requirements for the scientist are similar to those proposed by FELASA: a scientist is considered competent after having completed a graduate training in one of the biomedical sciences and, in addition, after taking a 3-week introductory course on laboratory animal science. These requirements are mandatory for all 'new' scientists. Researchers who were responsible for the design of animal experiments at the time that the provisions were issued were exempt.
Since 1986 the introductory course has been organized at several universities and is centrally coordinated by the Department of Laboratory Animal Science – Utrecht.

From the beginning, the three Rs (Replacement, Reduction, Refinement) have been the guiding principles in the design of the course (Russell & Burch, 1959). The contents of the course cover various aspects of laboratory animal science, e.g. biology and husbandry of frequently used laboratory animals; microbiology and diseases; genetic standardization and monitoring; health hazards in the animal house; design of animal experiments; anaesthesia, analgesia and experimental procedures; alternatives to animal use; ethical aspects and legislation; analysis of scientific literature. A full outline of the course is given by Van Zutphen (1988, 1989, 1991). During the course, lectures are alternated by practical sessions. Working groups are formed in order to stimulate a cooperative problem-solving attitude. In support of the problem-based learning exercises the services of the department's information and documentation centre (PREX) is available for the students. PREX has been established with the objective to collect, classify and make available relevant information in the field of laboratory animal science, including welfare issues, alternatives, ethics and legislation. This information is not only available for students but also for animal welfare officers and scientists designing animal experiments. At present, databases on several aspects are covered, e.g.:

- Laboratory animal science literature: literature references of papers published in the core journals in the field of laboratory animal science (from the first issue published onwards);
- Catalogue of inbred strains: characteristics of inbred strains (with literature references) and addresses of suppliers. This index has been developed by Dr M.F. Festing and has been made available to PREX for on-line distribution;
- Biological reference values: blood parameters and other biological data of laboratory animals;
- Alternatives: literature references on alternatives to animal experiments.

In addition to specialized databases PREX is also offering access to several CD-ROM databases (e.g. Medline; Agricola; Vet-CD).

From 1994 PREX will be accessible on-line via computer networking (Internet) or modem connections. Students are using PREX to solve problems that occur while elaborating tasks, e.g. preparing a protocol for an experiment or researching an alternative for a given procedure.

As an additional support to the course a textbook, containing basic facts and principles covering the main theoretical aspects, has recently been published (van Zutphen *et al.*, 1993).

Since 1986 more than 2000 persons have taken this introductory course. Based on the students' evaluation it may be concluded that the course is seen as a valuable contribution to the humane use and care of animals, and to the quality of experimental results. After having taken this course more than 98 per cent of the students indicated that if the course were not compulsory they would still recommend it to every scientist who is intending to use animals for research.

It should be emphasized that, although the completion of a biomedical graduate training programme including a course on laboratory animal science may provide a basis for the responsible use of animals, it certainly does not provide full competence. The wide range of experiments in the various fields of biomedical sciences implies that much must be learned in practice, e.g. in close cooperation with experienced researchers or animal technicians.

Laboratory animal scientist

Vocational training in the field of laboratory animal science is also needed for the recruitment of persons who are able to take the lead in the further developments of the discipline, but also for persons who are responsible for the quality control of animals in centralized animal facilities or who are responsible for the welfare of the animals.

These persons are mainly veterinarians who have taken a postgraduate professional training in laboratory animal science.

In the Netherlands, a 1-year postgraduate training programme has been made compulsory by law for veterinarians (or persons with an equivalent training) who wish to qualify for a position as animal welfare officer. These persons have the task to assist the scientist in the humane use and care of laboratory animals. They act as an advisor of the scientist but at the same time, and if necessary in the first place, as the advocate of the animals.

The programme consists of several modules and a period of research training. The modules usually cover the following topics:

- short introductory course on laboratory animal science (3 weeks);
- genetic standardization and genetic quality control (1 week);
- good laboratory practice (1 week);
- health monitoring and pathology (5 weeks);
- behaviour; welfare and stress (6 weeks);
- anaesthesia; analgesia; experimental procedures (5 weeks);

- alternatives to animal experiments (1 week);
- ethics and legislation (2 weeks).

The research project takes 6 months and is finished with a report or publication in a scientific journal.

This postgraduate training programme started in 1988. Annually no more than two or three persons are starting this course. For each of them a special programme is established, depending on the previous experience of the applicant. Until now (1993) ten persons have graduated.

Conclusions

In several countries training in the field of laboratory animal science has been made a compulsory component of the education of persons involved in animal experimentation. In the Netherlands training programmes have been made compulsory for animal caretakers, animal technicians, scientists and animal welfare officers. These training programmes are considered to be a cornerstone of responsible animal use and for quality in animal experiments.

References

Council of Europe Explanatory Report on the European Convention for the Protection of Vertebrate Animals used for Experimental and other Scientific Purposes (1985): Council of Europe, Strasburg.

Dennis, M.B. & Van Hoosier, G.L. (1989): The research animal management problem as a training tool for investigators. *Lab. Anim. Sci.* **39**, 477–478.

De Greeve, P.C.M., Hampson, J. & Van Zutphen, L.F.M. (1993): Legislation and animal experimentation. In: *Principles of laboratory animal science: a contribution to the humane use and care of animals and to the quality of experimental results*, eds. L.F.M. van Zutphen, V. Baumans & A.C. Beynen, pp. 9–16. Amsterdam: Elsevier Science Publishers.

EC Council Directive of 24 November 1986 on the Approximation of Laws, Regulations and Administrative Provisions of the Member States regarding the Protection of Animals used for Scientific Purposes (1986). *Official J. Eur. Comm.* 29, 1–6.

Olfert, E.D. & Flowers, F.H. (1983): Laboratory animal science education for the scientist: the Canadian experience. In: *Proceedings 8th ICLAS/CALAS Symposium*, Vancouver, pp. 23–26. New York: Gustav Fischer Verlag.

Report of the Working Party on Courses for Animal Licenses (1984). *Lab. Anim.* **18**, 209–220.

Russell, W.M.S. & Burch, R.L. (1959): *The principles of humane experimental technique.* London: Methuen.

Sarbourdy, M. (1987): Les enseignements relatifs aux animaux de laboratoire en France. *Sci. Tech. Anim. Lab.* **12**, 311–326.

The harmonization of training in laboratory animal science within Europe. *Proceedings of the Joint EFPIA/EC Workshop*, 17–18 June 1993, Brussels.

USA Animal Welfare Act. Improved Standards for Laboratory Animals Act (1985). Washington, DC: Office of the Federal Registry.

Van der Gulden, W.J.I., Van Hooijdonk, C.L., De Jong, P. & Kremer, A.K. (1972): *Proefdierkunde.* Nijmegen: CDL.

Van Hoosier, G.L. & Dahm, L. (1983): Education in laboratory animal medicine in the U.S. In: *Proceedings 8th ICLAS/CALAS Symposium*, Vancouver, pp. 41–48. New York: Gustav Fischer Verlag.

Van Hoosier, G.L., Dennis, M.B., Pekow, C. & Scott, C.S. (1993): Education and training through the use of problem-based-learning exercises. *Lab. Anim.* (in press).

Van Zutphen, L.F.M. (1988): Towards a qualified biologist: a proposal for a curriculum. In: *Competence of biologists for experiments on animals*, eds. H.M. van Emden, Tj. de Cock Buning & F.H. Lopes da Silva, pp. 41–46. Amsterdam: European Biologists Association.

Van Zutphen, L.F.M. (1989): Training programmes for biomedical scientists. In: *Animal experimentation: legislation and education*, eds. L.F.M. van Zutphen, H. Rozemond & A.C. Beynen, pp. 83–93. Rijswijk: Veterinary Public Health Inspectorate.

Van Zutphen, L.F.M. (1991): Education and animal experimentation. In: *Animals in biomedical research, replacement, reduction and refinement: present possibilities and future prospects*, eds. C.F.M. Hendriksen & H.B.W.M. Koëter, pp. 119–125. Amsterdam: Elsevier Science Publishers.

Van Zutphen, L.F.M., Baumans, V. & Beynen, A.C., eds. (1993): *Principles of laboratory animal science: a contribution to the humane use and care of animals and to the quality of experimental results.* Amsterdam: Elsevier Science Publishers.

The ethics of animal and human experimentation, edited by P.P. De Deyn.
©1994 John Libbey & Company Ltd., pp. 115–130.

11

The solicitude of the animal experimenter

Rudi D'Hooge[*] and Peter P. De Deyn[*†]

[*]*Laboratory of Neurochemistry and Behaviour at the Born-Bunge Foundation, University of Antwerp, Universiteitsplein 1, B-2610 Wilrijk, Belgium;* [†]*Department of Neurology at Middelheim General Hospital, Lindendreef 1, 2020 Antwerp, Belgium*

Summary

Animal experimentation has contributed to the advancement of human and veterinary medicine, and thus to the alleviation of pain and suffering in animals and human beings. Many phenomena studied by biomedical and behavioural scientists demand the use of living animals, and *in vitro* alternatives with the same reliability and validity as the animal models frequently do not exist. Depending on the stand one is prepared to take, one may or may not assign certain rights to animals. Neither analytical ethics, nor modern rights theory, is able to provide us with an unequivocal answer. Human beings perform experiments on animal subjects to achieve two goals they hold dear: human safety and freedom from disease. All the same, the authors of the present paper plead for a responsible science. It is firmly stressed that discomfort or suffering in experimental animals should be avoided as much as possible. Animal experimentation involves a balancing of benefits in terms of useful empirical knowledge against costs in terms of animal distress. It may be difficult though, to assess the importance of a piece of scientific research since the importance of a finding will often only become apparent long after its first publication. The need for public information and dialogue is emphasized. Scientists never really cared about their public image before, and they failed to discuss their activities in an open and straightforward way. They have been largely unprepared to meet the negative propaganda of animal rights extremists. It must be realized that the future of scientific endeavour can only be guaranteed in a society which realizes fully the importance of research, and which has good reasons to feel certain about a scientific community comprising reliable and morally responsible professionals.

Different views

The inquiry into structure and function of the brain is without any doubt one of the most ambitious and impressive of all human endeavours. Great stamina and zest is characteristic of the researchers involved, and their story reads like a novel (e.g.

Stevens, 1974; Worden *et al.*, 1975). It is the story of men and women whose life's work has been dedicated to the careful description of small constituents of the nervous system; to the unravelling of the network of nerve fibres and synaptic contacts; to the measurement of minute electric currents and potentials; to the analysis and the determination of tiny amounts of chemicals used by nerve cells to communicate with one another. With ingenious techniques and measuring instruments they have tried to reveal the brain's mechanism, and to understand the relationship between brain function and behaviour. And, although many questions still remain unanswered, truly spectacular successes have been achieved as well. Knowledge obtained through the work of these neuroscientists has been put to our common use, and has helped us to combat human suffering and disease. We have, moreover, every reason to believe that this kind of research will play a crucial role in our effort to alleviate pain, suffering, and human drama in the near future.

Undoubtedly, the study of visual perception is one of the most intriguing pieces of scientific research of our century. Visual perception does not happen as the old philosophers believed: our eyes do not project an image of our surroundings onto our mind's screen. Unlike in a *camera obscura*, a complicated neuronal process is involved, in which the brain composes an image based on signals from cells in the eye's retina, responding only to dark and light – flashing on-off. In this process, nerve cells in the visual cortex of the brain pass increasingly abstract information to one another – lines of different orientation, contours, etc. (Hubel, 1963). Eventually, the brain manages to put together a coherent image of our surroundings which appears to us to be wonderfully real and detailed.

Two American neuroscientists, David Hubel and Torsten Wiesel, have contributed significantly to our present day understanding of visual perception. Their work, which is still much cited by scientists all over the world, won them the 1981 Nobel Prize for Medicine or Physiology. Their efforts, and those of other eminent scientists like Colin Blakemore, have shown us how the particular structure of the brain enables processing of information, how this complicated structure develops, and how it is shaped by environmental stimulation (see e.g. Blakemore & Cooper, 1970). Hubel and Wiesel have always stressed the importance of their work for the understanding of the function and ontogenesis of the visual cortex, as well as for a more general insight into the relationship between brain and behaviour, and between brain structure and experience. Thus, Hubel, (1967, p. 43) writes: 'Perhaps the most exciting possibility for the future is the extension of this type of work to other systems besides sensory. Experimental psychologists and psychiatrists both emphasize the importance of early experience on subsequent behaviour patterns – could it be that deprivation of social contacts or the existence of other abnormal emotional situations early in life may lead to a deterioration or distortion of connections in some yet unexplored parts of the brain?'

Scientists are brought down to earth with a bump upon finding out that the general public is hardly prepared to participate in their enthusiasm when the use of animal subjects is mentioned. Woe betide the unfortunate scientist who persists in stressing the scientific importance of the work, regardless. He will not be heard, and will certainly not be understood. In fact, the accomplishments of biomedical and behavioural science are admired as long as they are discussed and explained in an aloof or abstract way. When scientists talk about the use of animal subjects, however, their work is greeted with denunciation, even when it is evident that all necessary precautions have been made to reduce animal suffering to a minimum.

Durant *et al.* (1989) carried out two national surveys to assess the American and British public interest in and knowledge of science. They found that although the public interest in science, medicine and technology is high, the knowledge of each area is surprisingly low. The public understanding of processes of scientific inquiry is especially disappointing. For example, when asked what it means to study something scientifically, only 10.5 per cent of the answers referred to the experimental method, and when respondents had to choose between three ways scientists could use to study the efficacy of a drug to treat high blood pressure, little more than half of them (56.3 per cent) picked the card with the right answer.

Many authors think this apparently low public understanding of science could be an important factor to explain the ambivalent public attitude in the animal research issue. 'The fascination that the fruits of medical research hold for [the general public] seems unending, as reflected in the space devoted to such developments in daily newspapers and on television, but this interest does not extend to the scientific process itself. Thus, many people deal with the animal use issue on an emotional level, feeling sympathy for the creatures that are a key part of research without recognizing their critical link to medical progress' (Iglehart, 1985, p. 400).

Far too often, the one-sided opinions of animal rights extremists strike home with the general public. In some instances, reaction to the use of animals in research has gone beyond mere incomprehension when scientists have become the target of hostile and violent campaigns (Loeb *et al.*, 1989; Breo, 1990; Cherfas, 1990; Matfield, 1991). In particular, research on the effects of environmental stimulation upon central nervous system development has suffered severely from negative propaganda. The famous Oxford University scientist Colin Blakemore, introduced earlier, has been targeted in a hostile and personal anti-vivisectionist campaign of many years' standing. When the British sensational paper the *Sunday Mirror* also accused Blakemore of animal abuse, the British Press Council decided to look into the matter. Soon it was established that the campaign was groundless, and adjudication ensued (Saunders, 1989).

On the other side of the Channel, colleagues of Blakemore were being chastised as well. The scientific journal *Nature* published, in quick succession, two papers by the French INSERM group Unité 94 on the development of the visual cortex in monkeys, and on the influence of visual stimulation upon this development (Dehay *et al.*, 1988, 1989). Shortly after publication of the second paper, a letter appeared in *Nature* from the well-known animal rights activist Clive Hollands on behalf of the Committee for the Reform of Animal Experimentation (Hollands, 1989). In his letter, Hollands stated that the experimental animals in the study of Dehay *et al.* (1989) experienced an unacceptable amount of distress, and that the study would not have been allowed in the UK. The letter provoked the umpteenth polemic with regard to the use of animal subjects in scientific research, where the different viewpoints were passed under separate review once more. A French animal liberation group did not, however, waste any time by participating in the discussion, but rather took offensive action: in the night of 20 May 1989, they forced their way onto the premises of (amongst others) Unité 94, stole a large number of animals, and damaged equipment, setting back research by at least 5 years (Coles, 1989).

Blakemore (1989) vigorously defended his French colleagues, and two well-known animal research advocates, Charles Nicoll and Sharon Russell, applauded his doing so. They admired the courage of apparently the only British scientist prepared to defend one of the most basic social prerequisites for the advancement of science: 'the freedom to conduct research without unwarranted obstruction or meddling' (Nicoll & Russell, 1989). They were alarmed by the fact that Clive Hollands, an official advisor to the Home Office no less, signed his letter as a member of the Committee for the Reform of Animal Experimentation, and they wondered: 'Is it appropriate for members of animal research "reform" groups to serve on committees that regulate animal research? Do we really want foxes minding our research hen-houses'?

Also according to Nicoll and Russell (1989), Hollands passed moral judgement on research he hardly knew anything about. Blakemore (1989) stated that the results of the French group were scientifically important, and performed by skilled scientists using sophisticated techniques and appropriate analgesics and anaesthetics. The French INSERM group is one of the best research institutes in the world with a leading role in research on biomedical subjects like AIDS, Alzheimer's disease, rehabilitation following brain damage, and basic neurosciences. 'I have collaborated with scientists there for many years in a study of the causes of childhood blindness and have found the animal house and laboratory facilities, as well as the quality of research, among the best I have seen anywhere', Blakemore (1989) writes. Or, as Norman Saunders (1989) of the University of Southampton stated: 'Their work on the development of the visual system is of the highest order and has led to important advances in the understanding of both basic mechanisms and clinical problems that may arise in the young'. Saunders pleads for more public support for pilloried scientists by their governments and the organizations that finance them.

Shortly after Blakemore's letter, Michael Balls (1989) declared on behalf of the influential and sincere Fund for the Replacement of Animals in Medical Experiments (FRAME): 'Terrorism in any form angers us no less than it angers Professor Blakemore'. Balls finds Blakemore's reaction a bit hysterical, and writes in the same letter that, 'This kind of emotional exaggeration damages the case which can be made for properly controlled experimentation on animals'. According to David Morton (1989), whose letter is published together with that of Balls, Blakemore does not elaborate properly on the justification of the French study, and he does not explain how these results advance understanding of the mechanism of development of the visual cortex of the brain. Morton feels that the ethical considerations with regard to animal experimentation are being considered *anti-scientific* by researchers far too often. 'There are real and difficult practical dilemmas involved in carrying out animal research and most scientists take these seriously' (Morton, 1989).

David Porter (1989), the outspoken Canadian animal issue moderate, was also disturbed by the amount of animal suffering in the French study. He believes the ethical dilemma in the use of animals in research originates from the difficulty in balancing the benefits accruing from research against the suffering involved. 'The extent of this dilemma is arguably proportional to the capacity of the animal to suffer and is thus particularly acute when the overlap with human attributes is greatest, as in the higher primates' (Porter, 1989). Porter justly argues that we share many or our cognitive and perceptual abilities with our animal relatives, and that we have the obligation to take this fact into sufficient account.

Undervalued importance of animal research

We leave it to well-informed readers to decide whether or not the research of the French group was justified; they have been swung back and forth between pros and cons more than enough. The scientists who defended their French colleagues so vigorously may have been too vague in their statements about the scientific importance of the work. The problem is however, that it is extremely difficult sometimes to assess the real importance of a piece of scientific research, and thus, at least in this respect, the comments of David Morton (1989) on Colin Blakemore's letter were uncalled-for. Unfortunately, one cannot always anticipate how a certain finding will advance our knowledge of a complicated natural phenomenon like, for example, the development of the cerebral cortex. The point is that the real importance of a finding will often only become clear long after its first publication, and this importance may not correspond at all with the original intentions or motivations of the researchers.

The research of Dehay *et al.* (1988, 1989) on their macaques may or may not have been justified – it all depends upon the kind of justification one is prepared to accept. Of course, it may well be that many years are needed to reveal the crucial insights the study has provided or to show the impetus the study has given in prompting other important studies. In his review article on the mechanism of development of the cerebral cortex, O'Leary (1989) refers to both papers of Colette Dehay and associates, and this could be an indication of the scientific importance of these studies, but it still leaves one question unanswered: Does scientific merit justify the sacrifice of animal subjects?

Regrettably, we have no quick and easy answer to this difficult question. Animal experimentation is neither unconditionally right, nor unconditionally wrong. As scientists, we are inclined to speak in favour of the advancement of scientific knowledge, and to hand out bouquets to the accomplishments of biomedical and behavioural science. All the same, we want to plead for a responsible science. Most explicitly, we do not want to join the ranks of the unconditional animal research advocates, and we have taken a firm stand against this position elsewhere (D'Hooge, 1991).

All the same, we cannot deny the crucial role animal experimentation has played and is still playing in biomedical and behavioural science. A great many authors have illustrated the contribution animal experimentation has made to the advancement of human and veterinary medicine, and thus to the alleviation of pain and suffering in animals and human beings (Nicoll & Russell, 1991; Paton, 1993; Miller, 1985). In an expensive campaign, the American Medical Association (1993) has tried to give greater publicity to the importance of animal experimentation. They give an impressive list of disorders and diseases modern medicine is able to prevent or cure thanks to knowledge obtained through animal experimentation. According to their data, the larger part of all biomedical advances has been due, in one way or another, to experimentation on animal subjects.

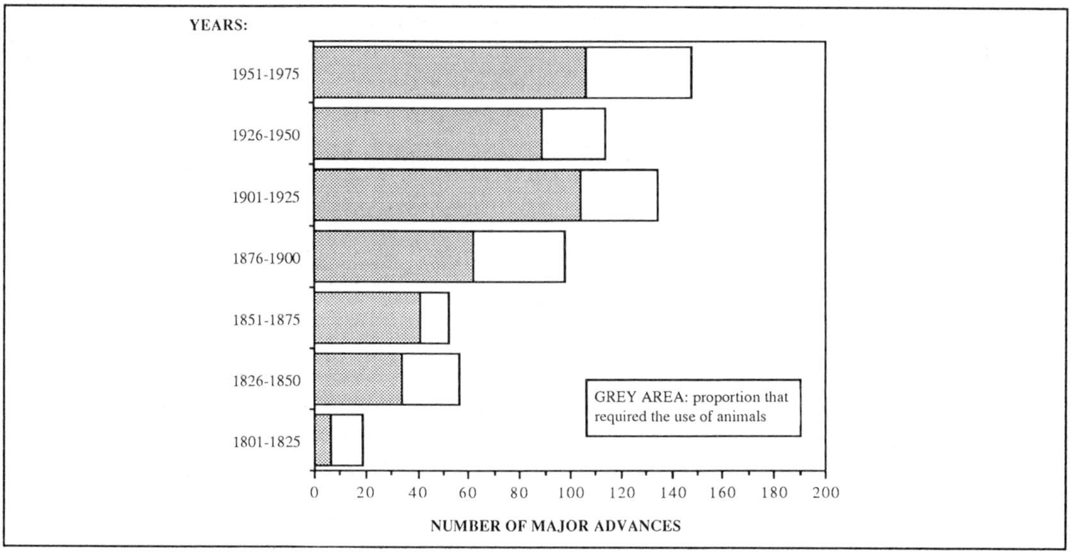

Fig. 1. Numbers of major biomedical advances during successive quarter-century periods. The proportion of advances that required animal research is indicated as a grey area. (Redrawn from Nicoll & Russell, 1991, p. 2889.)

Nicoll and Russell (1991) also found most biomedical advances to be due to work performed on animals (see Fig. 1). Between 1901 and 1975, animal experimentation contributed to 74 per cent of all important biomedical advances, and of the 82 Nobel Prizes for Medicine or Physiology awarded between 1901 and 1982, 71 per cent were based upon animal experimentation. Thus, Nicoll & Russell stress the key position animal experimentation occupies in the spectacularly successful history of biomedical science.

All around the world, scientific or medical associations and journals support this thesis, and emphasize the crucial role played by experiments on animal subjects. Moreover, most major animal welfare organisations, including the Belgian *Koninklijke Maatschappij voor Dierenbescherming* (i.e. our Royal Society for Animal Welfare), acknowledge the importance of animal experimentation as well. As two representatives of the British Royal Society for the Prevention of Cruelty to Animals (RSPCA) succinctly stated: 'Although we share with others a distant vision of a world free from animal exploitation, we take a pragmatic approach to animal experimentation. [. . .] We concede that some biomedical and scientific questions cannot be answered without the use of animals' (Jennings & Silcock, 1990).

These facts notwithstanding, animal rights extremists maintain that animal experimentation has played a highly dubious role in the history of the biomedical and behavioural sciences. Accordingly, they state that experiments on animal subjects cannot be justified and have to be halted since they have never contributed substantially to medical treatment anyway, and since alternative methods exist that do not require the use of animals.

Such derogatory statements bring some scientists to despair, and make them fear for the future of biomedical science. The former president of the American Society for Clinical Investigation, Robert Good, was up in arms about the use of his 1968 presidential address by animal rights activist Brandon Reines (1989) to prove the historical insignificance of animal experimentation. 'The major discoveries and insights of modern immunology would have been impossible without animal research', Good (1990) writes, and assures the reader that, 'Our search would be disastrously slowed, if not stopped altogether, if we could not study animals as well as human beings'.

The phenomena studied by biomedical and behavioural scientists demand, more often than not, the use of living animals, and *in vitro* alternatives with the same reliability and validity as the animal models frequently do not exist. It goes without saying that the study of behaviour requires the use of living animals, but many other branches of science also need the complexity of the intact organism. Pain research, especially on chronic pain (Casey & Dubner, 1989), is fraught with ethical controversy since one has to inflict pain, even if minimal, to study this dramatic phenomenon, but valid alternatives to the living animal often do not exist. In toxicology as well, researchers are frequently disappointed by the limited validity of the *in vitro* alternatives. In some cases, *in vitro* systems do not react to toxins at all like intact organisms do, and occasionally compounds that are apparently slightly toxic in *in vitro* testing are found to be highly toxic to the living organism (see e.g. Moss *et al.*, 1991). The infamous Draize eye irritation test is another example (Holden, 1988). Despite serious research efforts, a valid *in vitro* alternative to this test still remains to be found. Consequently, Pardes *et al.* (1991a, p. 1642) contend: 'The prospect of substituting known alternatives for many essential animal studies in the near future is greatly exaggerated by some animal-rights leaders. [. . .] The development of alternatives to using animals in research is desirable and is being carried out where possible. At this time, however, there is often no realistic substitute for living organisms, and human illnesses cannot wait'.

In all fairness, we all have to admit that animal experimentation is an essential part of biomedical and behavioural science. Suffice it to quote the unbiased words of David Porter (1992, p. 101): 'Contrary to allegations made by some critics of modern medical research, "good" things have come from animal experimentation, and, although their significance might be exaggerated by researchers, even in good faith, they have been fundamental to the understanding of biological mechanisms and to improvements in medical care'.

Unintended benefits accruing from animal research

Some scientists are so absorbed in their work, they can only see the scientific objective, and become blind to its general relevance in solving medical, psychological, social or ecological problems. Sometimes it may be even that a scientist is not at all interested in such problems, and is only concerned about his basic research questions. A famous example is the 17th century British scientist and discoverer of blood circulation, William Harvey. Even during his lifetime, he was a renowned scientist, and although we no longer agree with his research methods, he is still considered to be one of the founders of modern biomedical science. Yet Harvey was also known in his day as an incompetent and insensitive physician (Platt, 1967).

Based on a survey with specialists in these fields, Comroe and Dripps (1976) listed the ten most important clinical advances in cardiovascular and pulmonary medicine. Cardiac surgery, of course, topped their list, followed by vascular surgery and drug treatment of hypertension. According to the specialists Comroe and Dripps consulted, each of these ten advances yielded dramatic improvements in the medical treatment of patients suffering from cardiovascular or pulmonary disorders.

Each one of these advances relied on a large body of empirical knowledge in many areas of biomedical science. Cardiac surgery, for example, requires knowledge of preoperative diagnosis of cardiac defects (electrocardiography, angiocardiography, etc.), intraoperative management (asepsis, anaesthesia, resuscitation and surgical techniques, etc.), and postoperative care (analgesia, intensive care, infection, wound healing, etc.). Such knowledge stems to no small extent from animal experimentation. However and moreover, Comroe and Dripps found that 41 per cent of the studies which eventually led to a clinical innovation, had had no clinical objective at all. In other words, '41 per cent of the investigators, when they did their work, expressed no interest in a clinical problem – their goal was knowledge for the sake of knowledge. These data indicate clearly that planning for future clinical advances must include generous support for innovative and imaginative research that bears no discernible relation to a clinical problem at the time of peer review' (Comroe & Dripps, 1976, p. 109). Obviously, as Patrick Brunett (1989) stated most succinctly in his review of 20 years of biomedical research efforts, 'medicine remains primarily an empirical science in which advances take place through slow evolution, one person's discoveries building on the findings, both accidental and intentional, of countless predecessors'.

Adrian Morrison (1991) describes an example where the medical (in this case, neurological) relevance of the animal results were not anticipated by the researchers involved and only became apparent years later. He uses this case to conclude that 'biomedical research requiring the use of animals is necessary and justified even when the practical long-term gains cannot be seen . . . The trained mind must be allowed to pursue research – humanely, but with as few impediments as possible. That mind's curiosity is enough, and exercising that mind will almost inevitably pay off'.

More often than not, however, basic research without clear application possibilities is scorned. It is attributed to the perverse curiosity of the basic scientist, interested only in measurement and useless knowledge. But, in his *Advice to a Young Scientist*, Sir Peter Medawar looks at it from another angle. '"Curiosity killed the cat" is an old nanny's saying', he writes, 'though it may have been that same curiosity which found a remedy for the cat on what might otherwise have been its deathbed' (Medawar, 1981, p. 7).

Balancing benefits against costs

Although we might have the best of reasons to perform animal experiments in biomedical and behavioural science, one may still wonder whether or not these reasons justify the use of animal subjects at all. In his reaction to the article of Pardes *et al.* (1991a), an anti-vivisectionist writes: 'Regardless of the personal feelings or the motivation of the experimenters, the act of experimentation itself is inhumane' (Miller, 1991). But Pardes *et al.* (1991b) feel they voice the opinion of the larger part of the medical community when stating: 'We believe that we speak for most of the medical community when we say that humane treatment of research animals is imperative, and inhumane treatment unacceptable. We believe that we also speak for the majority when we say that if the argument is indeed forced into black-and-white terms – i.e. Is it defensible to sacrifice animal life in the effort to save human life? – the answer is yes'.

Animal rights activists, on the other hand, state that animals, like human beings, have certain rights that cannot be violated. Discriminating between living beings on the basis of the species to which they belong, they call *speciesism* by analogy with racism or sexism. Some analytical ethicists like Peter Singer or Tom Regan plead for the assignment of interests or even rights to animals by which they render some or all animal experimentation morally inadmissible (Vance, 1992). Their philosophical thesis has however been challenged by ethicists using the same utilitarian model (e.g. Frey, 1980), and thus analytical ethics obviously fails to provide us with a unequivocal answer to the question of whether or not people are allowed to use animals in scientific inquiry.

Depending on the stand one is prepared to take, one may or may not assign rights to animals, and even modern rights theory is unable to pronounce upon this dilemma unequivocally (Freeden, 1991). In his much-cited 1986 article, Carl Cohen dismisses the idea of animal rights, and defends animal experimentation vigorously. Cohen feels that the holders of rights should at least be able to grasp the concept of rules and obligations that apply to everybody. They must also be able to pass moral judgement on certain matters, or as Cohen puts it, they must possess the *capacity for moral judgement*. Clearly, some human beings lack this capacity (e.g. disabled individuals or young children), but according to Cohen it is not a test to be administered to each individual separately. 'What humans retain when disabled', Cohen (1986, p. 866) writes, 'animals have never had'.

Some authors are outraged when animal rights activists compare the abilities of mentally retarded human beings with those of apes, and use this comparison to assign the same rights to both. One of them firmly writes: 'There seems to be something almost malicious in debasing the issue of human rights by making this irrelevant comparison with animals' (Lansdell, 1988, p. 172). A multidisciplinary working party at the British Institute of Medical Ethics, consisting of activists as well as scientists, also agreed that 'In general there is no future in arguing for enhanced concern for animal welfare by lowering the moral status of human beings and the strength of our obligations to humanity' (Smith & Boyd, 1991, p. 311).

Countless authors have tried to distinguish human beings from animals on the basis of the unique characteristics that humans possess (e.g. Lieberman, 1991). The unfortunate point is that not all human beings possess these unique characteristics, and that we may thus be drawing a rather arbitrary line between human beings and the rest of the animal kingdom. Therefore, we do not believe this to be a very convincing criterion on which the assignment of rights may be based, or to be employed as justification for the use of animals by human beings. Some advocates of animal experimentation see no problem in this (e.g. Cohen, 1986), but we rather support the remarks of Robert Masta (1987) in his reaction to Carl Cohen's article: 'The philosophical argument that capacity for moral judgement is necessary for entitlement to rights could be viewed by some as merely a rationalization and the special exception for the mentally dysfunctional as a further weakness'. He proposes a way to get out of the impasse: 'Through simple awareness that society itself is the source of the rights within it, we can take care that such rights reflect the goals and values of the society, not those of zealots or demagogues. Freely discussing these goals and values during the decision-making process eliminates the need for later rationalization, and special cases are seen as uniform applications of the same principles to differing circumstances'. As Masta sees it, we perform experiments on animal subjects to achieve two goals we hold dear: *human safety and freedom from disease*. This is the reason why we do not assign to animals the right to self-determination. Over and above, we value human life more than that of animals, and we should not apologize for doing so.

Writes Kaplan (1988): 'It may appear strange that the busiest area of animal rights activism, and the area of its greatest success, has been the campaign against biomedical research. After all, the actual number of animals used in research is insignificant compared to those used in providing food or clothing, and the goals of the research – cure of disease, alleviation of the most painful conditions – must be judged vastly more estimable by any rational account'.

If one objects against the use of animal subjects in scientific inquiry, one can neither have a favourable opinion of the use of animals for companionship, transportation, food or clothing. Accordingly, some animal rights activists object to every use of animals by human beings. Some would rather see human beings not benefit at all from natural resources, and some of them appear to hold views about the natural world inspired by Walt Disney. Ingrid Newkirk of the animal rights group People for the Ethical Treatment of Animals (PETA) has a dream of 'a world where the lion will lie down with the lamb, where man will live in harmony with nature, where when two animals fight, human beings will intervene' (quoted by the American Medical Association, 1993). The untenability and utter absurdity of these extreme positions are sublimely caricatured by Stephen Norris (1990), and by *Science* editor Daniel Koshland (1988).

For indeed, we cannot be anything else but selfish or anthropocentric. Even animal rights extremists cannot persist in their refusal to benefit from animal experimentation, and in fact, as Kaplan (1988) notes, few animal research objectors have asked their physicians to deny themselves or their loved ones the benefits obtained through experiments on animal subjects. In a wider context, even James Lovelock (1988, p. 489) admits: 'To be selfish is human and natural. But if we chose to be selfish in the right way, then life can be rich yet still consistent with a world fit for our grandchildren as well as those of our partners in Gaia'.

Many authors do not mind being called speciesists. Carl Cohen declares whole-heartedly his being a speciesist. 'Speciesism is not merely plausible', Cohen (1986, p. 867) writes, 'it is essential for right conduct, because those who will not make the morally relevant distinctions among species are almost certain, in consequence, to misapprehend their true obligations'.

According to Stephen Post, 'interspecies egalitarianism leaves us with a badly distorted model of the real world of rights and obligations' (1993a, p. 133). Elsewhere Post writes: 'Our species kinship is a family-like phenomenon creating special obligations of beneficence that take precedence over our obligations to members of other species' (Post, 1993b, p. 295). Nicoll & Russell (1991, pp. 2890–2891), on the other hand, present a more sociobiological view on our speciesistic nature: 'Of course we are speciesists, as are all other animals, particularly social animals, which show a clear preference for their own kind in various ways . . . Any species that did not show preference for its own kind would soon become extinct'.

Like Post, we propose a *reasonable anthropocentrism*. When forced to choose, we must save the life of our fellow human being first; but in particular animals with a high level of consciousness and an ability to experience pain, deserve as much moral consideration as possible. Out of sheer necessity or moral responsibility people must choose in favour of people, and using animal subjects in some branches of science is one of the consequences of this choice. All the same, scientists are obligated to take the practical dilemmas with regard to animal experimentation seriously.

Most scientists would agree that discomfort or suffering in experimental animals should be avoided as much as possible. Many scientists also agree that animal experimentation involves a balancing of benefits in terms of useful empirical knowledge against costs in terms of animal distress. As a reaction to the public concern about the welfare of animal research subjects, legal rules and restrictions have been issued in many countries. These rules, however, remain vague with regard to the exact form and content of animal experiments (and probably justly so), and they certainly do not tell scientists exactly how the balancing in question should be done.

A number of authors try to fill this gap, and suggest concise methods to perform this balancing more systematically. The working party of the Institute of Medical Ethics, mentioned earlier, proposes some schemes to assess foreseeable and likely benefits accruing from an animal experiment, as well as costs for the animal subjects involved, and they work out some practical examples (Smith & Boyd, 1991). David Porter (1992) proposes an interesting scoring system that accounts for the objective of the experiment (aiming at direct alleviation of animal or human suffering, or basic research) and the chances of reaching the objective, as well as the characteristics of the experimental animal (its ability to suffer), extent and duration of the painful conditions involved (pain alleviation techniques considered), the relative duration of the experiment for the animal, the number of animals, and the quality of their lodging and care.

Leonard (1992), however, wonders about the exact purpose of Porter's scoring system. Indeed, when Porter's system is intended to impose legal restrictions on the use of animal subjects in scientific inquiry, it should also apply to the use of animals on farms or breeding facilities. There is, of course, no good reason why animal experimentation should be under more ethical scrutiny than other uses of animals for human benefit. According to Leonard, ethics are extremely idiosyncratic, and it is therefore, practically speaking, only important whether a particular human activity is legal or not. We think that advocates as well as opponents of animal experimentation should reasonably agree that legal rules must result from democratic dialogue.

Public information and dialogue

'As I see it, the only guarantee of relative freedom for scientific research is an enlightened public in a democratic society' (Eisenberg, 1973, p. 430).

Nowadays, science can no longer count upon the same unconditional and naive fascination it used to hold for the general public in the past. This is a relatively new phenomenon, but then of course in the meanwhile we have been confronted with the dangers of splitting the atomic nucleus and the disastrous effects modern technology can have on the environment. These and other unfortunate consequences of scientific knowledge have seriously damaged the belief in science. Although global science-fiction hits like *Jurassic Park* promote the image of the unreliable scientist, true stories of the irresponsible behaviour of some scientists have been made public as well. Every once in a while, new cases of really immoral experiments on humans or animals are revealed. Only recently, the American Energy Secretary Hazel O'Leary publicly divulged all the details of a disgraceful study on the effects of radioactivity on non-informed human subjects, performed in the years following World War II by scientists of famous US universities, and supported by the then government (Tisdall, 1994). Only acquainted with such spectacular cases and reading the ensuing press reports, no wonder ill-informed spectators have an unfavourable opinion of modern science.

Twenty-five years ago, following the publication of their article on genetic manipulation in bacteria, some Harvard Medical School scientists became involved in the moral discussion regarding this then new branch of science. They did not, however, hesitate to stress firmly the need for increased public involvement in these matters. 'As we see it', they wrote (Shapiro *et al.*, 1969), 'scientists are obligated to inform the public about what is happening in their secluded fields of research so that people can demand control over decisions which profoundly affect their lives. If our arguments mean that "the progress of science itself may be interrupted", that is an unfortunate consequence we will have to accept. It certainly should not inhibit us from speaking out on crucial issues'.

Now, most scientists are convinced that they can no longer hide in their laboratories from the criticism of the 'ignorant' public. When Floyd Bloom (1992) summarizes the skills the 21st century neuroscientist should be trained in, he distinctly mentions the ability to defend his case to the general public. Besides the necessary techniques and research strategies, Bloom feels the scientist will increasingly need such what he calls 'survival skills' in the struggle for scarce research funding. 'The ambivalent attitude of the public to science is extremely fragile' Bloom writes (pp. 385–386). 'Our chances for success are likely to be improved by connecting the research efforts to health and society, and by more effective communication of our science through the media'.

Animal rights extremists often win approval with their campaigns against animal experimentation, and this might puzzle or disappoint the enthusiastic men and women of science. However, this sad fact may well be the result of the reluctance or incompetence of scientists to discuss their activities in an open and straightforward way, and to engage in public dialogue. Scientists never really cared about their public image, and now they may have to pay for it. Andrew Rowan of the Tufts University's Center for Animals and Public Policy says it is about time scientists did something about their unfavourable public image: 'a scientist must break the standard public stereotype of being a dispassionate, objective and relentless seeker of the truth. Such individuals are respected but are not loved and they are certainly not perceived as good or reliable caregivers' (Rowan, 1991).

In the United States, scientific and public health organizations like the American Psychological Association, the American Medical Association, the National Institutes of Health (NIH) and the Alcohol, Drug Abuse and Mental Health Administration (ADAMHA) stand

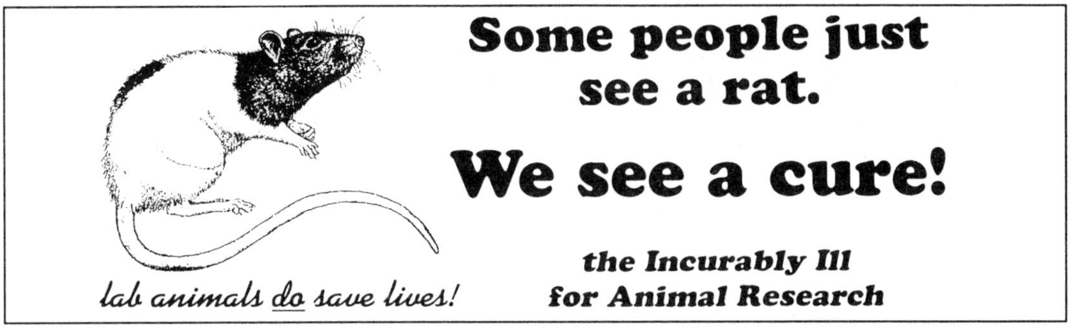
Some people just see a rat.
We see a cure!
lab animals do save lives!
the Incurably Ill for Animal Research

Fig. 2. A slogan of the American group the Incurably Ill for Animal Research. All around the world, people with different views and interests emphasize the benefits of animal experimentation and worry about the future of this branch of science.

up for animal experimentation. Like many other scientific journals, the influential journal *Science* has repeatedly made a stand for experimentation on animal subjects, and its editor encourages scientists to speak out and defend their cause to the public (Koshland, 1989). At a number of American universities, coalitions have been formed to defend animal experimentation (Holden, 1989).

In the United States as in many other countries, people with different views and interests feel they must take action to emphasize the benefits of animal experimentation, and express their worries about the future of this branch of science (see Fig. 2). ADAMHA administrator Frederick Goodwin stresses the importance for scientists to engage in this discussion also. 'Researchers must be encouraged to do something other than sit back, write white papers, and preach to the converted. We need to provide incentives for researchers to become actively involved in this struggle, and we need to equip them with useful tools. That involves media training as well as peer and institutional support'. (Goodwin, 1989, p. 2456.)

Some animal rights activists have not refrained from spreading slanderous information about animal experimentation. Coile and Miller (1984) tried to find out whether there was any truth in the accusations of the animal rights organization Mobilization for Animals with regard to the use of animal subjects in psychological research. However, not a single one of the extreme statements about the research methods used by experimental psychologists agreed with the description of these methods in the 608 animal research articles which appeared in the leading psychological journals during a period of 5 years prior to the announcement of the accusations.

Scientists have been largely unprepared to meet the negative propaganda of animal rights extremists. 'This propaganda has been doubly effective because the scientific community was unprepared to defend itself from media campaigns and the public was unequipped to assess the validity of the propaganda', confirms Scott Bernstein (1989) of the University of Illinois.

'We must respond in a forthright and honest way about what we do. We must continue to ensure that animal use in research is humane and appropriate', Richard Vance writes (1992, p. 1718). This includes two things: public dialogue to discuss the necessity of animal experiments in a straightforward way, and unconditional condemnation of animal abuse. Coile and Miller write (1984, p. 701): 'Nobody wants to see animals suffer needlessly, nor do they want progress toward the elimination of suffering in humans to be halted. Therefore, it is essential to be totally honest in the representation of facts concerning animal welfare in research'.

The future of scientific endeavour can only be guaranteed in a society which realizes fully the importance of research, and which has good reasons to feel certain about a scientific community comprising reliable and morally responsible professionals.

Acknowledgements. The authors obtained financial support from the Born-Bunge Foundation, the OCMW Medical Research Foundation, and the University of Antwerp. R. D'Hooge holds a Flemish Community IWONL scholarship.

References

American Medical Association (1993): *Medical progress. A miracle at risk.* New York: American Medical Association.

Balls, M. (1989): Use of animals in research. *Nature* **340,** 10.

Bernstein, S.L. (1989): Animal rights activists distort issues. *J. Am. Med. Assoc.* **261,** 784.

Blakemore, C. (1989): Misguided thinking on animals. *Nature* **339,** 414.

Blakemore, C. & Cooper, G.F. (1970): Development of the brain depends on the visual environment. *Nature* **228,** 477–478.

Bloom, F.E. (1992): Training neuroscientists for the 21st century. *Trends Neurosci.* **15,** 383–386.

Breo, D.L. (1990): Animal rights *vs* research? A question of the nation's scientific literacy. *J. Am. Med. Assoc.* **26,** 25.

Brunett, P. (1989): Twenty years of medical advances. *J. Am. Med. Assoc.* **261,** 782–783.

Casey, K.L. & Dubner, R. (1989): Animal models of chronic pain: scientific and ethical issues. *Pain* **38,** 249–252.

Cherfas, J. (1990): Two bomb attacks on scientists in the U.K. *Science* **248,** 1485.

Cohen, C. (1986): The case for the use of animals in biomedical research. *N. Engl. J. Med.* **315,** 865–870.

Coile, D.C. & Miller, N.E. (1984): How radical animal activists try to mislead humane people. *Am. Psychol.* **39,** 700–701.

Coles, P. (1989): Raids cause French workers to take stock. *Nature* **339,** 407.

Comroe, J.H. & Dripps, R.D. (1976): Scientific basis for the support of biomedical science. *Science* **192,** 105–111.

Dehay, C., Kennedy, H., Bullier, J. & Berland, M. (1988): Absence of interhemispheric connections of area 17 during development in the monkey. *Nature* **331,** 348–350.

Dehay, C., Horsburgh, G., Berland, M., Killackey, H. & Kennedy, H. (1989): Maturation and connectivity of the visual cortex in monkey is altered by prenatal removal of retinal input. *Nature* **337,** 265–267.

D'Hooge, R. (1991): Animal experimentation (but without man at the centre of the universe). *J. Med. Ethics* **17,** 213–214.

Durant, J.R., Evans, G.A. & Thomas, G.P. (1989): The public understanding of science. *Nature* **340,** 11–14.

Eisenberg, L. (1973): Human behavior, instinct, and aggression. *Science* **179,** 429–430.

Freeden, M. (1991): *Rights.* Milton Keynes: Open University Press.

Frey, R.G. (1980): *Interests and rights. The case against animals.* Oxford: Clarendon Press.

Good, R.A. (1990): The value of animal research. *Science* **248,** 538.

Goodwin, F.K. (1989): Animal research *vs* humane use: the struggle to sustain our research advances. *FASEB J.* **3,** 2455–2456; 2563–2564.

Holden, C. (1988): Much work but slow going on alternatives to Draize test. *Science* **242,** 185–186.

Holden, C. (1989): Universities fight animal activists. *Science* **243,** 17–19.

Hollands, C. (1989): Animal experiments. *Nature* **339,** 248.

Hubel, D.H. (1963): The visual cortex of the brain. *Sci. Am.* **209,** 54–62.

Hubel, D.H. (1967): Effects of distortion of sensory input on the visual system of kittens. *Physiologist* **10,** 17–45.

Iglehart, J.K. (1985): The use of animals in research. *N. Engl. J. Med.* **313,** 395–400.

Jennings, M. & Silcock, S. (1990): The invisible middle ground. *Lancet* **336,** 1512.

Kaplan, J. (1988): The use of animals in research. *Science* **242,** 839–840.

Koshland, D.E. (1988): Homo photosyntheticus. *Science* **239,** 449.

Koshland, D.E. (1989): Animal rights and animal wrongs. *Science* **243,** 1253.

Lansdell, H. (1988): Laboratory animals need only humane treatment: animal 'rights' may debase humane rights. *Int. J. Neurosci.* **42,** 169–178.

Leonard, P.A. (1992): Of animals and men. *Nature* **357,** 187.

Lieberman, P. (1991): *Uniquely human. The evolution of speech, thought, and selfless behavior.* Cambridge: Harvard University Press.

Loeb, J.M., Hendee, W.R., Smith, S.J. & Schwarz, M.R. (1989): Human *vs* animal rights. In defense of animal research. *J. Am. Med. Assoc.* **262,** 2716–2720.

Lovelock, J.E. (1988): The earth as a living organism. In: *Biodiversity*, eds. E.O. Wilson & F.M. Peter, pp. 486–489. Washington: National Academy Press.

Masta, R.I. (1987): The case for the use of animals in research. *N. Engl. J. Med.* **316,** 551.

Matfield, M.J. (1991): Animal liberation or animal research? *Trends Pharmacol. Sci.* **12,** 411–415.

Medawar, P.B. (1981): *Advice to a young scientist.* London: Pan Books.

Miller, B.L. (1991): Physicians and the animal rights movement. *N. Engl. J. Med.* **325,** 1581.

Miller, N.E. (1985): The value of behavioral research on animals. *Am. Psychol.* **40,** 423–440.

Morrison, A.R. (1991): Research on animals: unforseen benefits. *Science* **245,** 176.

Morton, D.B. (19890: Use of animals in research. *Nature* **340,** 10.

Moss, J.N., Hsu, A., Lange, B. & Scribner, H.E. (1991): The need for animal testing – report of a case. *Fd Chem. Toxic* **29,** 475.

Nicoll, C.S. & Russell, S.M. (1989): Freedom to conduct research. *Nature* **342,** 220.

Nicoll, C.S. & Russell, S.M. (1991): Mozart, Alexander the Great, and the animal rights/liberation philosophy. *FASEB J.* **5**, 2888–2892.

Norris, S.H. (1990): The last GASP. *J. Am. Med. Assoc.* **263**, 378.

O'Leary, D.D.M. (1989): Do cortical areas emerge from a protocortex? *Trends Neurosci.* **12**, 400–406.

Pardes, H., West, A. & Pincus, H.A. (1991a): Physicians and the animal-rights movement. *N. Engl. J. Med.* **324**, 1640–1643.

Pardes, H., West, A. & Pincus, H.A. (1991b): Physicians and the animal-rights movement (reply). *N. Engl. J. Med.* **325**, 1583–1584.

Paton, W. (1993): *Man and mouse: animals in medical research* (Second edition). Oxford: Oxford University Press.

Platt, Lord (1967): Medical science: master or servant. *Br. Med. J.* **4**, 439–444.

Porter, D.G. (1989): Animal experiments. *Nature* **340**, 180.

Porter, D.G. (1992): Ethical scores for animal experiments. *Nature* **356**, 101–102.

Post, S.G. (1993a): Baboon livers and the human good. *Arch. Surg.* **128**, 131–133.

Post, S.G. (1993b): The emergence of species impartiality: a medical critique of biocentrism. *Perspect. Biol. Med.* **36**, 289–300.

Reines, B.P. (1989): Animal experimentation. *Science* **245**, 583.

Rowan, A.N. (1991): Wrong on animal rights. *Nature* **354**, 101.

Saunders, N.R. (1989): Policing animal experiments. *Nature* **341**, 99.

Shapiro, J., Eron, L. & Beckwith, J. (1969): More alarums and excursions. *Nature* **224**, 1337.

Smith, J.A. & Boyd, K.M., eds. (1991): *Lives in the balance. The ethics of using animals in biomedical research.* Oxford: Oxford University Press.

Stevens, L.A. (1974): *Explorers of the brain.* London: Scientific Book Club.

Tisdall, S. (1994): US admits radiation test on citizens. *The Guardian Weekly* **150**, 6.

Vance, R.P. (1992): An introduction to the philosophical presuppositions of the animal liberation/rights movement. *J. Am. Med. Assoc.* **268**, 1715–1719.

Worden, F.G., Swazey, J.P. & Adelman, G., eds. (1975): *The neurosciences: paths of discovery.* Massachusetts: The MIT Press.

The ethics of animal and human experimentation, edited by P.P. De Deyn.
 pp. 131–142.

12

On the necessity of animal experimentation in the search for effective therapy of peripheral nerve disorders

Willem Hendrik Gispen and Frank P.T. Hamers

Department of Medical Pharmacology, Rudolf Magnus Institute, Utrecht University, Universiteitsweg 100, 3584 CG Utrecht, The Netherlands

Summary

In the present paper we discuss the necessity of animal experimentation in the search for an effective therapy of peripheral nerve disorders. Although *in vitro* studies may aid this search by primarily focusing on mechanisms of actions, the *in vivo* approach is often the only way to gap the bridge to the clinic. The complexity of nerve as a tissue and the unique function of the nervous system warrant an approach at the organismal level. The usefulness of animal models is illustrated by three examples: recovery of function following mechanical trauma, experimental diabetic neuropathy and cisplatin-induced neurotoxicity. It is argued that the underlying pathologies are such that *ex vivo* experimentation cannot meet the complexity of the pathogenesis. Hence it is to be expected that only the use of *in vivo* models will provide new leads in the search for effective therapy of peripheral nerve disorders.

Introduction

Neurological disorders are an important cause of human suffering and invalidity. Although many are not directly life-threatening, they profoundly influence the well-being of an afflicted individual, for diseases of the nervous system directly influence the ability to react to internal and external stimuli and thus the ability to exert control over one's environment.

The aetiology and pathophysiology of many nervous system disorders are incompletely known or understood; this is due both to the very intricate structure of the nervous system itself, with different cell types and different cells of a given type influencing each other, and to the intimate relationship with and dependence upon other organs and tissues (e.g. blood).

The causes of neurological disease are manifold. Genetic, metabolic, toxic, traumatic, immunological and degenerative (a term often used when the cause is not well known) factors all play a role. In the case of diseases of the central nervous system of such importance (in terms of incidence in the general population, especially in the elderly) as Parkinson's disease and Alzheimer's dementia the cause is largely unknown and therapeutic measures, if at all possible, are largely directed at reducing symptoms.

Many peripheral nervous system disorders are collectively known as neuropathies and include diseases that may remain subclinical, as well as severe manifestations of disabling motor, sensory and autonomic disturbances. Their cause is as polymorphic as their clinical manifestation and includes toxins (industrial products such as acrylamide, overdoses of otherwise essential compounds, e.g. pyridoxine, anti-cancer drugs such as cisplatin, vinca-alkaloids and taxol), malignant disease, and metabolic disease such as diabetes mellitus. Although current aims are to ameliorate the underlying disorder (if known) complete remission may never be reached.

Last but not least, physical trauma of the central and peripheral nervous system may lead to permanent dysfunction. One well-known trauma of the central nervous system is the compression lesion of the spinal cord, whereas nerve transection or laceration are prominent examples in the peripheral nervous system.

In view of the above considerations, it is clear that a better understanding of, and adequate therapies for nervous system disorders in general may greatly contribute to the quality of life in many people and diminish the burden these disorders cause for society as a whole.

The necessity of animal models in the search for therapies of nervous system diseases

In view of the complexity of nerve as a tissue, and of nerve function, it is difficult, if not impossible, to design an *in vitro* experiment using cells or tissue that would have sufficient bearing on the *in vivo* pathology of nervous system disorders. Such a condition does not imply that *in vitro* technologies are of no relevance to the search for new therapies. *In vitro* models have the advantage that they allow the controlled study of a limited set of events in the pathogenesis or in the putative therapy. They often precede or parallel *in vivo* experimentation that aims to study the disorder in its full complexity. It is the proper combination of approaches that eventually may lead to success. In the following paragraphs we will discuss some of the progress made in the search for an effective therapy for peripheral nervous system disorders that will illustrate the complexity of the issue and underscore the necessity of animal models.

Peripheral nerve trauma

The neuron is a highly differentiated cell and is most vulnerable in the brain as well as the peripheral nervous system. In general it is assumed that damage to cell bodies of neurons results in irreversible degeneration and cell death. Depending on the severity, size and location of the lesion in the nervous system such cell death may lead to permanent loss of function. At the other hand, if the damage is restricted to the neuronal processes (dendrites and axons) regeneration with successful reinnervation of the target is in principle possible.

Current thinking about the development of new pharmacotherapies that aim to promote successful reinnervation and recovery of function is influenced by the notion that neurotrophic factors that are active during the development of the nervous system may also play a role in the maintenance and repair of mature neurons. Since the discovery of nerve growth factor (NGF) in 1953, a whole family of more or less related factors has emerged, collectively called neurotrophins. On the one hand, knowledge of their function is paramount for understanding developmental neurobiology, on the other, it is hoped that that knowledge will lead to new neurotrophic therapies of compromised neuronal function. To date, the vast majority of neurotrophin history lies in tissue culture dishes and not in studies employing animals; albeit that more recently specific animal models of degenerative diseases are being introduced to investigate the efficacy of neurotrophins.

The advantage of experiments with cultured cells is obviously the possibility of studying mechanisms of action and of identifying the various cell types and their responses involved. The disadvantage is that the majority of studies concern foetal cells in optimal cultured conditions that *per se* will be very different from the conditions following damage to a mature neuron *in vivo*. Furthermore the repair process *in vivo* most certainly involves a complexity of cellular activities and factors that only in concert lead to proper recovery of function. Hence proven activity of neurotrophins in cell cultures is often difficult to demonstrate *in vivo*.

In order to cope with these serious experimental problems, experimental neurology often employs different animal models of a given human peripheral nerve disorder. In combination these models should resemble as much as possible the clinical situation. Depending on the disorder, such animal models are available and reliable. Assuming that the pharmacology of a given neurotoxin in the experimental animal is similar to that in the human, a great resemblance in neuropathological parameters may be expected. However, the seemingly simple mimicking of human mechanical trauma to nerves in animals might be much more difficult in view of the variability of traumas between individuals (location, severity, involvement of blood vessels etc.). Therefore we have employed various types of mechanical trauma of peripheral nerves of rats to study the putative efficacy of neurotrophic peptides of the ACTH/MSH family. These models also allow the evaluation of procedures that are commonly used to improve nerve repair such as advanced microsurgery, topical application and physical therapy.

Using a foot reflex withdrawal test and a free-walking pattern analysis test to monitor the return of sensorimotor function following crush lesion of the sciatic nerve in rats, we found that neurotrophic fragments and analogues of melanocortins, including the ACTH-(4–9) analogue ORG 2766, exhibit an inverted U-shaped dose–response relationship and are maximally active in a dose range of 7.5–75 μg/kg when given daily or every other day subcutaneously (s.c.). Oral doses of 125 mg/kg are ineffective, but it is possible to facilitate recovery of function by topical delivery of the peptide or by slow release from osmotic minipumps implanted s.c. or from biodegradable microspheres. Peptide treatment must begin within a short period of induction of the lesion – there is a 'critical period' of 1 week – but its beneficial effects on histological and neurophysiological parameters are still apparent after several months. The precise location of the amino acid sequence that confers neurotrophic activity on the peptides is uncertain. It is clear however that, as for many of the other effects of melanocortins on the nervous system, the critical information for stimulating neurite outgrowth is contained in the amino acid sequence between positions 4 and 10; the peptide ORG 2766 is frequently used in studies of these effects (Gispen, 1990).

Histological and functional studies strongly support the notion that the melanocortins do not enhance the rate of outgrowth but rather increase the number of newly formed sprouts at the site of lesion. It has been suggested that the peptides mimic or amplify an endogenous signal that operates early in the regenerative response of the damaged neuron (reactivation of expression of proopiomelanocortin (POMC) or neurofilament breakdown; Bär *et al.*, 1990).

Edwards *et al.* (1984) have shown with a bioassay for α-MSH that α-MSH-like bioactive material is present in degenerating nerve stumps. During the development of the rat spinal cord, POMC mRNA and POMC-derived neuropeptides were shown to be expressed transiently from E13–E15 days of gestation, suggesting a specific role for POMC in the development of the peripheral nervous system (Carr & Haynes, 1988). Furthermore, immunocytochemical evidence of enhanced amounts of α-MSH in the motor neurones of mice with inherited motor neurone disease or muscular dystrophy, conditions in which the maturation of the end plates is delayed into adulthood and continued formation of new neuromuscular junctions is an ongoing process, suggests that enhanced production of melanocortins is associated with stages of active axonal growth (Hughes & Smith, 1988, 1989). However, in a recent study, we were unable to establish that up-regulation of POMC gene expression does occur in the neurons of the damaged sciatic nerve or locally in proliferating Schwann cells or in infiltrating mononuclear blood cells at the site of the nerve crush. Thus, the previously demonstrated induction of POMC-related immunoreactivity in damaged nerves is not due to increased POMC mRNA levels. Although we were not able to show an increase in POMC gene expression, we cannot exclude the possibility that there is increased production of biologically active peptides caused by (1) a more efficient translation of the low levels of POMC mRNA present in both neuronal cell bodies and non-neuronal cells at the crush site or (2) altered precursor processing. However as we were not able to detect α-MSH in crushed peripheral nerve with a radioimmunoassay, we favour the view that the previously shown immunoreactive α-MSH-like material in peripheral nerve is unrelated to POMC and could represent crossreactivity of α-MSH antibodies with as yet unidentified molecules (Plantinga *et al.*, 1992).

As indicated above, the use of an animal model allows the study of factors involved in neuronal repair other than humoral target-derived factors that promote outgrowth following damage. Such factors relate to the significance of proper blood flow (oxygen, glucose, blood borne trophic factors) and to the putative efficacy of controlled exercise of the damaged neuromuscular system under study. In this context, recent studies in our laboratory aim to evaluate the beneficial effect of physical exercise on functional recovery following a crush lesion of the rat sciatic nerve. Control rats were kept under standard housing conditions. One experimental group was kept in an enriched environment consisting of a large cage in which food and water were supplied at opposite sides of the cage. These delivery points were only accessible following an obstacle course set at different height. As the eating of dry chow is interrupted by the drinking of water, rats were forced to master the obstacle course in order to satisfy their needs. The other experimental group consisted of rats that were kept on a limited supply of water rendering them sufficiently thirsty to stand on their hind legs in order to obtain extra water from a drinking spout that was adjustable in height. In this way, controlled exercise of the hindlegs was obtained. Evaluation of walking patterns (functional motor behaviour) and reactions to a mild electric stimulus to the sole of the foot (sensory function) were used to quantify the recovery of function. Both the 'enriched environment' and 'drink-trained' groups of rats showed enhanced recovery as compared to the control group. The results of this experiment suggest a relevant neurotrophic effect of physical exercise in peripheral nerves after mechanical trauma (van Meeteren *et al.*, 1993). The conditions mimic those that are routinely employed in the clinic (i.e. controlled physical therapy) and could only have been created by using an animal model.

Diabetic neuropathy

Diabetic neuropathy is a frequently diagnosed and underestimated complication in patients with type 1 and type 2 diabetes mellitus. Prevalence figures vary between 5 and 80 per cent, depending on the duration of the disease, screening methods and heterogeneous criteria. Neuropathy is a syndrome that presents itself in different ways: the most common neuropathy is the combined sensorimotor–autonomic neuropathy. Frequently occurring symptoms are burning pain, paraesthesias and numbness, usually beginning in the distal parts of the lower extremities. Muscle weakness sometimes develops in the distal parts of the leg. The combination of sensory loss together with muscle weakness can cause problems with walking (Dyck *et al.*, 1987).

Diabetic neuropathy is chosen as an example of a peripheral nerve disorder where the primary cause of the pathogenesis lies outside the nervous system, being the result of disturbed metabolic homoeostasis of the individual as a whole. It has been argued that the noxious influence of these metabolic disturbances cannot be monitored in tissue culture but only in an animal with experimentally or genetically induced disturbances reminiscent of those seen in patients with diabetes mellitus.

There is a considerable amount of literature on the pathogenesis of diabetic neuropathy (Dyck *et al.*, 1987). One can roughly divide the various theories into three categories. First, there is the so-called 'metabolic' theory. Chronic hyperglycaemia causes an increased activation of the polyol pathway by which glucose is converted into sorbitol by the enzyme aldose reductase, and subsequently into fructose. The accumulation of sorbitol causes a depletion of the glycolipid, myo-inositol. Myo-inositol is an important glycolipid for normal neuronal functioning. Depletion of myo-inositol causes a decreased activity of Na^+, K^+, ATP-ase and thereby a decrease in impulse conduction. Inhibition of aldose reductase and supplementation of myo-inositol at an early state of experimental diabetic neuropathy (EDN) has proven that functional and morphological changes in diabetic nerves can be postponed. The second theory is the so-called 'vascular hypothesis'. Chronic hyperglycaemia causes structural changes (thickening of basement membranes) in the endoneural vessels, causing a decrease in blood flow to the peripheral axons and Schwann cells. This leads to chronic hypoxia and a decrease in all oxygen-dependent processes, resulting in nerve degeneration.

A third theory is based on the glycosylation of neural proteins, which results in neuropathy. Analogous to the formation of glycosylated haemoglobin (HbA1), glucose can irreversibly attach itself to functionally important neuronal proteins. This can ultimately lead to a loss of function of these proteins. It has been reported that glycosylated myelin can increase the activation of macrophages, thereby inducing an excessive turnover of myelin. It is probable that not one single mechanism is involved in the pathogenesis of diabetic neuropathy, but rather a combination of various factors.

A simple and effective treatment of diabetic neuropathy does not exist although it is generally assumed that proper metabolic control may prevent or ameliorate the diabetic peripheral neuropathy. In two experimental models of diabetic neuropathy, we tested the putative efficacy of chronic treatment with a calcium antagonist of the dihydropyridine type known to block L-channels. Studies in developmental neurobiology revealed the significance of intraneuronal Ca^{2+} homoeostasis in neuronal plasticity (Katchaturian, 1989). The Ca^{2+}-hypothesis suggests that neurite outgrowth during development and repair can only proceed when intracellular Ca^{2+} levels lie within a specific outgrowth-permissive range. Cessation of outgrowth or reduction in neuronal plasticity can be induced by signals that elevate Ca^{2+} concentration above that range. Extreme excitatory imbalance in transmitter input leading to a marked elevation of intracellular Ca^{2+} is neurotoxic and eventually may lead to cell death (Kater *et al.*, 1989). In view of the apparent significance of Ca^{2+} homoeostasis to neuronal plasticity during development, repair and ageing, many attempts have been made either to influence neuronal repair or to provide neuroprotection by the administration of drugs that are known to affect intracellular Ca^{2+} levels. One line of research focuses on the putative efficacy of the so-called Ca^{2+} antagonists that block the voltage-sensitive L-channels.

Following demonstration of specific binding sites for dihydropyridine in neural tissue it is becoming clear that these Ca^{2+} antagonists have profound neuro- and psychopharmacological effects (Traber & Gispen, 1989). In this respect special attention has been focused on nimodipine (isopropyl(2-methyl-ethyl)1,4-dihydro-2,6-dimethyl-4(3,5-pyridine dicarboxylate) as this compound penetrates the blood-brain barrier relatively well. Recent studies from various laboratories revealed a potent neuroprotective action of nimodipine. As the dihydropyridines also block L-channels in the vascular system, in addition to its neuropharmacological effects, nimodipine might promote neuroprotection by affecting nerve blood flow as well. As the pathogenesis of diabetic neuropathy most likely involves neuronal and vascular components, nimodipine therapy might be of singular significance.

In the first model, rats received a single intravenous injection with streptozotocin. This drug is known to kill the β-cells in the islets of Langerhans. As a consequence, the animals developed high blood glucose levels as no insulin was injected. These animals showed pathology similar to that seen in human diabetes mellitus. Measurement of peripheral nerve conduction velocity is often used as a tool to monitor longitudinally the onset and development of a peripheral neuropathy. In the first series of experiments immediately following the streptozotocin injection, rats received either saline or nimodipine treatment (10 mg/kg i.p./48 h) that lasted throughout the experimental period of 7 weeks. At various intervals, the functionality of motor and sensory nerve fibres was measured by means of transcutaneous stimulation of the sciatic nerve and recording of the M- and H-responses. Three weeks after the induction of the diabetes mellitus all streptozotocin-saline treated rats displayed the expected significant reduction in both sensory (SNCV) and motor nerve conduction velocity (MNCV). This decrease gradually increased until the end of the experimental period. If nimodipine instead of saline was given, following the initial decrease, a gradual restoration of both SNCV and MNCV was observed, indicative of a neuroprotective effect (Kappelle *et al.*, 1992).

In the next series of experiments we examined the effect of nimodipine treatment on an already existing neuropathy in streptozotocin-diabetic rats. Five groups of rats were studied: group 1 consisted of age-matched, non-diabetic controls and groups 2, 3, 4 and 5 of diabetic rats. Four weeks after the streptozotocin injection, the SNCV and MNCV were decreased and treatment was started: group 2 was treated with placebo, group 3 with 5 mg/kg i.p. nimodipine, group 4 with 10 mg/kg and group 5 with 20 mg/kg every 48 h. The animals which were treated with the high nimodipine doses showed a significant improvement in both SNCV and MNCV from week 6 onwards, whereas this beneficial effect was not found in rats treated with the low dosage. Thus we concluded that nimodipine can ameliorate existing diabetic neuropathy in streptozotocin-induced diabetic rats (Kappelle *et al.*, 1993).

Prior to clinical testing of the putative efficacy of nimodipine for patients suffering from diabetic neuropathy, the neuroprotective efficacy in experimental diabetes mellitus was studied using another animal model of diabetic neuropathy in which, as in the clinic, insulin treatment is standard. This model uses the BB/Wor rat first described in 1974. Approximately 80 per cent of these rats develop diabetes mellitus at 55–120 days of age. The onset of the diabetic syndrome is acute and characterized by hyperglycaemia, hypoinsulinaemia, polyuria and glycosuria. Auto-antibodies are produced against the 64 kD islet cell protein preceding the onset of spontaneous diabetes (Kappelle, 1993).

We studied the effect of nimodipine on already existing neuropathy in the BB/Wor rat. After the development of diabetes, insulin treatment was started immediately. SNCV and MNCV were measured at weeks 0, 6, 8, 10 and 12. The BB/Wor rats that did not develop diabetes were kept as age-matched controls. After 6 weeks, when a significant slowing of SNCV and MNCV had developed, the diabetic animals were divided into two treatment groups: one group was treated with vehicle i.p. every 48 h, and the other was treated with nimodipine (20 mg/kg) i.p. every 48 h. The level of metabolic control, as assessed by measuring glucose and HbA1 levels, was not different for the latter two groups. After the start of treatment at week 6, rats treated with nimodipine showed a significant improvement in SNCV and MNCV. Since the impairment of blood flow seems to be an important factor in the pathogenesis of diabetic neuropathy, sciatic nerve blood flow was measured at the end of the experiment by laser-Doppler technology. Indeed diabetic rats showed a marked reduction in nerve blood flow which again was counteracted by chronic nimodipine treatment (Bravenboer *et al.*, 1993). Collectively the data suggest that nimodipine is able to ameliorate the experimental diabetic neuropathy. The mechanism of action presumably involves a combination of at least two different factors. One is direct neuroprotection by blocking L-channels on neurons, since it has been shown that intracellular free calcium levels are elevated in the nerves of diabetic rats. However, the enhancement of nerve blood flow points to an effect on vascular L-channels which in itself may have contributed to improved nerve function. Such a complex mechanism of action would be very difficult indeed to study *ex vivo* and therefore the data underscore the significance of an animal model for diabetic neuropathy. On the other hand it still remains to be determined of what predictive value the models are to the clinical situation, as no effective therapy of human diabetic neuropathy has yet been developed.

Cisplatin neuropathy

Peripheral neuropathies due to oncolytic treatment were briefly mentioned earlier in the introduction. These neuropathies are among the most menacing side effects encountered in the treatment of cancer. With improvements in supportive care, the administration of higher cumulative dosages of oncolytic drugs is now a reality and as a consequence the incidence of neurotoxic side effects increases. At present, peripheral neurotoxicity is almost always considered as the dose-limiting toxicity. Discontinuation of oncolytic treatment, however, may profoundly interfere with adequate treatment of the malignancy. It will be clear that prevention of this side effect is important both in order to increase oncolytic efficacy and to establish a better quality of life.

Cisplatin is an important drug in the treatment of various malignancies, most notably those of the genito-urinary tract. The drug is rated as one of the most active oncolytics available for the treatment of ovarian cancer. Its major long-term side effects are nephro-, oto- and neurotoxicity. Since reduction of nephrotoxicity has become feasible, neurotoxicity is nowadays regarded as the major dose-limiting side effect. Cisplatin neurotoxicity is limited in almost all cases to the peripheral nervous system and to ototoxicity. Only sporadically are central nervous system or autonomic dysfunctions attributed to cisplatin (Hamers *et al.*, 1991b).

The peripheral neuropathy induced by cisplatin is characterized by numbness, tingling, loss of vibratory sensation and diminished propriocepsis. Spinal ataxia resulting in disability may ensue. The motor system does not seem to be affected at all (Roelofs *et al.*, 1984; Thompson *et al.*, 1984). The first symptoms are those of a bilateral sensory neuropathy with numbness and tingling, often in a stocking and glove distribution. As the neuropathy continues, position sense becomes progressively impaired. In severe cases this may lead to wheelchair dependency because of a severe sensory ataxia. These symptoms are often accompanied by uncomfortable and painful paraesthesias. The neuropathy becomes more severe with increasing cumulative doses of cisplatin (frequently reached with high-dose treatment regimens) and although cisplatin-based chemotherapy is discontinued if severe neurological disabilities develop, the neuropathy is irreversible in 30–50 per cent of patients (Hamers *et al.*, 1991b).

Thus far the pathogenesis of this neuropathy remains obscure. Post-mortem histological examination of peripheral nerves reveals a primary axonal degeneration and loss of thick fibres. As cisplatin preferentially affects the sensory part of the peripheral nervous system, the primary lesion is rather at the level of the dorsal root ganglia as it is here that the cell bodies of the sensory nerves are located. They lie outside the central nervous system and are therefore not protected by the blood–brain barrier that constitutes a very effective defence against cisplatin; cisplatin concentrations in dorsal root ganglia are similar to those in tumour tissue, whereas cisplatin concentrations in brain and spinal cord are at least a ten-fold lower (Thompson *et al.*, 1984). How cisplatin affects the neurons is unclear: Peyrot *et al.* (1983) reported that hydrolysed cisplatin (the active form) may inhibits tubulin microtubule polymerization *in vitro*, albeit less efficiently than established microtubule poisons such as colchicine and vinca-alkaloids. If this interaction with tubulin is one of the damaging mechanisms *in vivo* as well, cisplatin might interfere with cytoskeleton synthesis and maintenance and impair neuronal function in this way. Terheggen *et al.* (1989) investigated the occurrence of cisplatin-DNA adducts (responsible for the anti-tumour action of cisplatin) in dorsal root ganglia and could only find these adducts in satellite cells, but not in the sensory neuron somata themselves. These results indicate that *in vivo* cisplatin perhaps does not reach the neurons themselves but rather exerts its action through the satellite cells. Based on present knowledge, it seems impossible to produce a valid *in vitro* model for cisplatin-induced neuropathy. In tissue culture studies, our group has been able to show that cisplatin inhibits neurite extension and cell migration from cultured foetal whole chicken dorsal root ganglia. Administration of cisplatin to Schwann cell cultures reveals that cisplatin is very toxic for these cells *in vitro* (Hol *et al.*, unpublished observations). The relevance is not clear, however, as *in vivo* cisplatin pathology of Schwann cells (demyelination) seems to be secondary to disease of the axon, and because it cannot explain the preference for sensory neurons as opposed to motor neurons (both fibre types are myelinated). Although these studies provide additional information, they do not explain the clinical picture.

Therefore, De Koning *et al.* (1987) developed a rat model for cisplatin neuropathy. Although not all signs and symptoms present in the human clinic of cisplatin neuropathy are accessible in the rat (e.g. paraesthesias are very difficult to test, if at all), one of the key symptoms, ataxia, can be investigated in the animal model, albeit indirectly. The sensory ataxia observed in patients with cisplatin neuropathy is due to disease of the so-called I_a-fibres, the nerve fibres that innervate the muscle spindles. The information these fibres convey is essential for coordinated movements. Moreover, these nerve fibres are the thickest and thus fastest-conducting fibres in the body. Thus, when one measures the sensory nerve conduction velocity in a mixed peripheral nerve one measures the conduction velocity of these I_a-fibres. A decrease in the sensory nerve conduction velocity thus indicates disease or loss of these fibres. By means of a simple technique it is possible to measure reliably both the maximal motor and sensory nerve conduction velocities in the sciatic nerve of the rat repeatedly. In rats subjected to chronic cisplatin treatment the sensory nerve conduction velocity decreases whereas the motor nerve conduction velocity is not affected (De Koning *et al.*, 1987). This is exactly what one expects, based on knowledge of the human clinic. Based on our encouraging results with the melanocortin-like peptide ORG 2766 in the model for mechanical nerve lesions we tested the hypothesis that this peptide might also diminish or even prevent a neuropathy in the cisplatin-treated rats. Indeed, the peptide treatment ameliorated the neurotoxic signs and symptoms (Gerritsen van der Hoop *et al.*, 1988a,b). Stimulated by these preclinical findings, a randomized, double-blind, placebo-controlled study was initiated to assess the efficacy of ORG 2766 in the prevention of cisplatin neuropathy in women with ovarian cancer. A dose of 1 mg/m^2 injected subcutaneously directly before and 24 h after cisplatin and cyclophosphamide infusion (75 and 750 mg/m^2 every 3 weeks) proved to prevent the increment in vibration perception threshold observed in placebo co-treated patients. Moreover, fewer neurological signs and symptoms were recorded than in the placebo group. The rates of clinical response to chemotherapy were similar in all groups.

The results of this clinical pilot study suggest that ORG 2766 can prevent or attenuate cisplatin neuropathy in the human clinic without adversely affecting the cytotoxic effect of the drug (Gerritsen van der Hoop *et al.*, 1990).

Despite the apparent effectiveness of ORG 2766 in preventing cisplatin-induced neuropathy in the human clinic, many questions remained unanswered. For example, it is unknown whether the peptide might be expected to prevent neuropathy with the more intense cisplatin treatment schedules studied in the clinic. We tried to answer this question in the animal model by subjecting the animals to more intense cisplatin treatment. The results of this animal study indicated that ORG 2766 prevents the neuropathy with high-dose cisplatin treatment as well as with low-dose treatment (Hamers *et al.*, 1991a). Follow-up of several patients previously treated with ORG 2766 indicated that some began to complain of neuropathological symptoms after both cisplatin and peptide treatment were discontinued (Hovestadt *et al.*, 1992). Increase or even first occurence of neuropathocological symptoms during the first months after the last cisplatin dose is a well-known phenomenon (Hamers *et al.*, 1991b). One might assume that this phenomenon could be studied in the animal model in more detail, and eventually test whether continued ORG 2766 treatment might help to prevent the occurrence of these symptoms. However, we failed to find evidence for a delayed occurrence of cisplatin-induced neuropathic changes in rats previously co-treated with cisplatin and peptide (Hamers *et al.*, 1993).

Nonetheless, the results obtained with the studies on cisplatin neurotoxicity indicate that animal experiments can play an important role in the investigation of putative neuroprotective therapies for the human clinic.

Conclusion

In this paper we have focused on laboratory experiments that are of significance in the study of peripheral nerve lesions and their therapy. In view of the complexity of the problem we are confronted with, it seems impossible to rely solely on *in vitro* experimentation. Although *in vitro* models are powerful for studying aspects of pathogenesis or therapeutic mechanisms, they are inherently simple and thus apt to fail at predicting the reaction of the organism as a whole. In this paper we discussed several human peripheral nerve disorders that require *in vivo* rather than *in vitro* experimentation. For example in the nerve crush model we present beneficial effects of physical exercise on nerve regeneration. Although outgrowth of regenerating axons occurs to a certain extent, controlled exercise of the neuromuscular system enhances this process, possibly by stimulating nerve blood flow. The nerve blood supply is also an issue in the second model, diabetic neuropathy, where it is one of several factors that is of importance in the pathogenesis of the disorder. Experiments with nimodipine, a drug that both protects neurons and ameliorates blood supply, illustrate the power of the animal model in this disorder. The third model, cisplatin-induced neuropathy, illustrates the significance of results obtained in the animal model for the human clinic. These studies underscore the value of the animal model for predicting the clinical action of a putative neuroprotective agent.

References

Bär, P.R.D., Schrama, L.H. & Gispen, W.H. (1990): Neurotrophic effects of the ACTH/MSH-like peptides in the peripheral nervous system. In: *Neuropeptide concept*, ed. De Wied, D., pp. 175–211. Amsterdam: Elsevier Science Publishers BV.

Bravenboer, B., Kappelle, A.C., Biessels, G., van Buren, T. & Gispen, W.H. (1993): Improvement of nerve conduction velocity and sciatic nerve blood flow by nimodipine in the BB/Wor rat. Third meeting of the Diabetic Neuropathy Study Group of the EASD, 3–5 September 1993, Istanbul, Turkey.

Carr, A. & Haynes, L.W. (1988): Transient appearance of proopiomelanocortin (POMC) messenger RNA and N-terminal peptides in rat embryo spinal cord. *Neurosci. Res. Commun.* **3**, 31–39.

De Koning, P., Neijt, J.P., Jennekens, F.G.I. & Gispen, W.H. (1987): Evaluation of *cis*-diammine-dichloroplatinum(II) (cisplatin) neurotoxicity in rats. *Toxicol. Appl. Pharmacol.* **89**, 81–87.

Dyck, P.J., Thomas, P.K., Asbury, A.K., Winegrad, A.I. & Porte, D. (1987): *Diabetic neuropathy.* Philadelphia: WB Saunders Co.

Edwards, P.M., Van der Zee, C.E.E.M., Verhaagen, J., Schotman, P., Jennekens, F.G.I. & Gispen, W.H. (1984): Evidence that the neurotrophic actions of α-MSH may derive from its ability to mimic the actions of a peptide formed in degenerating nerve stumps. *J. Neurol. Sci.* **64**, 333–340.

Gerritsen van der Hoop, R., De Koning, P., Boven, E., Neijt, J.P., Jennekens, F.G.I. & Gispen, W.H. (1988a): Efficacy of the neuropeptide ORG 2766 in the prevention and treatment of cisplatin-induced neurotoxicity in rats. *Eur. J. Cancer Clin. Oncol.* **24**, 637–642.

Gerritsen van der Hoop, R., Neijt, J.P., Jennekens, F.G.I. & Gispen, W.H. (1988b): Both in normal and high-dose cisplatin treatment ORG 2766 protects from neurotoxicity in rats: electrophysiological and histological results. *ENS satelite symposium, San Remo* p. 39. (Abstract)

Gerritsen van der Hoop, R., Vecht, C.J., Van der Burg, M.E.L., Elderson, A., Boogerd, W., Heimans, J.J., Els, D., Vries, P., Van Houwelingen, J.C., Jennekens, F.G.I., Gispen, W.H. & Neijt, J.P. (1990): Prevention of cisplatin neurotoxicity with an ACTH(4–9) analogue in patients with ovarian cancer. *N. Engl. J. Med.* **322**, 89–94.

Gispen, W.H. (1990): Therapeutic potential for melanocortins in peripheral nerve disease. *Trends Pharmacol. Sci.* **11**, 221–222.

Hamers, F.P.T., Gerritsen van der Hoop, R., Steerenburg, P.A., Neijt, J.P. & Gispen, W.H. (1991a): Putative neurotrophic factors in the protection of cisplatin-induced peripheral neuropathy in rats. *Toxicol. Appl. Pharmacol.* **111**, 514–522.

Hamers, F.P.T., Gispen, W.H. & Neijt, J.P. (1991b): Neurotoxic side-effects of cisplatin. *Eur. J. Cancer* **27**, 372–376.

Hamers, F.P.T., Pette, C., Bravenboer, B., Vecht, C.J., Neijt, J.P. & Gispen, W.H. (1993): Cisplatin-induced neuropathy in mature rats: effects of the melanocortin-like peptide ORG 2766. *Cancer Chemother. Pharmacol.* **32**, 162–166.

Hovestadt, A., Van der Burg, M.E.L., Verbiest, H.B.C., Van Putten, W.L.J. & Vecht, Ch.J. (1992): The course of neuropathy after cessation of cisplatin treatment, combined with Org 2766 or placebo. *J. Neurol.* **239**, 143–146.

Hughes, S. & Smith, M.E. (1988): Effect of nerve transection on β-endorphin and α-melanotropin immunoreactivity in motor nerves of normal and dystrophic mice. *Neurosci. Lett.* **92**, 1–7.

Hughes, S. & Smith, M.E. (1989): Proopiomelanocortin derived peptides in transected and contralateral motor nerves of the rat. *J. Chem. Neuroanat.* **2**, 227–237.

Kappelle, A.C., Bravenboer, B., Traber, J., Erkelens, D.W. & Gispen, W.H. (1992): The Ca^{2+} antagonist nimodipine counteracts the onset of an experimental neuropathy in streptozotocin-induced diabetic rats. *Neurosci. Res. Commun.* **10**, 95–104.

Kappelle, A.C., Bravenboer, B., van Buren, T., Traber, J., Erkelens, D.W. & Gispen, W.H. (1993): The Ca^{2+} antagonist, nimodipine, and existing neuropathy in the streptozotocin-induced diabetic rat model. *Br. J. Pharmacol.* **108**, 780–785.

Kappelle, A.C. (1993): Thesis: On the pathogenesis and treatment of experimental diabetic neuropathy. Utrecht University, Utrecht, The Netherlands.

Katchaturian, Z.S. (1989): The role of calcium regulation in brain aging: reexamination of a hypothesis. *Aging* **1**, 17–34.

Kater, S.B., Mattson, M.P., Cohan, C. & Connor, J. (1989): Calcium regulation of the neuronal growth cone. *Trends Neurosci.* **11**, 315–321.

Peyrot, V., Briand, C., Crevat, A., Braguer, D., Chauvet-Monges, A.M. & Sari, J.C. (1983): Action of hydrolyzed cisplatin and some analogues on microtubule protein polymerization in vitro. *Cancer Treat. Rep.* **67**, 641–646.

Plantinga, L.C., Verhaagen, J., Edwards, P.M., Schrama, L.H., Burbach, J.P.H. & Gispen, W.H. (1992): Expression of the pro-opiomelanocortin gene in dorsal root ganglia, spinal cord and sciatic nerve after sciatic nerve crush in the rat. *Mol. Brain Res.* **16**, 135–142.

Roelofs, R.I., Hruskesky, W., Rogin, J. & Rosenberg, L. (1984): Peripheral sensory neuropathy and cisplatin chemotherapy. *Neurology* **34**, 934–938.

Terheggen, M.A.B., Gerritsen van der Hoop, R., Floot, B.G.J. & Gispen, W.H. (1989): Cellular distribution of *cis*-diaminedichloroplatinum(II)-DNA binding in dorsal root spinal ganglia: effect of the neuroprotecting peptide Org 2766. *Toxicol. Appl. Pharmacol.* **99**, 334–343.

Thompson, S.W., Davis, L.E., Kornfeld, M., Hilgers, R.D. & Standefer, J.C. (1984): Cisplatin neuropathy. *Cancer* **54**, 1269–1275.

Traber, J. & Gispen, W.H. (1989): *Nimodipine and central nervous system function: new vistas.* Stuttgart-New York: Schattauer.

van Meeteren, N.L.U., Brakkee, J.H. & Gispen, W.H. (1993): The effect of physical exercise on functional recovery following a peripheral nerve lesion in the rat. *Physiotherapy Theory and Practice* **9**, 77–85.

The ethics of animal and human experimentation, edited by P.P. De Deyn.
©1994 John Libbey & Company Ltd., pp. 143–148.

13

Ethical justification: to whom?

Tjard de Cock Buning

Department of Animal Problems, Faculty of Medicine, University of Leiden, PO Box 9602, 2300 RC Leiden, The Netherlands

Summary

In this paper the following question is addressed: to whom is ethical justification directed? Most commonly, justification is formulated as a statement towards society, and more precisely towards critical animal welfare groups within society. Ethical review committees certify these justifications and tend to act as safeguards to protect valuable research interests against violent agents from outside. However, this formal justification does not guard many researchers in their personal life. They still find themselves in a position that they avoid talking about their experiments to their own children.

The thesis is advanced that another, more personal, justification should be added to relieve the researcher's conscience about the moral load induced by the employer. Three arguments are discussed within the context of the philosophy of justification: a personal argument, a historical argument and a systematic argument.

Finally, the author makes a plea for changes which will enable the next generation of biomedical researchers to show their experiments to their children with pride.

Introduction

Which will create more problems for the researcher: justification of animal experiments against pressure groups or against his or her own children? The former is most commonly pictured as the main problem of researchers, while the latter situation is often ignored. Although it is, psychologically speaking, understandable that one projects negative aspects towards other people, as Frijda (1986) formulated one of his basic laws of emotion, it distracts attention from the principal moral issue, as demonstrated by the following argument. When a researcher succeeds in convincing a pressure group of the necessity of offering animals to the conquest of a life-threatening disease, he will not necessarily succeed in convincing his own child of the inevitability of experimenting on 'lovely' mice. On the other hand, when one performs experiments in such a way that they are approved by one's own child, pressure groups will also join in. The point I am putting forward here is that justification in terms of necessity of a particular *goal* is a rational discourse, whereas the justification of the actual *act* to perform (i.e. handling, operating, housing) evokes a direct moral response of aversion or acceptance. As for the rational side, my co-workers and I elsewhere described the procedures to structure this discourse (Theune & de Cock Buning, 1992) and the pitfalls (de Cock Buning *et al.*,1993; Smit,1988). In this paper I will discuss the hidden trap which will sooner or later catch all who are engaged in animal experiments: personal moral conscience.

Moral conscience

The genesis of moral conscience is described by psychologists in various contexts. Piaget (1977) and Kohlberg (1976) describe the maturation of the moral being in successive stages. During the first stages the parents dictate right and wrong to their children. This stage is called 'heteronomous' (laws from the other). When the child grows up, he or she will 'internalize' the moral notions given by outsiders. In the next stage, the norms are felt and executed as one's 'own' personal moral rules. Others are corrected by this person with explicit reference to these moral rules. This stage is called the 'autonomous' (own laws) stage. In the following stages the person reconsiders the moral rules and evolves to a truly moral being detached from personal gain. Behaviourists discard such a descriptive approach; they try to elucidate the basic mechanisms behind this 'behaviour'. They focus on the mechanism of 'internalization', which to them appears to be nothing but learning by means of reward and punishment (Eysenck, 1976). In their view, mice can be taught (shaped) to behave morally. Conscience turns out to be conditioned fear.

Both approaches emphasize that the environment is an important factor in the genesis of conscience. As Levinas, according to Key (1992), would add, a single isolated human being can never attain the notion of morality. At least one other person is needed to experience the restricting of one's own sense of freedom in order to create a space of respect to 'meet' the other.

Indeed, curiosity for the other person induces a chain of phenomena that constitutes the basic outline of morality: having an open mind towards the other, accepting time to listen, trying to understand, projecting oneself in the position of the other. Anyone who has ever fallen in love, experienced having a child, became a parent, or just got friendly with an animal, knows what I mean. So, one of the roots of morality is the sense of caring. There is a strong, almost instinctive, notion to care for beings in whom one becomes interested after a personal meeting. This is one of the main reasons why physicians have a difficult time deciding whether a therapy should be stopped. Once a relationship is established, it is hard to give up the sense of caring. On a more abstract level this notion is described as 'ethical responsibility'.

The personal argument

Scientists engaged in animal experiments have to face unique problems which isolate them as a group from society and the daily notion of morality. They either start as clinicians with a strong existential experience of the suffering of human patients, or as biologists curious to unravel the wonders of nature. In the first case the moral commitment towards patients forces them into the field of animal experiments. To avoid a moral dilemma their life is organized in such a way that the lab animals are not 'met' in the above-mentioned sense of Levinas. Lower-ranking staff members are ordered to execute the animal experiments and the animals are depersonalized as much as possible (Visser & Grommers, 1986; Arluke, 1988). In the second case, basic and profound knowledge of a species leads to a growing feeling of respect for that species. In order to avoid the unescapable spiral of self-limitation of research, curiosity is redirected beyond the animal towards a higher and more abstract level of knowledge: the animal becomes a means, a so-called model. Again, the animal is depersonalized (Arluke, 1988).

Although this strategy is successful in the sense that one survives in one's profession, it creates an immense gap between the researcher and those who participate in the non-professional part of his or her life. Every day family and friends are met who might ask the researcher questions about his experiments which the researcher would rather like to avoid (Arluke, 1992).

In a way, traditional role patterns, i.e. the hard-working father who earns the money and does not speak about his work, provide a suitable cover for the scientist. Modern couples, often educated in the same field of research, might develop a relationship where an unspoken rule dictates that the topic of animal experience is not to be raised. The question is, however, how long this problem can be hidden. And do we want this situation to carry on?

Some will argue that the situation is unnecessarily dramatized. The best approach is suggested to be the following one: be honest and tell everybody what you do. There is nothing to be ashamed of in the search for cures of dreadful diseases. Indeed, the goals are honourable, but just limiting a description of one's profession to the goals is one of the best strategies to circumvent the sensitive point: the actual experiment. This can easily be observed when the argument is turned around: describe the experiment without telling the goals. Even the simple procedure of a subcutaneous implantation of tumour tissue will evoke an aversive gut reaction among any audience of laymen. This aversion arises from the afflicted basic notion of caring. It is afflicted by a being endowed with the power to mutilate innocent healthy animals. Thus the aversion is directed towards the researcher who is the embodiment of this power. His or her deeds are considered shameful because of this unequal match of power. I will recommend any researcher convinced of the ethical way he handles animals to invite his own young children to the operation room. Why young children? Because they will not be distracted by a rational description of the goals and because they are the next generation and will judge you at the end of the day. Those who pass this test successfully will live with a clearer conscience.

The historical argument

When our children grow up and expand as new generations into the next century, they may look back to history and formulate a final judgment about our high-tech scientific enterprise. What will they say? Of course, they will be grateful for our efforts to expand the body of knowledge and for our efforts to conquer fatal diseases. But I doubt whether they will think mildly about the way we performed animal experiments.

I base this negative prediction on current 20th century perception and moral judgement of the physiologists of the 19th century. Is it not odd that the great comparative physiologist Francois Magendie (1783–1855) is now condemned because of his experiments on unanaesthetized living animals, even though the use of ether was applied after his death? Still, nobody likes to be compared with Magendie. However irrational, we as the next generations tend to measure the moral status of our ancestors with our current state of technology. We admire Magendie's pupil Claude Bernard because of his efforts to find an anaesthetic before continuing experiments on living animals. In other words, the background of our criticism of Magendie is that he did not wait, or that he did not investigate technical solutions to limit animal suffering. The same will be true for future generations who will judge our ways of gaining knowledge and conquering diseases. Why are we putting so little effort into the development of high-tech alternatives? Why do we not incorporate advanced nutrition-dependent switch-on genes in the exploration of genetic diseases in animals? Is it too complicated? Remember, this argument was often used by Magendie. From the perspective of future generations, 'complicated' only means a transient state of acquiring routine and skills. There is no morally valid argument to postpone the application of new inventions in order to limit the suffering of animals.

Even now children might ask you one day why you still used animals ten years ago, while plenty of tissue cultures had already been developed.

The historical distortion also surfaces with respect to the economical argument. Although money plays an important part in current discussions about the development of alternatives (especially those alternatives which are more expensive than the traditional animal models), all relevance seems to vanish from a historical distance. Only those persons or industries who invested efforts and capital in alternatives will receive moral applause from the next generation.

The systematic argument

Within the context of consequentialistic ethics it is vital to anticipate possible consequences of an ethical decision. In the case of animal experiments this is usually understood as the estimation of the health benefits to be gained and the suffering inflicted upon the laboratory animals. The first appears a hopeful wish which sometimes comes true and the second is a harsh reality. From the perspective of the directly involved, well-motivated researcher it is understandable that consequences are synonymous with the research goals aimed at. From a less biased outsider's perspective other aspects also appear relevant for the analysis of consequences. For example, what are the consequences of animal experiments which fail to produce consistent results? The animals will then have suffered without leading to results that may justify these experiments. The scientist in question will object that even so-called failures are instrumental to guide the research process to a different direction. This is, however, a fallacious, circular argument that can be represented as follows: 'All experiments add to the body of knowledge; those which do not are interesting and therefore add something to the body of knowledge.' In other words, no experiment can ever be useless. The logical impossibility of designing a hypothetical situation to falsify this argument demonstrates the circularity of the argument.

Instead, consequences should be analysed by imagining an unbiased person living in the future looking back in time to the research project in question. He or she will certainly notice the excellent projects that will have led to scientific breakthroughs. From that perspective all other, less significant, results and failures will seem to lack ethical justification.

I agree that this hypothetical 'next generation' cannot provide us with the necessary clairvoyant information to avoid dead ends, but it elucidates that the current habit of interested researchers and managers who justify every 'promising' research project, is controversial. In order to get closer to a more realistic estimation of the success rate of animal experiments an imaginary next generation's perspective is recommended to researchers as an antidote against their understandable optimism.

Conclusion

The current procedure of justifying animal experiments by getting approval from ethical review committees is effective as a business ethic (an ethical code for staff, a safeguard against society), but it fails to protect the conscience of the individual. At least two aspects need serious consideration in order to improve the mental stability and the satisfaction of the creative researcher. This can be achieved by a fast introduction of high-technology techniques to refine biological research in such a way that the procedures could equally well be performed in front of one's own child, or even at one's own child (in principle). Secondly, alternatives to animal experiments should be developed to replace animal models by non-animal models. One day in the future I hope to enter a laboratory together with my (grand)children without feeling ashamed towards the young ones about the state of dignity of scientists and animals.

Acknowledgements. With respect to the moral problems discussed in this paper I like to thank the participants of the workshop in ethics (one full day, 20 times a year, 20 participants) for their courage and willingness to discuss these personal and confidential matters. This workshop is given by the author and is a part of the 3 week course on laboratory animal science. This course is compulsory by law in The Netherlands for graduated biomedical students who like to obtain a licence to design and to supervise animal research (see also Ch. 10, *Education and training in laboratory animal science*).

References

Arluke, A.B. (1988): Sacrificial symbolism in animal experimentation: object or pet? *Anthrozoos* **2.2**, 98–117.

Arluke, A.B. (1992): Trapped in a guilt cage. *New Scientist* **134**, 33–35.

de Cock Buning, T., Heeger, F.R. & Verhoog, H. (1993): Ethical aspects of animal experimentation. In: *Principles of laboratory animal science*, eds. L.F.M. van Zutphen, V. Boumans & A.C. Beynen, p. 389. Amsterdam: Elsevier.

Eysenck, H.J.(1976): The biology of morality. In: *Moral development and behaviour*, ed. Thomas Lickona, pp. 108–131. New York: Holt, Rinehart & Winston.

Frijda, N.H. (1986): *The emotions*. Cambridge: Cambridge University Press.

Key, J. (1992): *Structuur van Levinas' denken, in het perspectief van een ontwikkelingsgang*, p. 254. Kampen, Kok-Angora.

Kohlberg, L. (1976): Moral stages and moralization. In: *Moral development and behaviour*, ed. Thomas Lickona, pp. 31–53. New York: Holt, Rinehart & Winston.

Piaget, J. (1977): *The moral judgement of the child*. Harmondsworth: Penguin Books.

Smit, C. (1988): *Dierproeven, 100 jaar discussie.* Kampen: La Riviere & Voorhoeve.

Theune, E.P. & de Cock Buning, T. (1992): Grenzen aan dierexperimenteel onderzoek. (report) *Proefdier & Wetenschap* 4, Leiden.

Visser, M.B.H. & Grommers, F.J. (1986): *Dier of Ding, objectivering van dieren.* Wageningen: Pudoc.

The ethics of animal and human experimentation, edited by P.P. De Deyn.
 pp. 149–157.

14

Animal experimentation in the United States: the challenge and response

Jerod M. Loeb

Director of Research and Evaluation and Chief Scientific Officer, Joint Commission on Accreditation of Healthcare Organizations, One Renaissance Blvd, Oakbrook Terrace, Illinois 60181, USA

Summary

The animal activist movement has a revealing history and began in earnest in 19th century England with the rise of anti-vivisectionism. Today, anti-vivisectionism has been replaced by animal rights and the movement has become world-wide. More than 1000 activist groups operate in the US alone with annual revenues that certainly exceed $50 million, though some estimates place those revenues as high as $200 million.

While the animal activist movement has a singular goal – the abolition of the use of animals in all contexts – there are both fundamental philosophical and secondary 'practical' arguments used against the medical research community. The impact of the animal protection movement was initially to heighten concern among the scientific community about appropriate animal welfare issues; however, today the animal rights movement is having a definite deleterious effect upon medical research progress and technological innovation. One of the most discouraging aspects of the organized efforts against medical research has been the involvement of a small number of physicians and scientists. Historically these physicians often agitated against the germ theory of disease, against vaccination and other prudent public health measures. Today, these few science and medical professionals within the animal rights movement suggest that animal research has never been the foundation of medicine, that effective alternative technologies are available and that research using animals is unnecessary.

Many challenges have been raised to the use of animals in research from questioning the value of basic research to emotional issues such as the use of primates, 'alternatives' to animals, and purported painful experiments. While nearly 90 per cent of the animals used in medical research are rodents, the activist literature rarely portrays that fact. Virtually every device, drug, and procedure used in human and veterinary medicine owes its development in whole or in part to experiments conducted in animals, but activist literature continues to misrepresent the facts. More than two-thirds of the Nobel prizes awarded in Physiology or Medicine since 1901 have involved experiments that utilized animals.

The animal activist movement has succeeded in winning the minds and purse strings of many for a variety of reasons. Growing science illiteracy, the poor image of science and the scientist, a lack of public understanding of the scientific process and cultural anthropomorphism all contribute to the winning of converts. Many activist groups attempt to couch their messages in the cloak of credibility by using seemingly authoritative voices. For example, the Physicians Committee for Responsible Medicine, an animal rights group, is neither physician nor responsible. The pseudo-scientific messages promulgated by groups such as this have been used with increasing frequency and success by animal rights movement.

Animal rights has been seen as a sharp two-sided controversy with staunch antagonists at both extremes – those who support animal research (and thus purportedly believe in the mistreatment of animals) and those who oppose animal research (and thus purportedly believe in animal welfare). The fallacy inherent in this analysis is continually fostered by media coverage. The biomedical research community supports responsible and humane animal care and use. Theodore Roosevelt once noted that '. . . conscience without common sense breeds folly . . .' For medicine to progress, we must demonstrate conscience and promote common sense.

Introduction

Controversy surrounding the use of animals in biomedical research and education is not new. Since the Victorian era, animal activists have been urging the cessation of animal use in many contexts, most notably, in medical research. In recent years however, the tactics and strategies of contemporary animal rights groups have grown in scope and intensity and now clearly pose an increasingly direct threat to the future of medical progress. Proponents of animal rights appeal to the emotions and attempt to raise seemingly complex ethical and social issues as a veiled means of reinforcing their belief that any human use of animals, in any context, constitutes 'speciesism'. Intimidation and harassment have become routine among many animal rights organizations and the contemporary scientific and medical communities have been slow in responding.

Many challenges to medical research using animals have been raised during the past century. For example, activists have suggested that 'alternatives' to animals already exist and that only inertia and tradition on the part of research investigators prevents any change in the status quo thereby failing to reduce the number of animals used. However, a significant reduction in the number of animals used in research has been noted within the last decade, due in large part to the diligent efforts of scientists to find adjunctive models. The number of animals used in biomedical research in the United States has been estimated by the United States Office of Technology Assessment (a branch of the US Congress), to be about 20–25 million per year. The American Association for the Advancement of Laboratory Animal Care reports that in the period 1980–1990, the number of dogs used in research dropped by 42 per cent and the number of cats dropped by 51 per cent. In 1990, the number of dogs and cats used in research, teaching and testing combined represented less than 1 per cent of the total number entering animal pounds and shelters. The American Humane Association estimates that, in 1990, 63 per cent of the dogs and 81 per cent of the cats entering pounds and shelters were euthanized. It is important to note that approximately 18–20 million of the total number of animals used in research are rats and mice bred specifically for research purposes. These numbers may be placed into proper context by realizing that each year about 5 billion animals are used for food in the United States alone. Similarly, more than 400 million animals are estimated to be killed on roadsides each year, 20 million cats and dogs are abandoned by their owners and 20–30 million cats and dogs are killed yearly in animal pounds and shelters. In fact, for every 10–20 dogs and cats killed in pounds, one is used in medical research.

Few of the arguments used by animal rights organizations today are new. Animal activist groups have argued for years that basic biomedical research has no clinical value and that animal experiments are duplicated needlessly, primarily to foster the careers of research investigators. While the public continues to overwhelmingly support the responsible use of animals in medical research, activists nevertheless continue to successfully convince unsuspecting legislators of the need for new restrictive rules and regulations governing research. While a host of federal, state and institutional regulations have been instituted that strictly regulate medical research, the implementation and governance of those rules are attacked by animal activists. Although the litany of advances in human and veterinary medicine over the last several generations clearly documents the importance animals have played in medical research and testing, animal rights groups negate that history. Activists look to improvements in public health and nutrition as the major reasons why morbidity and mortality have decreased. The improved nutrition and better public health measures promoted by activists certainly represents prudent advice. Unfortunately however, acceptance of this advice by society cannot be legislated. Moreover, diseases like coronary heart disease, cancer, genetic diseases, and many others cannot be eradicated by simple changes in lifestyle alone.

The current animal rights movement excels in portraying itself as new, growing and occupying a distinct moral, ethical and intellectual high ground. Perhaps in view of this, the animal activist community has managed to recruit a small number of health care professionals into their ranks. This is not a new phenomenon and has existed for generations. Although seemingly antithetical to their education and training, a few physicians and scientists have always been associated with the animal activist movement, both as classical antivivisectionists and today, as contemporary animal rights activists. Many of the early physicians associated with the anti-vivisectionist movement were homoeopaths trained in proprietary medical schools. These same physicians often spoke against the germ theory of disease, against vaccination and practised on the fringes of current medical thinking. Today, physician animal activists seem to share many of the same fundamental beliefs about medical research being promulgated by lay members of these groups, most notably, that research using animals is unnecessary, duplicative, cruel, unregulated and outdated. They state that effective alternatives to animal use are available but that custom favours use of animal models. They argue that funding of animal-based research continues at the expense of disease-prevention strategies, that animal research misleads investigators and that little substantive progress in medicine has ever been made (or ever will be made) using animal models of human disease. The public often tends to think of physicians as authoritative on virtually all medical topics. They often fail to distinguish among the medical specialties. To a scientist, a psychiatrist's comments on the work of a thoracic surgeon may carry limited weight. However, to the public, the 'Dr' title creates an almost instant credibility across all medical specialties.

It is instructive to analyse how the medical community nearly 100 years ago responded to challenges raised by a small group of vocal anti-vivisectionist physicians who spoke out against research using animals (and in some cases, humans). The attitudes and statements in the literature and speeches of anti-vivisectionist physicians of decades ago have changed little among the few physicians today who subscribe to the animal rights philosophy. It is important for the medical community to gain some historical perspective on physician involvement in this movement since the moral, scientific and philosophic arguments have deviated little over the years; more importantly, neither has the rhetoric used by such physicians to attempt to convince the public of the credibility of their views. Their approach is extremely clever and highlights a few small grains of truth intermixed with apocryphal data, the use of material taken completely out of context from its original meaning and denial or misrepresentation of scientifically valid facts.

In 1909, Angell, a professor of psychology at the University of Chicago and a staunch defender of medical research, argued that anti-vivisectionists '. . . assert that needless pain is an unmitigated evil and that its gratuitous and intentional causation is a sin and a crime ... they allege that animal experimentation is: (1) not justified by any results it has yet attained, and (2) that it is demoralizing and brutalizing in its influence both on those who conduct it and those who observe it . . . certain more conservative critics urge that, although its occasional employment has resulted in justifying benefits to both man and the animals, it is done too extensively, is done when results cannot possibly justify it, done carelessly and with indecent disregard of all the humanities . . . the case is somewhat complicated in the public mind by the appearances among the extreme critics of not a few gentlemen who sign themselves MD and who claim a professional knowledge of the details of the case . . .'

In the current controversy, at least two animal rights groups in the United States are run by physicians. These organizations are the Physicians Committee for Responsible Medicine (PCRM) and the Medical Research Modernization Committee. The PCRM has close ties with People for the Ethical Treatment of Animals (PETA), the most prominent and largest animal rights organization in America. PETA has at least 350 000 members and an annual budget of $9 million. The President of PCRM serves as scientific advisor to PETA and has testified on behalf of PETA before the Congress of the United States. Membership in the PCRM is believed to be about 50 000 of which less than 0.5 per cent are believed to be bonafide physicians. Physician members of PCRM use the techniques noted by Angell on a regular basis. For example, in a recent speech at Indiana University, the President of PCRM, himself a psychiatrist, noted that biomedical researchers who used animals in laboratory work were exhibiting signs of what he termed 'psychotic behaviour'. PCRM 'experts' regularly make public statements that are highly critical of specific research programmes. They have criticized important work in cardiovascular and cerebrovascular medicine, neuroscience, anaesthesiology and many other areas. In each case, PCRM has taken original material out of context and presented an erroneous portrayal of the research in question. Members of PCRM have defamed the reputations of institutions and individuals in an effort to convince the public that animal research is cruel, immoral, ineffective and/or inappropriate. This approach has proven to be a very effective fund-raising tool. Under scrutiny, one finds that when PCRM speaks to the uninformed, it tends to manipulate the truth. PCRM often presents oversimplified analyses to complex issues. Comments and research are taken out of context. Facts, issues and, most important, the true goals and beneficiaries of medical research are ignored and forgotten. In June of 1990, the American Medical Association (AMA) House of Delegates passed a resolution denouncing PCRM for implying that physicians who support the use of animals in biomedical research are irresponsible, for misrepresenting the critical role animals play in research and teaching and for obscuring the overwhelming support for such research which exists among practising physicians in the United States.

In 1909, Charles Eliot, the President Emeritus of Harvard University and himself a staunch medical research defender, noted that three main doubts had surfaced over the preceding 40 years concerning the value of animal experimentation. These doubts were '. . . (1) the connection between medical research and medical practice; (2) what is the use of trying to ascertain the nature of disease in animals when it is not known that the same disease occurs in man, or that the treatment successful for an animal would be successful for men; and (3) is truth seeking in biology commendable, even with the help of anaesthesia and aseptic technique, if the research be conducted at the expense of the comfort, joy or life of animals? . . .' These general tenets were shared by Meltzer, who noted in 1910 that the accusations against medical research using animals generally were raised by two distinct groups '. . . high science and low ignorance; the former frequently insinuating that the results are not sufficiently exact to be ranked as scientific work, and the other that animal experimentation has never been of any use either to science or to the practice of medicine . . .' It is interesting to note that here too, the PCRM argues from a similar vantage point nearly 100 years later. The public is easily misled because of the credibility and visibility provided to such physicians and organizations that suggest significant physician involvement.

The misappropriation of medical authority is another common technique used to denigrate medical research. This approach was used by the early anti-vivisectionist physicians and is still used today. In 1920, William Keen, a prominent turn-of-the-century American surgeon, noted that Sir Frederick Treves, the eminent English surgeon, was often misquoted by anti-vivisectionists as an opponent of animal research. In spite of denials that were published on several occasions, the misquotation still continued to appear in antivivisectionist literature for decades. Apparently the misquotation of scientists and physicians has always been a favourite technique of animal activists. These misquotations, omissions of relevant material and even fabricated quotations, while often refuted in multiple ways by the original authors, are never corrected in subsequent material produced by the animal activist community. In a recent letter to the editor of the *Medical Tribune*, Neal Barnard, the President of the PCRM, used selective quotations from a report of the AMA Council on Scientific Affairs to imply that carcinogenicity testing using animals was an outmoded and inappropriate method of determining exposure risk to various toxic compounds. Not quoted in Barnard's letter was the next sentence in the AMA Council report which stated that, while the technique might be outmoded, no other equally useful techniques had been developed that might supplant the use of animal testing to determine carcinogenicity; therefore, such testing was deemed to be quite appropriate.

One must ask why the public is seemingly receptive to the rhetoric of animal activists.

The scientific enterprise

There are many ways in which the scientific enterprise is at risk in our society today. In terms of public-policy development, science is often seen as a lesser priority. Rather than science driving the formulation of appropriate public policy, public policy is often developed in direct opposition to scientific fact. Recent calls for prospective HIV testing for all health care professionals is a prime example. The economic competitiveness of any nation can be severely compromised by decisions made by a government that has little appreciation for, or understanding of, the scientific method. Scientific terrorism has become a regular part of the agendas of any number of activist groups. This has been most common within the animal rights and environmental movements. The destructive tactics of various activist groups seriously threaten scientific progress. Anti-biotechnology activists often join forces with animal rights activists to target specific research programmes or research investigators. This vocal minority has been an effective force in helping to shape public opinion. In the United States, controversy has arisen regarding the potential use of bovine somatotropin as a stimulant to milk production in cows. At the root of this argument is a general distrust for governmental regulatory mechanisms, a disdain for recombinant technology and a perception that animals are being exploited by science. At the same time, the public is ill-informed and, perhaps understandably, displays distinct hostility toward the unknown. Several well-publicized environmental disasters have created a distrust in nearly all technology. In a recent survey conducted at an animal activist protest march, when queried, nearly half of all protesters thought that science had done 'more harm than good' and only about one-fourth felt that science had done 'more good than harm.'

Spectacular scientific and technological discoveries have been made over the last several years but understanding of the ethical dimensions underlying these discoveries has been slower in coming. Perhaps the best example involves our ability to offer testing for a wide array of genetic abnormalities, including Huntington's disease and cystic fibrosis, without the concurrent ability to yet offer a cure. The scientific community is often uncomfortable in speaking out on issues and, occasionally when scientists do speak in public, because of an inability to communicate about complex issues, more harm is done to the cause. There has also been a definite reluctance on the part of the scientific community to be accountable to the public. Finally and perhaps most significant is the growing trend towards science illiteracy among the public. According to a recent study by the National Science Foundation, only about 13 per cent of the American public understands the basic tenets of the scientific method. While there might be great interest in scientific topics, and public surveys do show high interest, the dichotomy between interest and understanding is enormous. This is particularly apparent in the attitudes expressed by precollege students regarding their image of the scientist.

From an early age virtually all children are inquisitive and seek to understand the unknown. Indeed, it has been said that all children are born scientists; it is only when these children enter school that they perceive science to be dull, uninteresting and boring. Too often science is taught as a body of facts rather than as a way of thinking. The image of the scientist to young children is often coloured by the portrayal of scientists on television cartoons or in magazines. The spectre of the 'mad scientist' is rampant in children's minds. When it comes to animals, anthropomorphism is common. The transformation of Mickey Mouse from 'Steam Boat Willie' to a lovable creature that in no way looks like a mouse would undoubtedly be puzzling to our ancestors who considered rodents as vermin, a source of disease, and an animal to be destroyed. Animals are portrayed in the media as child-like, playful, trusting, honest, adventurous and innocent. Animals have been made almost more attractive than the children from whom their inspiration was drawn originally. This hypothesis becomes more tenable when one considers that several animal rights activists have argued that it would be better to allow children to die from illness rather than proceed with the animal research needed to find cures. Animals should be respected as animals; not recreated as people. Even inanimate objects such as robots have been endowed with character. The day may soon arrive when we will be reluctant to dispose of an old computer because of a fear that we might destroy its soul.

Why are animals used in research?

Scientists justify the use of animals in biomedical research on essentially two grounds – the contribution that the information makes to human and animal health and the lack of any viable means of gaining similar information through other technologies. While animal activists contest experiments that utilize animals on many grounds, the fact remains that, historically, animals have played a critical role in virtually every important medical development. More than two-thirds of the Nobel Prizes in Physiology or Medicine since the inception of the award in 1901 have been given for experiments in which animals were used. In fact, the first Nobel Prize in Physiology or Medicine was given to von Behring for his discovery of diphtheria antiserum, a discovery that could not have been made without the use of guinea-pigs. A brief chronological review of some of the more well-known advances in medical science supports the view that animals have been imperative. In the pre-1900 era, the treatment of rabies, anthrax, beriberi and smallpox, the basic principles of infection control and pain relief and the early management of heart failure using digitalis required the use of animals. In the early 1900s, the treatment of histamine shock, nutritional diseases such as pellagra and rickets and the development of electrocardiography required the use of experimental animals. The discovery of insulin and thyroxin and the development of intravenous feeding were major advances of the 1920s that were made possible because of basic experiments that required animal use. In the 1930s, therapeutic use of sulfa drugs, prevention of tetanus and the development of anticoagulants, modern anaesthesia and neuromuscular blocking agents were pioneered. The 1940s brought treatments for rheumatoid arthritis, leprosy and whooping cough, the beginning of the therapeutic use of antibiotics, discovery of the Rh factor and the prevention of diphtheria. The Salk and Sabin vaccines for polio were developed in the 1950s as was cancer chemotherapy, open heart surgery and cardiac pacemakers. In the 1960s a vaccine for rubella was developed, and corneal transplantation, coronary bypass surgery and radioimmunoassays were perfected. The prevention of measles, the development of non-addictive pain medications and the modern treatment of coronary artery disease were major developments in the 1970s that required animal use. In the 1980s the use of cyclosporine and other anti-rejection drugs, artificial heart transplantation, identification of psychophysiological factors in depression, anxiety and phobias, the use of monoclonal antibodies and the discovery of HIV as the causative agent for AIDS all required the use of animals. Finally, in the current decade, pancreas and liver transplantation, thrombolytic therapy for acute myocardial infarction and human gene therapy were developed. Advances in veterinary medicine have also been spectacular. These have included the development of immunizations against such diseases as distemper, rabies, parvovirus and infectious hepatitis, the treatment of animal parasites, orthopaedic surgery for horses, surgery to correct hip dysplasia in dogs, experimental radiation techniques and cancer treatment in dogs, treatment for brucellosis in cattle, improved nutrition for pets and the treatment of feline leukaemia. The common denominator in each of these discoveries that improved animal and human health was the responsible use of animals in biomedical research.

The result of these experiments in medical science has been the elimination or control of many infectious diseases and the development of many life-saving techniques. For many, this has meant a longer, healthier and better life with much reduced pain and suffering. For some it has meant life itself. While healthy life-styles and better public health measures undoubtedly have contributed to the improvements noted in morbidity and mortality, still more basic and clinical research needs to be done. Investigations are now underway in human gene therapy, molecular biology of inherited disease and disease susceptibility, growth factors and signalling, the molecular basis for disease pathogenesis, molecular targets for therapy (cancer and environmentally-induced diseases), gene and cell structure and function, gene mapping, development of molecular probes to detect disease, molecular biology of alcoholism and drug abuse, basic biology of sensory processes and drug delivery mechanisms. Little progress will be made in any of these areas without the use of animals.

It is important to understand that the issue of animals and research is not simply an academic debate. It is not merely scientists' rights or science itself that is at risk. If medicine loses this battle, we will all be the ultimate victims. Already activist groups have succeeded in halting research that was designed to help alleviate human and animal suffering. The scenario is familiar. Animal activist groups target a particular researcher or project. They demonstrate and manipulate the media. They bring out the same old photos of laboratory animals and use them out of context. The researcher, usually unskilled in public relations, falls behind in the quest to help shape public opinion. The PCRM (or a similar group) will lend seeming credibility to the animal rights arguments and protests. Soon, in the eyes of the public, it becomes physician against physician. Next the funding is withdrawn and the research programme is terminated. The possible understanding of basic mechanisms, cures, techniques and treatments are never found. The real victim, the public, is never mentioned. The list of triumphs of medical research involving animals reads like a history of medical achievement. Each one of us can be a victim on an individual basis as we suffer the effects of ageing, birth defects, congenital disorders or accidents. Despite the claims of the PCRM, and what we would all like to believe, not all diseases are preventable. We are all at risk.

In June 1992, more than 100 American professional and voluntary health organizations signed a statement of support for animal research. The statement noted in part '. . . We . . . wish to reaffirm our support for the continued humane use of animals in biomedical and behavioural research, testing and education. We ask that the point of view of the patients, the health care provider and the researcher be considered in the public discussion on the use of animals in biomedical research. We reject the characterization of animal research as unnecessary, for we have seen the life-saving and life-enhancing benefits of such research. We recognize that there is much to be learned from animal experimentation that cannot be achieved in other ways. Thus, we take strong exception to the position of those people who would impede medical progress towards relieving human and animal suffering by halting medical research. The abandonment of animal research would be an abrogation of our primary responsibility – to try to save human lives – and of our responsibilities to save and improve animal lives as well. Should animal research be lost to the scientific community, the victims would not be the scientists. The victims would be all people; ourselves, our families, our neighbours, our fellow humans. Human life is at stake; human suffering is at issue. While great strides have been made in the understanding, prevention and treatment of diseases, there is still much to be learned. Much of that research relies on laboratory animals ...' What a wonderful legacy.

References

American Medical Association (1992): *Medical progress: a miracle at risk*. Chicago, IL: AMA.

French, R.D. (1975): *Antivivisection and medical science in Victorian society*. Princeton, NJ: Princeton University Press.

Loeb, J.M., Hendee, W.R., Smith, S.J. & Schwarz, M.R. (1989): Human *vs* animal rights. In defense of animal research. *JAMA* **262**, 2716–2720.

Loeb, J.M. & Runkle, D.C. (1990): Responding to animal activists. *Issues Sci. Technol.*, Summer 1990, pp. 31–34.

The ethics of animal and human experimentation, edited by P.P. De Deyn.
 pp. 159–172.

15

Ethical aspects of the use of laboratory animals in drug safety research

Herman Van Cauteren

Safety Assessment, Janssen Pharmaceutica NV, Turnhoutseweg 30, B-2340 Beerse, Belgium

Summary

The main purpose of pharmaceutical research is to find and develop new and better medicines for man, animals and plants. For each project the benefits of this research should be weighed ethically against its risks for the experimental animal. The main contribution of new medicines for man or animals lies in their ability to bring about an increase in life expectancy (more than 30 years has been added to the life expectancy of humans since the beginning of the century) and a substantial improvement in the quality of life, which is endangered by general or specific diseases in man and animal. For a responsible use of laboratory animals, these gains should be analysed against the odds by comparison within and between species.

The research and development process (R&D) of a new medicine is long and difficult, and requires a major investment. It starts with a computerized quantitative structure–activity analysis. After synthesis of a series of new chemical compounds, pharmacological screening starts, mainly by means of *in vitro* set-ups. Then, *in vivo* models are introduced for the investigation of activity, kinetics and safety in laboratory animals. Subsequently, clinical trials in man or target animals (e.g. farm animals or pets) are carried out and, if successful, the international registration file for marketing is prepared and presented to the authorities.

In this R&D process, account is taken of the strengths and weaknesses of the various *in vitro* and *in vivo* models.

The main reason for conducting experiments in laboratory animals in connection with new drugs lies in the ethical and regulatory aspects of exposure of man to a new active substance.

The Declaration of Helsinki (1964) in general, as well as national and international guidelines in particular, require, besides *in vitro* tests, a set of experiments on laboratory animals to demonstrate the activity, and more importantly, the safety, of a new drug. This process proceeds gradually, as a function of the extent and phase of the clinical research to be carried out. An overview of the set of toxicity studies currently used is given.

Adequate prediction of possibly harmful side-effects for man or target animal, as evaluated in toxicology trials, is achieved by application of a quantitative analysis (dose–response curve) and a qualitative risk assessment (presence or absence of unacceptable side-effects). Besides the ethical and regulatory responsibility of conducting an investigation of a new drug, toxicological research also supports the liability aspects of the medicine when it is on the market. After initial shortcomings leading to tragedies in the history of the use of medicines (e.g. thalidomide, diethylstibestrol), toxicology expanded greatly in the 1970s and 1980s and predictability for human safety has been adequate. In addition, the quality of toxicological research was boosted by the introduction of GLP (Good Laboratory Practices). Unpredictable, rare side-effects can still occur and post-marketing pharmacovigilance in patients remains essential. Toxicology research is charged with socio-economic obligations with reference to safety at school, in the workplace and in the environment. In this context, the importance of scientific research was recently underlined in the Declaration of Heidelberg (14 April, 1992). The challenges to find new and better medicines for both humans and animals are enormous, in both the West and developing countries. There is also a need for new chemicals in plant and materials protection.

In perspective, the research and development of new products point clearly to a further shift from *in vivo* to *in vitro* models and further application of 'the three Rs' (replacement, reduction and refinement). The recent harmonization of the international guidelines for drug research is crucial in this respect and should result in decreased use of experimental animals. As a future view, it is expected that toxicological studies will be initiated in a more flexible way, balancing ethical aspects between animal experimentation and testing in volunteers and patients.

Purpose and benefits of pharmaceutical research

The main goal of pharmaceutical research is to discover and develop new and better medicines. These medicines can be used to prevent or treat and, if possible or feasible, to cure diseases in man. Similarly, these or other medicines can do the same in specific animal species, be they pets, farm animals or wildlife. For the latter animals, they can be used to help to save endangered species. A typical example is the effect of mebendazole, a de-wormer, on the health and survival of the panda in China (Hanjiang Pharmaceutical Factory, 1985).

New medicines are needed for human diseases for which no or poor therapy exists, such as multiple sclerosis, dementia (Alzheimer's disease), several types of cancer, AIDS or a more common infection such as flu, which still is a cause of mortality. According to the World Health Organization (WHO), the challenge to find new medicines is large for both the industrialized and developing countries (Nakajima, 1992). New medicines can be not only more effective but also safer and economically more feasible or cost-effective. The term 'high effectivity' denotes an improvement in the percentage of responders to therapy and/or in the degree of response (e.g. partial or complete response). A new medicine can be called safer when the side-effect liability is smaller and/or when certain side-effects present with the predecessor medicine are less frequent or absent.

The contribution of pharmaceutical research for mankind has been impressive (National Research Council, 1988). The life expectancy has increased over recent decennia by more than 30 years and a major part of this prolongation is due to the availability of medicines such as antibiotics, anaesthetics, vaccines, insulin, antihypertensives and anti-cancer drugs. Moreover, the quality of life has also improved immensely because of new medicines. Pain or other disturbances can be reduced and patients can be partially or completely cured from specific diseases affecting their quality of life (e.g. psychotic disorders, epilepsy, diabetes). Preventive medicines (especially vaccines) have also reduced or even eliminated disabling infections. The best example is the almost complete eradication of polio with the international use of a polio vaccine. In addition, new medicines can also imply socio-economic advantages thereby improving the health care economic balance. In particular, the reduction in hospitalization and the increase in more ambulant therapy are very important in both industrialized and developing countries.

The research and development of a new medicine

The research and development process of a new medicine is long and difficult and requires a major investment (Fig. 1). The search for a new chemical entity starts with a literature search and a quantitative structure analysis using computerized data banks and three-dimensional drawing systems. The new chemical entities selected are identified and chemists synthesize them in small amounts in their lab. After chemical synthesis, the pharmacologist will examine the compounds for their primary and secondary effects in a set of *in vitro* models, called *in vitro* activity screening. These models can vary from isolated receptors or enzymes, membranes, cell or organ cultures or infectious agents grown *in vitro* (e.g. viruses, bacteria, yeasts, fungi, parasites). The compounds are tested at concentrations varying from low, subactive, up to high, eventually toxic, levels. The latter effects are measured particularly in cell culture and the ratios between effective and toxic concentrations are taken into account in the further selection of the new candidate drug, also called a lead compound. Lead compounds are then put through a series of *in*

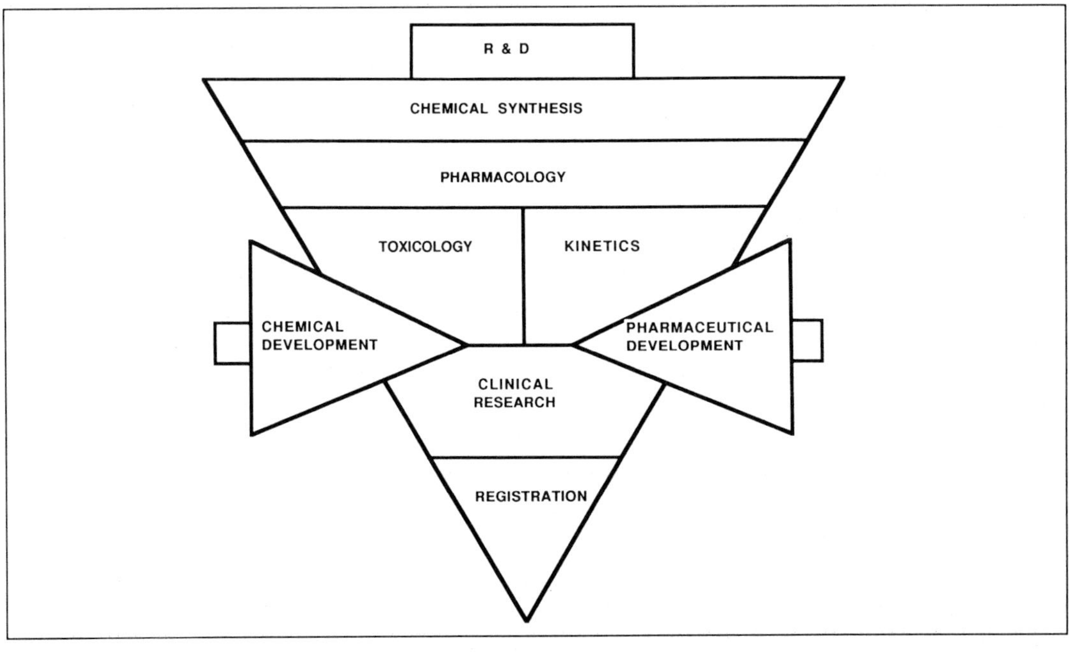

Fig. 1. Schematic representation of the research and development process of a new medicine.

vivo laboratory animal models, mainly in rats and mice. These models study the more complex mammalian organism and they will further define the primary (i.e. desired or envisaged therapeutic) activity, and the presence and degree of secondary effects (i.e. potential presence of non-desired, side-effects) are quantified. Subsequently, one or two new lead compounds are selected for further development. This development process (Fig. 1) consists of four main nonclinical activities and prepares the way for the start of the clinical trials.

The four activities are chemical, pharmaceutical, pharmacokinetic and toxicological development. Chemical development consists of the synthesis of a high quality, pharmaceutically acceptable grade of an amount of the candidate drug needed for the other development activities. Pharmaceutical development takes care of finding the optimal dosage forms for the laboratory animals and target patients (man or animals). The pharmacokinetic research studies the kinetics of the candidate drug in the body, including its absorption, distribution, metabolism and excretion in the various mammalian species. Toxicological development will define the safety of the candidate drug in a set of *in vitro* and *in vivo* models (see more discussion below).

When these four non-clinical activities have made sufficient progress, with acceptable and promising results, clinical trials in the target patients (man or animals) are initiated after approval has been granted by the responsible authorities (either ethical committees or the national ministries of public health or agriculture). In man, phase I, II and III are distinguished:

phase I: volunteers or patients (10–20 persons)
- → human pharmacokinetics
- → human pharmacodynamics
- → tolerance

phase II: open study in patients (tens of patients)
- → efficacy + dose-range finding
- → tolerance

phase III: extended, placebo-controlled, double-blind study in patients
(200 – ≥ 2000 patients)
- → efficacy
- → safety

Phase III clinical trials in particular are long lasting and involve many countries. Finally, when clinical efficacy and safety fulfil the expectations for a promising new drug, the international registration file is submitted to the (inter)national authorities for marketing application.

Rationale for the need of the use of laboratory animals in drug safety research

The main reasons to use laboratory animals in drug safety research are to be found in the ethical and regulatory aspects of exposure of man and the environment (Parliamentary Office of Science and Technology, 1992). Moreover, when the clinical development and registration process are completed and marketing authorization is granted, the liability issue (i.e. the legal responsibility) for the safety of the new medicine becomes a further factor necessitating safety studies *in vitro* and in laboratory animals.

Ethical aspects

The ethical aspects of human exposure to a new chemical entity are specified in the Declaration of Helsinki (1964) and the International Ethical Guidelines of the World Health Organization (WHO) (1992). These principles specify that new pharmaceuticals can be administered to man when an acceptable medical rationale and a risk *vs* benefit balance is available. This evaluation includes the safeguarding of the integrity of the research subject (volunteer or patient), and an informed consent is necessary. The reference to animal experimentation is listed in the first basic principle of the Declaration of Helsinki (WHO, 1992): 'Biomedical research involving human subjects must conform to generally accepted scientific principles and should be based on adequately performed laboratory and animal experimentation and on a thorough knowledge of the scientific literature'.

More recently, these guidelines have been redrafted in WHO guidelines for Good Clinical Practice (GCP) for trials in man on pharmaceutical products (WHO, 1992). In this document, good clinical practice is a standard for clinical studies which encompasses the design, conduct, termination, audit, analyses, reporting and documentation of the studies and which ensures that the studies are scientifically and ethically sound and that the clinical properties of the diagnostic/therapeutic/prophylactic product under investigation are properly documented.

Regulatory aspects

The national and international guidelines require that a research institute (pharmaceutical company, university) provides evidence of the safety of the new candidate pharmaceutical before the first clinical trial (i.e. a phase I study) in man or target animal can be initiated. Subsequently, the safety evaluation has to be extended gradually and in proportion with the extent of the further clinical (phase II and III) trials.

In general, one can state that these guidelines provide formal research models to evaluate the safety as required by the ethical principles mentioned above. For human pharmaceuticals, the guidelines derive mainly from the authorities responsible for public health and safety. For veterinary pharmaceuticals, the ministry of agriculture is involved but for food-producing animals the situation is more complicated, as public and environmental safety also have a large influence on the requirements.

A pharmaceutical company has to satisfy the authorities requesting studies in laboratory animals, while at the same time trying to minimize those studies, with a view to animal welfare.

The major reference sources for safety evaluation of human pharmaceuticals are the national guidelines of the major Western countries. The latter are most important because patent protection for marketing is guaranteed. Next to guidelines of countries such as Canada, Australia or Sweden and other Scandinavian countries (so-called Nordic countries), three major guidelines are used, i.e. those of Japan (Ministry of Health and Welfare, 1989), the United States Food and Drug Administration (US FDA, 1982) and

European Community (EC) (The rules governing medicinal products in the European Community:EC 1989). The Organization for Economic Co-operation and Development (OECD) has also published internationally accepted standard protocols for toxicity studies (1981). Common to all guidelines are the following requirements for safety evaluation (Speid *et al.*, 1990):

- single and repeated dose toxicity
- reproduction toxicity
- genotoxicity
- carcinogenicity.

Single dose toxicity studies evaluate the overdosing effects of a single dose in two animal species, usually the mouse and the rat. In the past, the lethal dose in 50 per cent of the animals tested had to be determined. However, following the first International Conference on Harmonization of Guidelines (ICH1) held in Brussels in 1991, the LD_{50} requirement was dropped and single-dose toxicity studies can be conducted that use other, more appropriate methods, such as the fixed-dose procedure. In addition, the dog as a non-rodent species is no longer required (Proceedings of the First International Conference on Harmonization, 1991).

Repeat-dose toxicity studies are carried out in a rodent (usually rat) and non-rodent species (usually dog) in order to evaluate any adverse effect in the body, focusing especially upon the pathological evaluation of all tissues and organs. The duration of these studies is proportional to the duration of exposure in man or target animal. For the route of administration, the clinical route is chosen.

As an illustration, the EC (1989) guidelines specify the following:

Intended exposure in man	Minimal duration of toxicity study
≤ 1 day	2 weeks
≤ 1 week	1 month
≤ 1 month	3 months
> 1 month	6 months

Interguideline differences in the duration of the toxicity studies do exist, since originally Japan and the US requested toxicity studies to last up to 12 months. However, the recent harmonization initiative between Japan, US and EC changed this and for rodents, 6 months is now accepted by the three parties (Proceedings of the First International Conference on Harmonization, 1991). For the duration of the dog studies, analysis is continuing.

Reproduction toxicology studies consist of:

- a segment I study, evaluating male and female fertility, usually in rats
- a segment II study, assessing the adverse effects on the developing embryo.

Embryotoxicity and teratogenicity (i.e. the induction of embryonal malformations) in particular, are examined in two animal species, usually the rat (rodent) and the rabbit (non-rodent) species.

- a segment III study, evaluating in rats the adverse effects on the developing foetus (i.e.

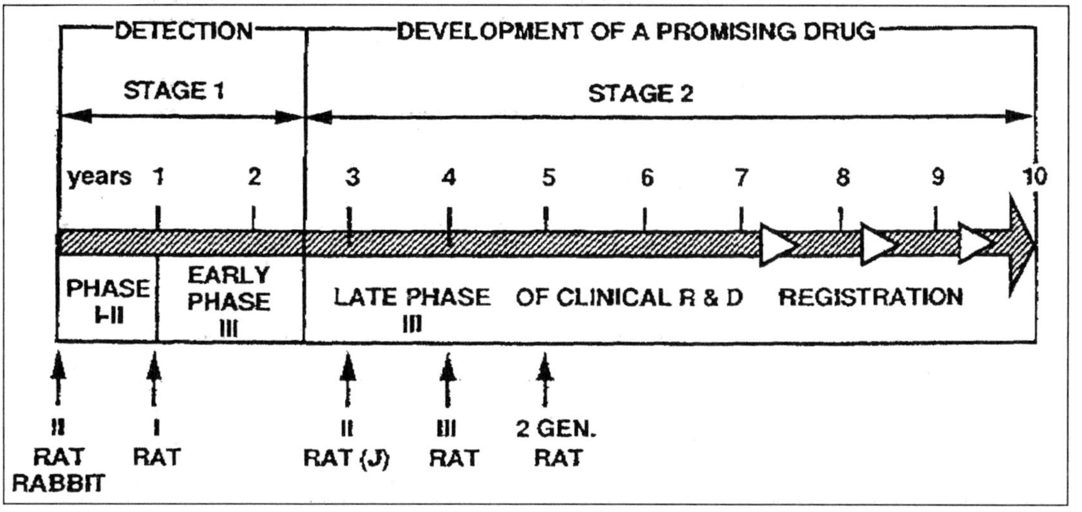

Fig. 2. Two-stage approach to follow the progress in the clinical research of a candidate drug.

in the last term of pregnancy), parturition and early postnatal, lactation phase.

In order to follow the progress in clinical research, a two-stage approach is followed (Fig. 2). In the first stage, embryotoxicity and teratogenicity studies (Segment II) are conducted in two species (usually the rat and the rabbit). These two studies are done when administration of the new candidate drug to pre-menopausal female volunteers in clinical trials (phases I and II) is planned. In addition, when repeated-dose toxicity studies (e.g. 3-month toxicity studies) indicate a specific effect on the gonadal tract of male or female animals, a fertility study (segment I) in rats is done as well during this first stage.

Reproductive toxicology testing during the second stage covers all other regulatory requirements and is initiated when clinical trials of phase II and early phase III have revealed promising results. Depending upon the proposed age population of patients and the indications of the new candidate drug, a fertility study (segment I) in rats is conducted, if not yet carried out. Subsequently, during late phase III clinical trials, a peri- and postnatal study (segment III) in rats is carried out to provide information on the risks of exposure of women during late pregnancy and lactation.

Finally, a total reproduction or two-generation study is conducted in rats fulfilling the requirements in reproductive toxicology of the major regulatory bodies (US, Japan and EC). In this two-stage approach, two segment II studies (rats and rabbits) and one segment I study in rats are made available at an early stage. The other reproduction studies conducted in a later stage of clinical development provide the reproductive toxicology information required for world-wide registration application.

Genotoxicity studies evaluate the potential effects of a new pharmaceutical on the genetic information system. A set of studies is conducted here, starting *in vitro*. The so-called Ames test in special strains of *Salmonella typhimurium* (an enterobacterium) and the mouse lymphoma cell test (a cell-culture test) are commonly used to evaluate possible effects on point or gene mutations. Another endpoint *in vitro* is the chromosome aberration test in human lymphocytes (also a cell-culture test), evaluating possible effects on chromosomes. In a later stage of development, genotoxicity tests are also conducted in *in vivo* models, of which the micronucleus test in rats or mice is the most commonly used, studying possible effects on chromosome in bone marrow cells. Genotoxicity testing is a good example of the shift to conduct, when feasible and validated, *in vitro* studies instead of *in vivo* models.

Carcinogenicity studies are the longest lasting studies since they cover the greatest part of the lifespan of the rodent strain used. Currently two species have to be evaluated, usually rats, tested for at least 24 months, and mice, tested for at least 18 months.

Carcinogenicity studies are required for human pharmaceuticals when the expected duration of exposure in man is prolonged (e.g. more than 3 months continuously or 6 months intermittently). Studies are also needed when suspicion of carcinogenicity is raised from the chemical structure or from findings in other toxicity studies. For veterinary pharmaceuticals, carcinogenicity studies are usually required for products used in food-producing animals.

Other toxicity studies also might be required in particular cases. For pharmaceuticals used topically, topical toxicity studies are required. For example, a dermal application drug requires appropriate repeated-dose toxicity studies with a dermal application. Other endpoints such as sensitization or phototoxic potential have also to be studied in an appropriate animal species (usually the guinea-pig is used). However, it should be mentioned that during recent years, tests for human pharmaceuticals have been increasingly conducted directly in human volunteers. This evolution is an interesting example in the ethical interplay between animal and human experimentation.

Liability aspects

Once the regulatory issues for approval have been cleared, the product liability stays with the manufacturer of the new medicine (Dukes & Swartz, 1988; Broekhuijzen-Molenaar & Stolker, 1986). This implies that the side-effect liability has to be optimally covered. In this respect, package information for patients and doctors, including the relevant toxicity findings *in vitro* and in laboratory animals must be present. Also postmarketing surveillance of larger patient populations might reveal more rare side-effects to be mentioned here. For this purpose, each company has an international pharmacovigilance programme and so-called phase IV studies, i.e. clinical trials after marketing of the medicine, are conducted in patients.

Predictability of toxicology studies for the safety of pharmaceuticals

The *in vitro* and *in vivo* toxicology studies assess the safety of the medicine in a quantitative and qualitative way (Fig. 3). By application of low dose levels in the therapeutic range up to high dose levels in the toxic range, the safety margin is estimated. In this respect, the principle of Paracelsus (1493–1541) 'All substances are poisons; there is none which is not a poison. The right dose differentiates a poison and a remedy' is still valid. For certain modern medicines, safety margins (i.e. the ratio of therapeutic *vs* toxic dose, and exposure levels) are very large, implying a very low risk for overdosing. Quantitatively, potential adverse effects on reproduction, genetic material and cancer can be

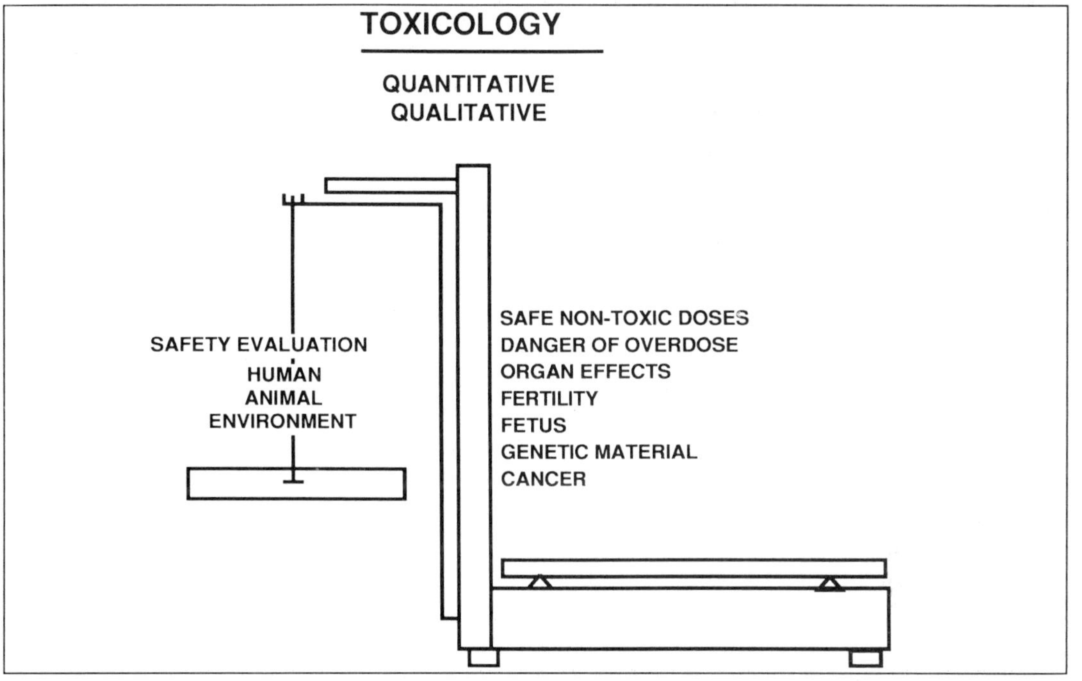

Fig. 3. Quantitative and qualitative assessment of the safety of a candidate drug by *in vitro* and *in vivo* toxicology.

estimated.

In modern toxicology, the various toxicology studies are considered to be sufficiently sensitive and sufficient scientific understanding is present to interpret the findings observed. In the past, a few tragedies of clinical side-effects occurred, of which thalidomide (1960) is the best known (Manson, 1986). Thalidomide was used to relieve nausea and vomiting during pregnancy in women and resulted in teratogenic effects (especially phocomelia or shortened limbs) in a fraction of the newborns. Subsequently, this finding was examined in laboratory animals. Whereas the mouse and rat were resistant, hamster and especially the rabbit were very sensitive. From this case onwards, it was therefore decided to have teratology studies done not only in a rodent species, but also in the rabbit as a non-rodent. As a matter of fact, it was this case, and other cases such as diethylstilbestrol (DES) that boosted the extent of toxicology research and largely contributed to the currently existing set of toxicity studies.

The current level of predictability is considered high because of the well developed and sensitive methods of evaluating non-clinical and clinical safety during the drug development process. This predictability can be calculated, based upon studies that compare the number of drug discontinuations with that of the total number of drugs registered (Bakke *et al.*, 1984). Ten drugs have been discontinued in the US and the UK for safety during the period of 1964–1983 (Dukes & Swartz, 1988). When compared to the total number of drugs newly registered during this period, these 10 drugs only represent 2 per cent.

Only rare, unpredictable effects might remain undetected in toxicology and phase III clinical studies, but pharmacovigilance and phase IV studies can anticipate this issue to a large extent (see also discussion above). Let us not forget the words of Warren Burger, Chief Justice of the US Supreme Court: 'Perfect safety is a chimera: Regulation must not strangle human activity in a search for the impossible'.

Quality of the conduct of toxicological research

The conditions for conducting an experimental study in laboratory animals are well defined. National and international laws, directives and guidelines on the protection and welfare of the laboratory animal are available (e.g. EC directives, Official Journal of the European Communities, 1986) and, well applied, guarantee an optimal quality of life including housing, feeding and sanitation. The presence of diseases is excluded or kept to a minimum. Life expectancy is limited and laboratory animals are bred on purpose, completely separated from the external environment. During the experiment, there is veterinary supervision, and pain, suffering or discomfort are kept to a minimum. Euthanasia is applied when necessary.

In order to comply with the international guidelines and especially in order to have a toxicology study internationally acceptable on a worldwide basis, toxicology studies are conducted under Good Laboratory Practices (GLP) (US FDA, 1978; Official Journal of the European Communities, 1987, 1988). Similar to the above mentioned GLP for clinical trials, these guidelines guarantee that the study preparation, conduct and reporting is done at a high technical and scientific level, so that only one toxicology study conducted in one recognized laboratory is necessary for full acceptance by the regulatory authorities worldwide.

Other objectives for toxicological research

The challenges to find new and better medicines for both man and animals are enormous, when the existing diseases in these populations with no or insufficient treatment are taken into consideration. There is also a need for new chemicals in plant and materials protection. The prevention of human food decay and the preservation of valuable materials (e.g. wood) are particularly important. Besides drug safety evaluation, toxicological research is also charged with socio-economic obligations with reference to safety at school, in the workplace and in the environment. As a result of some initial shortcomings in toxicological research, it has expanded considerably, and now encompasses an entire battery of highly specific test models. The importance of scientific research was recently underlined in the Declaration of Heidelberg (14 April, 1992). In this declaration signed by 62 Nobel prize winners and more than 1400 scientists, scientific research and technology are placed centrally to guarantee the future of our planet and to overcome the changes caused by overpopulation, famine and diseases. An anti-research stance is dangerous for economic and social development.

Evolution of drug safety research

As mentioned earlier, the set of toxicological studies has been fully established over the past few decades and national and international guidelines have specified how each study should be conducted.

Two main evolutions are now occurring: first, a further shift from *in vivo* to *in vitro* models and second, international harmonization and rationalization of guidelines for toxicological research. Both evolutions will contribute to a decreased and more refined use of laboratory animals and they will contribute to the implementation of the three Rs (replacement, reduction, refinement).

Further shift from in vivo *to* in vitro *models*

In the future, a further shift from *in vitro* to to *in vivo* test models and also a further application of the three Rs, replacement, reduction and refinement are to be expected. The motivation for this is present in the drug research process itself because of the four Es, ethical considerations (animal welfare), economical aspect (*in vitro* studies are cheaper), increasing Effectivity of *in vitro* screening, and Evolution in scientific knowledge and insights.

Especially important here is the principle of unity in diversity (National Research Council, 1988). Despite there being millions of different species, there is a certain unity in anatomy, metabolism, cell biology and genetics. Increased knowledge makes a partial generalization possible in biology and has led to the development of certain alternatives to the use of laboratory animals. A few examples:

- teratology by *in vitro* embryo culture: in the past 150 rats, 150 guinea-pigs/compound
- heart toxicity in heart cell muscle culture: in the past 100 rats/compound
- pyrogens tested *in vitro* in *Limulus amaebocytes* lysate: formerly two rabbits/compound.

Before an *in vitro* test such as the *Limulus* test can replace a regulatorily required *in vivo* test, international validation should be finished and regulatory acceptance has to be completed (Balls *et al.*, 1990). Such a validation process, which can take several years, is now occurring in the EC for the Draize test for eye irritation of cosmetics in rabbits. The recent foundation of the European Centre for Validation of Alternative Methods (ECVAM) in Italy will certainly help to speed up the validation of acceptance of new *in vitro* tests (Balls *et al.*, 1993).

It should also be mentioned that *in vitro* safety research is an intrinsic part of *in vitro* screening during discovery research. Thus the more toxic candidates can be differentiated from the less toxic ones and eliminated before *in vivo* exposure in the laboratory animal is considered.

International harmonization and view of the future

In addition to replacement, a further reduction and refinement of the necessary use of laboratory animals must be striven for. The recent harmonization of the international guidelines for research on human pharmaceuticals is very important here (Proceedings of the First International Conference on Harmonization, 1991). A few examples:

- the pyrogen test/development and validation of the *in vitro Limulus* test (see above)
- the single-overdose study/no exact LD_{50} any more; no dog study (USA, Japan)

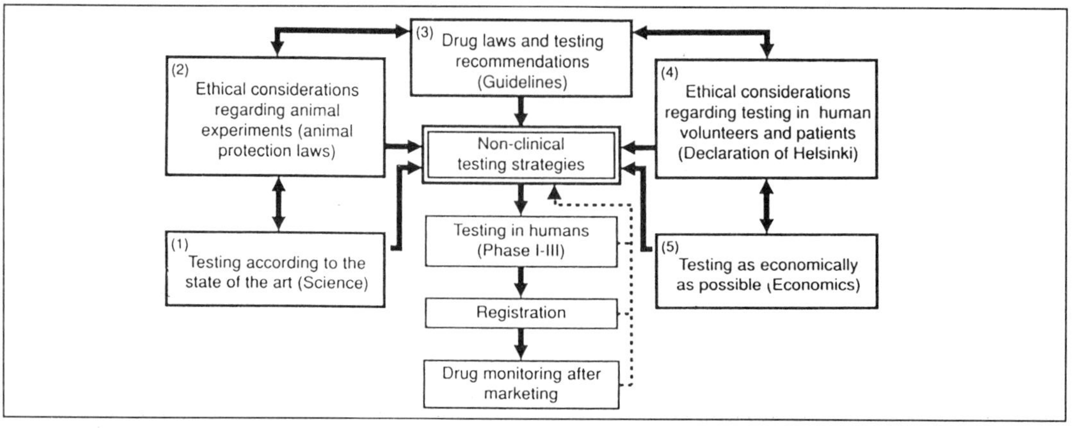

Fig. 4. In the rationale for the conduct of a toxicology study, ethical aspects of animal experimentation must be compared carefully with those of testing in volunteers and patients (Günzel & Bass, 1991).

– the repeated-overdose study/no 12 months study on rats any more (USA, Japan)

– fertility studies/no duplicate studies any more but tripartite protocol

– mutagenic studies/first *in vitro*; then *in vivo*

– carcinogenicity studies (rat, mouse)/choice of dose by exposure; dose not too high.

This harmonization process is not yet completed and further international rationalization is necessary. Future programmes will analyse the value of the 12- *vs* 6-month dog study and hopefully will eliminate one or both (preferably the 12-month duration as it is twice as long). Moreover, the ongoing evaluation of the value of two species (rat and mouse) *vs* one (preferably the rat) for the carcinogenicity studies might lead to a large reduction of the number of rodents used.

A further future view is presented in a drafted EC note for guidance (Günzel & Bass, 1991), where in the rationale for the conduct of a toxicology study, it is stated that the ethical aspects of animal experimentation must be compared carefully with those of testing in volunteers and patients (Fig. 4).

Further conduct of the study will merely depend upon the degree of estimated risk and available suspicion for potential side-effects. Another reduction in the number of laboratory animals used can be obtained if the optimal number of animals to be used for each type of study is specified. Indeed, most actual guidelines specify only the minimum number of animals. Similar to the recent activities for human pharmaceuticals, a reduction of animal use in safety testing for other products (veterinary pharmaceuticals, agricultural products, chemicals, food additives, cosmetics . . .) should also be envisaged. Future deregulation (i.e. the reduction and/or relaxation of strictly defined guidelines on safety testing) on a worldwide basis is the most direct approach to obtain this. In this process, special emphasis should be given to the more conservative and demanding countries.

References

Bakke, O.M., Wardell W.M. & Lasagna L. (1984): Drug discontinuations in the United Kingdom and the United States, 1964 to 1984: issues of safety. *Clin. Pharmacol. Ther.* **35**, 559–567.

Balls, M. (1993): Editorial. The foundation of ECVAM: a significant step towards the replacment of animal tests? *Alternatives Lab. Anim.* **21**, 123–124.

Balls, M. *et al.* (1990): Report and recommendations of an international workshop on promotion of the regulatory acceptance of validated non-animal toxicity test procedures. *Alternatives to Laboratory Animals* **18**, 339–344.

Broekhuijzen-Molenaar, A.M.L. & Stolker, C.J.J.M. (1986): *Geneesmiddelen en aansprakelijkheid.* Deventer: Kluwer.

Declaration of Heidelberg, April 14, 1992.

Dukes M.N.G. & Swartz B. (1988): *Responsibility for drug-induced injury.* Amsterdam, New York, Oxford: Elsevier.

Günzel P. & Bass R. (1991): Considerations regarding the development of individual nonclinical test strategies in the European Community. *Hum. Exper. Toxicol.* **10**, 297–304.

Hanjiang Pharmaceutical Factory (1985): How mebendazole saved a grand panda. Investigation report – V 5561.

Manson, J.M. (1986): Teratogens. In: *Casarett and Doull's toxicology, The basic science of poisons,* 3rd edn, eds. C.D. Klaassen, M.O. Amdur & J. Doull, pp. 195–220. New York: Macmillan.

Ministry of Health and Welfare – Japan (1989): Toxicity test guidelines.

Nakajima, H. (1992): Sixteenth Assembly of the International Federation of Pharmaceutical Manufacturers Associations (IFPMA), Singapore 9–11 September.

National Research Council (1988): *Use of laboratory animals in biomedical and behavioral research.* Washington DC: National Academy Press.

OECD (1981): *Guidelines for testing of chemicals.* No. 452. Paris.

Official Journal of the European Communities (1986): Council Directive, on the approximation of laws, regulations and administrative provisions of the Member States regarding the protection of animals used for experimental and other scientific purposes, November 24, No. L358. pp. 1–28.

Official Journal of the European Communities (1987, 1988): Council Directive, on the approximation of laws, regulations and administrative provisions of the Member States regarding the good laboratory practices and the survey of application to tests on chemical substances, December 18, 1986, No. L 15/29–30; Council Directive on the inspection and verification of good laboratory practices, June 9, 1988, No. L 145/35–37.

The Parliamentary Science and Technology Information Foundation (1992): *The use of animals in research development and testing.* UK: September 1992.

Proceedings of the First International Conference on Harmonization, Brussels (1991): eds. P.F. D'Arcy & D.W.G. Harron. Belfast: The Queen's University of Belfast.

Speid, L.H. *et al.* (1990): Harmonization of guidelines for toxicity testing of pharmaceuticals by 1992. *Reg. Toxicol. Pharmacol.* **12**, 179–211.

The rules governing medicinal products in the European Community (1989): Volume III: *Guidelines on the quality, safety and efficacy of medicinal products for human use.* Revised and completed edition, January 1989. Brussels.

US Food and Drug Administration (1978): Federal Register 21 CFR Part 58, *Good laboratory practice for nonclinical laboratory studies,* December 22, 1978.Washington DC: FDA.

US FOOD and Drug Administration (1982): *Toxicological principles for the safety assessment of direct food additives and color additives in food.* Washington DC : FDA.

WHO (1992): *International ethical guidelines.* Geneva: WHO.

Section IV:
Randomized clinical trials

The ethics of animal and human experimentation, edited by P.P. De Deyn.
©1994 John Libbey & Company Ltd., pp. 175–185.

16

Reflections on ethical aspects of drug development

Erik L. Noach

Professor Emeritus of Pharmacology, University of Leiden, Van der Valk Boumanweg 234, NL-2352 JG Leiderdorp, The Netherlands

Summary

Decisions to develop molecules with promising therapeutic properties into (medicinal) drugs are based on three categories of consideration, each with ethical implications:

Commercial: High development costs must be proportional to the expected size of the market. Ethical aspects: should drugs for 'unprofitable' diseases (few patients, or poverty of population, for instance endemic diseases in developing countries) remain undeveloped?

Scientific: Is this new drug a breakthrough, or, if not, does it contribute to better basic understanding of drug action? Is the scientific effort in proportion with the scientific reputation of the establishment? Ethical aspects: might the 'promising substance' also be used for inhumane applications (toxicology, biological warfare)? Does the manufacture cause environmental damage? Is the discomfort to test animals acceptable in view of the expected value of the drug?

Medical: Benefit/risk ratio; 'me too' drug or real innovation? Ethical aspects: is human experimentation sufficiently low-risk?

The following part of this survey is mainly focused on the present situation in the Netherlands.

Animal experiments: In the Netherlands, successful completion of special training courses is legally required for every person participating in animal experiments. Animal ethics committees are operative, at the moment still on a voluntary basis (accepted everywhere), in the near future to be required by law and supervised by a governmental agency. The committees assess submitted protocols and may withhold approval. Within every research establishment (university or industrial) one or more special functionaries are responsible for day-to-day supervision of ongoing animal experiments and function also as advisers for developing new research protocols. The animal ethics committees pay special attention to the feasibility of the animal experiment as seen from the three Rs viewpoint: replacement by *in-vitro* tests, refinement of procedure, reduction in numbers. Further topics for consideration are: species selection, anaesthesia, limitation of discomfort to test animals, methods of euthanasia. These points are weighed with regard to the medical importance of the drug under investigation.

Experiments in human subjects: In the Netherlands, no drug experiments involving human subjects may be performed without prior assessment of the protocol by a medical ethics committee; every establishment (laboratory, clinic) where such experiments are performed is legally required to have its own committee or access to an ethics committee elsewhere. In all, about 150 such committees are now operative. Care is taken that the committees are competent in ethical, juridical and scientific matters. Training courses for prospective committee members are provided by a number of academic and reputable non-academic institutes. A preliminary requirement for approval of protocols is adherence to the (international) rules for Good Clinical Practice. As elsewhere, in the assessment of protocols much attention is given to procedural matters such as informed consent, securing of voluntary cooperation and right of withdrawal. In addition, other aspects are constantly reviewed. Some examples are given:

(1) It is well understood that for final assessment of the value of new drugs, post-marketing surveillance is indispensable. Recent legislation concerning privacy is an impediment for collecting the necessary epidemiological data since access to medical records is heavily restricted. This gives rise to a principal discussion about the boundary between public and private interest in health matters.

(2) Another important ethical problem specific for drug research is connected to the question whether the drug under study may be expected to provide a significant advancement of therapeutic possibilities. In view of the always limited number of available volunteers and restrictions in available scientific manpower and hospital beds, competing industrial requests for drug studies should be weighed against each other. In other words: the investigator should consider his own motivation and should refrain from fallacious reasoning such as: 'I will participate in me-too-investigations in order to earn money for more fundamental research'.

(3) Finally, it should be realized that ethical problems in drug studies are of a short-term character. We are still far away from solutions for long-term problems concerning the special and economic consequences of continuous improvement of health and prolongation of life span, which, among other factors, are brought about by potent new drugs. Politicians specialized in matters of health care and drug cost management should acquire reasonable knowledge of medical ethics.

Introduction

In the past decades, major developments in ethical concepts have profoundly contributed to changed experimental procedures in medical research. Until the 1960s, scientists could, after having taken financial and other organizational hurdles within their institutions, rather freely decide about the design and execution of the experiments necessary for their investigations. Now, the scientific community has become used to submitting projects first to ethical screening committees to obtain moral approval of intended experimental procedures. Such ethical screening is performed separately for animal and human experiments, by independent committees, operating within the context of legal and internationally canonized moral rules. The delay caused by such committee interventions, although sometimes experienced as a nuisance, has in general been counterbalanced by marked improvement of experimental protocols and a sharpened awareness of researchers about their moral responsibilities. This is part of a general shift in attitude within society towards more responsibilities of individuals for their fellow-beings. It is beyond the scope of this review to go into details on the sociological, political and philosophical backgrounds of these developments. As far as medical experiments are concerned, many of the deliberations which ultimately resulted in the Declaration of Helsinki on the conduct of research with human experimental subjects (1989) found their roots in abhorrence of the abject cruelties committed as so-called 'medical experiments' to defenceless prisoners in concentration camps. In matters concerning conduct of animal experiments, general rules as required in many countries by legal provisions came forward when the perseverance of 'animal protectors' merged with public feelings about moral limits to the infliction of pain or hardships – even if done for the benefit of mankind.

It is in the light of these evolutions in public opinion that procedures in drug research also came to be adapted. This review is meant to be a reflection on the main ethical issues to be considered in the successive phases of drug research when decisions have to be taken about further steps. The *content* of such decisions will be covered by other contributions to this volume.

It should be well understood that in every decision in whatever area of human endeavour moral components are and always have been present, since 'morality' means: decent behaviour within the limits of norms which prevail in a certain society. However, in the past such moral issues were often more or less intuitively, and hence often incompletely and irrationally, handled. Since 'ethics' is to be defined as: the scientific study of morality, it follows that the content of ethical consideration of research projects is the systematic and rational investigation as to whether such projects fit into the current concepts of decency.

Unfortunately the term 'ethics' with its grammatical derivations is often misused. So, for instance, the designations of certain therapeutic agents as 'ethical drugs' is without any meaning in the scientific sense and should therefore be avoided, even if 'only' used for promotional purposes.

The following discussion will be limited to crucial points where major decisions have to be made about further progress in the transformation of an already available (old or newly synthesized) chemical compound into a medicinal drug and will end with some considerations about general aspects of future consequences of drug use in society.

The sequence of the discussion will be as follows:

(1) The primary decision to start biological investigations
(2) The start of animal experiments
(3) The start of human experimentation
(4) Post-marketing surveillance
(5) Ethical issues in medical progress.

It is obvious that modern drug development is largely an industrial activity. Although highly important, academic research as a basis for the pharmaceutical industry will not be discussed here.

The primary decision to start biological investigations

Without going into details it is evident that in the research laboratories of pharmaceutical industries much emphasis is placed on efforts to protect the safety of future users of their products. This claim on 'uniqueness' of safety investigations is often proudly mentioned in promotional publicity, but it may be viewed with some relativism: consider, for instance, the amount of energy, intelligence and money invested by automobile manufacturers to improve the safety of their cars! Protection of the community against possible harm caused by industrial goods is everywhere required by many laws and it is justifiable to place the burden of preventive measures on the manufacturer. In reflecting on the role of industry in general in society we should not forget that the very first and main aim of any enterprise is: to survive, to remain in business, to be able to compete and, if possible, to extend activities. This motive is by no means devoid of ethical dimensions: think of providing employment, preventing poverty, supporting the economy, stimulating human inventiveness. The pharmaceutical industry very obviously aims at her own survival by serving the public in providing powerful but safe medicines.

In the decision process about the development of new drugs the following moral components have to be envisaged:

(a) Economic considerations: as mentioned, these include moral issues such as employment and public welfare.

(b) Scientific interest: human creativity is a strong and ubiquitous force, often impossible to restrain and of widely divergent moral content. The creation of important new drugs may improve the moral status of a company, which may at times be more important than profits, whereas the development of another 'me too' drug sometimes causes some contempt, even pity from others since it may suggest a lack of creativity in the scientific staff. Creativity is not always primarily aimed at the development of new therapeutic agents, even in industrial pharmacological laboratories. As an example, the development of the β-adrenergic blocking agents may be mentioned. They were originally wanted in order to test Ahlquist's hypothesis that two kinds of adrenergic receptors exist, the α and β group. The existence of α-agonists and β-blockers as well as β-agonists had been shown already. Final proof of Ahlquist's theory (1948) required the demonstration of β-blocking drug action. Such drugs were found in an industrial laboratory by Powell & Slater (1958) and Black and Stephenson (1962). Once they had succeeded in designing the β-blocker dichloroisoprenaline, the scientific aim had been fulfilled and no urgent need was felt to use such substances therapeutically: it was deemed dangerous to use drugs which might decrease the force of cardiac contractions; only some years later clinical experiments (Black & Prichard, 1973) (performed before the days of ethical committees!) showed that the β-blockers were among the most important drugs for the treatment of cardiovascular disease. As a consequence, multiple 'me too' preparations were developed, many of which were better than the original prototypes.

In conclusion, pharmacological creativity, together with serendipity, may lead to new drugs for which the medical profession had not yet asked. After a bright idea about possible practical application the courageous moral decision may be taken to try a substance, for better or worse, in living creatures, or to abandon it.

(c) Medical requirements are, of course, rather 'undilutedly' morally founded: the desire to be of benefit to mankind is the main driving force for medical activities. Specific requests for the development of new drugs are a constant stimulus to the industry, but the decision to take action depends also on considerations of other aspects: are there enough patients to make the drug profitable? What is the market position of the enterprise as compared to that of competitors? This means that the cycle returns to its first item: the economic situation.

In summing up, the final decision to start the development of new drugs depends on a complicated interplay of many factors, all of which have moral aspects which deserve contemplation.

The start of animal experiments

After the decision to start development of a new drug or group of drugs has been taken, animal experiments have to be planned and submitted to the approval of an animal ethics committee. The function of such committees, in many countries by law required to operate in biomedical research institutions, is critical appraisal followed by acceptance or rejection of planned experiments, and much attention is given to pain protection, anaesthesia, post-experimental care and killing of test animals; among the criteria of judgement is also the question whether an experiment with living animals shall or can be substituted by *in vitro* procedures. The Dutch government, animal protection societies and the pharmaceutical industry together finance a multidisciplinary committee which has a special assignment to develop such substitutions. It is taken for granted – even by the animal protectionist members of this committee – that the validation of *in vitro* experiments as models for the *in vivo* situation may require many extra animal experiments.

Discussions in animal ethics committees are carried out on a professional, rational level so that *intra muros* purely emotional argumentations, such as were formerly held between experimenters and 'anti-vivisectionists', nearly always may be avoided. Nevertheless it is very important to keep the general public well informed about the scope and extent of animal experiments in academia and industry in order to counteract destructive forces such as 'animal liberators' whose actions very often result in lethal effects for the animal population they want to 'liberate'.

Discussions about animal experiments should start by taking for granted that in everyday life man acts as a 'ruler' over the life and death of animals, using them for food, clothing, transportation and also as 'best friend in the house'. In this context, the use of animals for improving human health is not to be condemned on ethical grounds, provided that handling of experimental animals is careful, respectful and humane. Such principles, supported by legislation, have helped to delimit acceptability as far as inflicting pain, discomfort and suffering are concerned. Legal measures have also resulted in improvement of living conditions for experimental animals and upgrading of the training of competent animal caretakers and biotechnicians.

However, even although animal ethics committees and researchers in most cases attain agreement on proposed investigations, there remain fundamental questions for which no answer is readily available; they are of sufficient importance to merit professional ethical consideration. Some of these basic problems will be mentioned here:

(a) It is unanimously accepted that the number of animals used in an experiment has to be as small as methodologically possible. However, the moral motivation of such a ruling idea is not quite clear: is, in any one experiment, the suffering of the total number of test animals the sum of individual sufferings and is the extent of individual suffering influenced by that total number? Is the moral burden for an investigator using 100 animals ten times as heavy as if only 10 animals were used? Or do we limit the number of animals because we then may restrict the number of animals especially bred, especially brought to life in order to be kept in captivity for future sacrifice? If so, does the discomfort of captivity depend on the number of animals?

(b) It is unanimously accepted that monkeys and other higher animals should only be used in experiments if the required results are of crucial importance for human (or veterinary) health problems and impossible to obtain otherwise. But why do special considerations exist for these animals (and some other species such as dogs, cats, horses . . .)? Why should a monkey's life be valued as more important than that of a rat? Or are we just 'sentimental' because we pretend to understand a monkey's discomfort better than a rodent's or do we think that it has a greater capacity to suffer? Is this a fallacy, just as for a long time it was thought that fish do not feel pain, because we don't see facial expression of their suffering? And what should be done if a monkey remains free of pathological symptoms after an experiment – for instance, after having been infected with HIV – but may not be used for other experiments, or could be infectious for humans? We gravely hesitate to sacrifice such animals, for instance in order to get more space in the colony; several animal ethicists propose to provide 'retirement homes' for post-experimental chimpanzees. This will be very expensive, because individual apes may survive for several decades. The financial burden on science budgets might even severely limit research!

Again: is that reasonable? In modern primate centres, chimpanzees are brought to life by human planning and for human benefit – does this justify their killing if they are no longer needed? Wouldn't that be merciful because we would thereby shorten a life of captivity?

Such discussions – for which in this essay no answers are given! – regularly take place in ethical committees for animal experiments, as is this author's personal experience. It would be worthwhile to plan consensus conferences for such questions.

(c) It is unanimously accepted that enough data from animal experiments should be collected before trials with human experimental subjects are started. But what does 'enough' mean? Here we often encounter two general approaches, each defended by two different parties: at one side are the ethicists together with the economists, who would like to restrict animal experiments for moral and financial reasons; at the other side are physicians and governmental health (for instance: registration) authorities who would like to have a maximal number of pharmacological and especially toxicological tests performed in order to warrant protection of future users. The scientists 'at the bench' are not infrequently somewhere between those two parties: they know that some experiments, required for a drug registration procedure, are without much sense and could be omitted or changed. Sometimes this happens: the famous LD_{50} test has been replaced by less drastic assessments of toxicity. On the other hand, every pharmacologist and toxicologist knows that no matter how 'complete' testing may have been, sooner or later there may appear new, unexpected and unpleasantly surprising effects which may gravely affect the practical use of a drug. Famous examples are the congenital malformations of children of mothers who had used thalidomide during their pregnancy, and the very late health hazards for adult daughters of mothers treated with diethylstilbestrol during pregnancy to prevent abortion. At the time of introduction of these drugs, nobody seriously could have thought of screening for such side effects! Unfortunately, without any doubt such tragic events will happen again in the future. The medical profession is well aware of such risks but it remains a problem that consistent legislation regarding product liability is still far from satisfactory. Especially the question remains whether a manufacturer or prescribing physician is morally responsible for as-yet unknown, hazardous aspects of drug use that appear much later. It would be reasonable to provide in such cases legal protection by taking into account what the 'state of the art' of science and medicine was at the time of marketing or prescription.

(d) It is unanimously accepted that experimental animals should be protected and handled with maximal care and experiments should be supervised by independent committees. In this light it is a matter of sarcastic spite among scientists that society maintains a double standard of morality as far as animals are concerned. Experimental animals are handled with care but we permit that cattle and livestock are often handled, kept and transported under most inhumane, cruel and miserable conditions. The excuse heard in the Netherlands is that this usually happens out of economic necessity in view of international commercial competition: for instance, Italians are presumed not to like canned meat but to prefer meat from freshly and locally slaughtered animals, even if heavily stressed animals are brought to death after having spent 36 h without food or water in a speeding lorry. Because of such experiences it has come to my knowledge that scientists in a major veterinary research institution are afraid of introducing into agricultural practice their findings on veterinary health improvement because they know by experience that farmers abuse such knowledge by putting more animals together in stables or transportation vans 'because the animals are healthier now and thus can stand more discomfort'. Conflicts of interest between governmental health ministries on the one hand, and ministries of agriculture and foreign trade on the other are obvious and long-lived; it seems to be extremely difficult to find a practical solution which is morally acceptable!

The start of experiments with human subjects

Before discussing decisions to be taken when considering human experimentation, some preliminary general remarks are opportune. First, no general rules can be given as to the minimal amount of data from animal experiments which has to be collected before human experimentation is morally acceptable; in every single situation this is the subject of deliberations between investigators and ethical committees; this point will not be dwelt upon.

Over the past three decades, great progress has been made in the design and performance of experiments in humans with potential new drugs. A large degree of standardization of procedure is available nowadays, which helps investigators in planning their experiments and Ethical Committees and Institutional Review Boards in their evaluations. Of course it may be stated soberly that for industry the main motive for human experimentation is the completion of the registration dossier in order to market a new product. It is up to the investigators to perform the legally required experiments in a morally acceptable way, protecting experimental subjects from danger and discomfort and carrying out the experiments only in informed experimental subjects who have given their consent (or proxy consent in mentally incapable subjects such as small children and psychiatric patients, if their participation in experiments is unavoidable). Details of such procedures, as covered by the Declaration of Helsinki (1989) and of the functioning of ethical committees are beyond the limits and purposes of this review.

An issue which deserves special attention in the discussion concerning experimental subjects is that by permitting and even legally requiring large-scale experimentation in human subjects, a great moral principle has been abandoned which has guided medicine over the ages: the Hippocratic oath that a doctor has to refrain from inflicting harm other than that required for therapeutic purposes to individuals who seek his advice. Our modern scientific procedure demands that a sample of the total population, namely the people participating in the test, is exposed to incompletely predictable chances of danger or discomfort so that the total population may profit from the results of such experiments. It is often argued that a physician, when participating in an experiment, does not act as a therapist but carries out a scientific task within the confines of a 'contract' with the experimental subject. However, this argument is only partly valid and perhaps somewhat hypocritical, sometimes in case of phase II (human pharmacology) and especially in phase III (therapy evaluation) experiments; in the latter, the treatment and control groups receive medical care as patients but may not be presumed to have equal chances of relief of distress or improvements in health. We encounter here not only an important deviation from classical medical ethics but a no less important evolution in public norms of morality: in matters of drug testing, the interests of society prevail over the well-being of the individual. We will come back to this switch in attitudes later in this review, because it is also present in political discussions on health care.

When the moment has come to start human experiments, the manufacturer will try to persuade capable clinical scientists to perform the trials. Provided that the financial side has been adequately provided for, the decision to accept this invitation to do research firstly depends on considerations concerning scientific competence, technical facilities, time available and number of experimental subjects to be expected. But in addition, moral problems may arise if a choice has to be made between different new drugs for clinical–pharmacological evaluation. Are there ethical criteria which are of use in such decision-making? The problem is limited for drug-testing commercial enterprises: they may follow commercial guidelines within the limits of their scientific competence and, provided the drug is not expected to present unusual hazards, no important restrictions are evident.

More difficult is the situation for clinical researchers in universities and hospitals. Their choice will have moral aspects, because other factors are at stake.

They will have to consider whether the drug to be tested will really be important in the practice of medicine, but in defining 'importance' many different aspects have to be taken into account: will many patients be helped by this drug? Will it contribute to a breakthrough in the treatment of a serious disease? Other aspects also deserve attention: especially serious reflection is needed in case of a proposal to investigate a *me too* drug. Is it supposed to have any real advantage over the existing '*me*'? In the absence of a good reason to assume so, should experimental subjects be exposed to it, and how should in all honesty the request for their voluntary participation be expressed? It certainly would not be helpful to convince prospective volunteers with phrasing such as:

'I would greatly appreciate your participation as an experimental subject, although I must admit that this drug is nothing new and of limited value'. The only morally acceptable motive for doing investigations with such drugs would be the expectation, derived from animal experiments, that it might be a great improvement in the specific domain of that category of drugs, for instance if the incidence or seriousness of common side effects might decrease: antihistamines without sedation, anti-hypertensive drugs without orthostatic hypotension, cytostatics without effects on bone-marrow, etc.

But in real life, other motives often also come into play which may induce an investigator to be not too critical in selecting a drug for testing: he may, by accepting money for drug testing, finance more important but unsponsored research projects or acquire technical facilities or staff expansion for his department – an important issue in the present difficult financial situation of universities! Alternatively, he may expect that perhaps his scientific status will increase by this research project – or, ultimately, more direct materialistic motives may be at stake. Ethical self-search, defining the limit between altruistic medical and more selfish motives should be part of the selection process. After a decision to participate in a drug trial has been taken, the institutional ethics committee should also be critical about this issue, because recruiting of experimental subjects is unacceptable if no real medical purpose is served: any inconvenience, irrespective of how small, would not be compensated by the benefit for society as a whole.

Post-marketing surveillance

Irrespective of how detailed requirements for drug registration may be, they will never be sufficient for a definitive judgement about the ratio between benefit and risk. Long-term post-marketing surveillance is the only available way to obtain a final assessment. The scientific methodology for this process is still in development; who should be obliged to report, what organizational and legal requirements are necessary? Will an industry reveal its sales figures so that the incidence of undesirable events may be fairly assessed? In the deliberations and negotiations on these matters ethical problems also emerge, especially concerning privacy in the epidemiological part of post-marketing studies. Epidemiologists need data which hardly can be obtained without intruding into the personal privacy of patients. However, in many countries privacy nowadays is protected by legislation and includes medical records. Therefore, here again public and private interests may clash in conflicting situations. This is even more evident if medical data of deceased persons will have to be studied. Such data may be of utmost importance to reveal side effects, but who is entitled to give permission to study hospital records? Evidently this is not only a matter of moral consideration for the epidemiologist, but also for legal and other governmental agencies to find a solution. Whatever consensus will be reached, it seems to me that for such epidemiological studies approval from a medical ethical committee should be obtained.

Ethical issues in medical progress

Costs for medical care are continuously increasing. Everywhere governments are attempting to curb such cost increases, while also trying to maintain an acceptable level of care. However, no political solution is as yet available for the expectation that in the long run good health care may have economic consequences which will make it impossible to preserve our present standard of living.

What are these expected deleterious developments? By human creative endeavour new methods and technologies for health improvement will continuously come forward resulting in a further prolongation of average life span. The shape of the population pyramid will change, old-age groups will increasingly preponderate over the younger generations. Hence, an increasing proportion of the population will absorb an ever larger portion of the national income for retirement pensions, during longer periods per capita. A decreasing fraction of the community will have to earn the income needed for this support. People of every age will demand optimal medical care with more effective drugs and complicated and expensive apparatus. Costs will rise to unbearable heights.

These gloomy prospects of the economically evil consequences of improving health are well understood and discussed at length in many circles. As to the consequences for health care proper, the general conclusion is that selection of priorities in health provisions are inevitable. Such priorities may be chosen in different ways: the World Health Organization's slogan 'Health for all in 2000' is a recommendation for attempting to diminish regional differences in the level of general health (Veatch, 1976). In the area of drug development this might mean: concentration of research efforts on the invention and adequate distribution of therapeutic agents specifically aimed at fighting epi- and endemic diseases in underdeveloped areas. Pharmaceutical companies combine their forces with WHO experts to realize such plans in a way which may be realized financially.

Within developed countries, a different concept is being considered: here, politicians recommend preferential attention for specified groups of illness such as AIDS, cardiovascular diseases and cancer. In the context of this review this might mean: priority for drug developments in these areas, for instance by assigning research grants or even by simplifying registration procedures. However, for practising physicians in our geographical region other consequences have also to be envisaged: if priorities in attention for specific groups of patients are chosen, other groups will evidently receive suboptimal care: independent of good medical attention of their physicians, financing of research for their sickness will be insufficient. This means that new medically underprivileged groups will develop. 'Charity for the poor' will obtain a new significance for the medical profession: 'the poor' are not only those afflicted by financial poverty but also patients whose treatment will not be at the best level which science could provide. In the context of this review this may mean: as a consequence of political decisions on health care, a chemical substance promising to be a good therapeutic for a certain disease will not be developed because preference has to be given to development of a different drug for a different disease.

Ethicists have only recently become interested in such situations: until now, in the area of drug development ethical assessments were mainly centred around short-term problems such as research projects for already selected drugs. The long-term consequences of governmental planning under conditions of limited resources still await serious and systematic studies.

Epilogue: towards new study areas in medical ethics

What should this new area of ethical research contain? In this, the final section of this review, some recommendations for study topics will be given which are of interest for planning the development of new drugs.

The starting point should be: generally accepted moral items such as justice for all (Rawls, 1971), equal access to health-care facilities, no discrimination of special groups (age, sex, colour, moral conduct). This includes: no preference for special areas of drug research other than mentioned in earlier sections of this review. However, in view of limited resources an *analytical assessment of selection criteria* should be given. For instance: if preferential illness care is envisaged, what are the norms used for defining a 'hierarchical' order of diseases (example: cardiovascular + cancer > rheumatism > respiratory disease . . .). What other factors besides financial consideration are guiding principles? As a next step, a similar *analysis* should be made *of selection norms for treatment methods* out of the larger supply of technical possibilities: where is the limit between what should be done and what would be possible? For instance: are such norms based on financial considerations only, or on special interest for specific categories of patients? But also: should limitations be placed on the availability of existing drugs or on the development of new ones, and what are the criteria?

A further important topic is an *assessment of the limits of solidarity in society* with regard to health care, research, risk coverage. What norms are at the basis of decisions concerning the preponderance of the community's over that of the individual's well-being? This problem has been mentioned already several times in this review, for example in view of selection of experimental subjects in drug testing.

And, finally, if a decision has been taken to make a division between 'privileged' over 'underprivileged' groups of patients (as defined earlier), the question remains whether the *care for the medically underprivileged*, earlier indicated as 'medical charity', is more than pastoral care in medical disguise for those who are condemned.

Only after a thorough ethical analysis of these topics it will be possible to arrive at rational decisions as to whether our norms need modification. Once more it should be realized that the role of the ethicist is not to be a judge over society's mores but to serve as a guide in a landscape with as-yet poor cartography.

References

Ahlquist, R.P. (1948): A study of the adrenotropic receptors. *Am. J. Physiol.* **153**, 586–600.

Black, J.W. & Prichard, B.N.C. (1973): Activation and blockade of adrenoceptors in common cardiac disorders. *Br. Med. Bull.* **29**, 163–167.

Black, J.W. & Stephenson, J.S. (1962): Pharmacology of a new beta-adrenergic receptor blocking compound. *Lancet* **ii**, 311–314.

Helsinki (version 1989): World Medical Association Declaration of Helsinki. Recommendations guiding physicians in biomedical research involving human subjects. Lately amended by the 41st World Medical Assembly, Hong Kong 1989.

Powell, C.E. & Slater, I.H. (1958): Blocking of inhibitory adrenergic receptors by a dichloro analog of isoproterenol. *J. Pharmacol. Exp. Ther.* **122**, 480–488.

Rawls, J.A. (1971): *Theory of justice.* Oxford: Oxford University Press.

Veatch, R.M. (1976): What is just health-care delivery? In: *Ethics and health policy*, eds. R.M. Veatch *et al.* Cambridge: Ballinger Publishing Company.

The ethics of animal and human experimentation, edited by P.P. De Deyn.
©1994 John Libbey & Company Ltd., pp. 187–192.

17

Good clinical practice: burden or blessing?

Remco Donker and Marc H.A.P. Broeren

Ciba-Geigy B.V., Raapopseweg 1, 6824 DP Arnhem, The Netherlands

Summary

In 1990 a guideline on Good Clinical Practice (GCP), issued by a working party of the European Community, came into force. The objective was to establish a standard for protecting the rights and safety of subjects involved in clinical investigations and for assuring the quality and the integrity of the data generated. A similar concept had been operative in the USA since about the 1960s. The European Guidelines started a process of worldwide harmonization and implementation of the principles of Good Clinical Practice. All parties involved in this process, and especially the investigators and the pharmaceutical companies, were forced to adapt and change their usual practice accordingly. In general this has meant that they have to invest more time and resources for the benefit of the assurance of scientific and ethical credibility of clinical trial data. The question remains whether this is worthwhile.

Basic concept of good clinical practice

Not so long ago, performing a clinical trial was rather easy. When the pharmaceutical industry wanted to initiate a trial, the investigator usually presented an outline from which a study design was made. Approval from an ethics committee was acquired after a small talk with the committee's chairman, and sometimes informed consent was not more than a recommendation to the patient that the trial was in his best interest. The protocol and case report form usually were very simple; sometimes they did not take more than one piece of paper. The trial was completed in a short period of time and the final report was published easily in a reputable journal. The investigator did most of the work, the pharmaceutical company was hardly involved.

Results from such a trial were generally considered to originate from good quality research. However, since most of the time a lot of information was not reported during the trial or even got lost, this could not be verified efficiently.

However, clinical research in Europe has changed drastically with the introduction of the Good Clinical Practice (GCP) standards. The main reason for developing these standards was the need to harmonize the regulations and requirements for worldwide registration of new drugs. Mainly in the USA, but in some European countries as well, research data obtained in foreign countries were accepted reluctantly. In these countries, some clinical trials had to be repeated in order to get a drug registered.

On the other hand, important ethical principles, such as a patient's informed consent and approval of a trial by an ethics committee, required a more global approach and definition. At the time the European Community (EC) became aware of this need and decided to set new standards, the American health authorities – the Food and Drug Administration (FDA) – had already quite advanced and well maintained regulations in operation. With the global vision in mind, it is therefore very well understandable that the GCP Guidelines eventually developed by the EC were to a great extent based on the FDA's principles (Moran, 1991).

These now generally accepted principles of GCP involve: protection of subjects, scientific standards, statistics and methodology. Leading to the following definition of GCP: 'A collection of rules and procedures aimed at protecting the rights and safety of subjects involved in clinical investigations and assuring the quality and the integrity of the data generated'.

Historic outline of Good Clinical Practice Regulations

A summarized review the history of GCP runs as follows:

1947: Nuremberg Code: safeguarding of the integrity of the research subject; introduction of voluntary consent.

1964: 18th World Medical Assembly, Helsinki: recommendations guiding physicians in biomedical research involving human subjects (Declaration of Helsinki).

1990: Committee for Proprietary Medicinal Products (CPMP) of the European Community: Note for Guidance: Good Clinical Practice for Trials on Medicinal Products in the European Community.

1991: Council for International Organizations of Medical Sciences (CIOMS), initiated by the WHO and UNESCO: International Guidelines for Ethical Review of Epidemiological studies.

1993: CIOMS: International Ethical Guidelines for Biomedical Research Involving Human Subjects.

Why Good Clinical Practice?

The thalidomide tragedy in the early 1960s was an important stimulus to set up regulations for development, testing and marketing medicinal products. In addition, a number of serious abuses of the rights of particularly vulnerable groups such as prisoners, elderly and mentally handicapped people were reported in the USA around the 1950s. A shameful example is the abusive study in which poorly educated black men were used to investigate the natural course of syphilis at a time when effective treatment was already available.

In the USA, the FDA reacted in 1962 with the Drug Amendment Act, including a procedure for obtaining approval for undertaking clinical trials, which became known as the Investigational New Drug (IND) procedure. Pharmaceutical companies wishing to license their products in the US were from then on obliged to conduct their clinical trials in keeping with the guidelines of the FDA's IND procedure. In 1964, the World Medical Assembly endorsed the Declaration of Helsinki. Ever since this Declaration has been the accepted basis for clinical trial ethics and must be fully known and followed by all persons engaged in research on human beings.

Both the US IND procedure and the Declaration of Helsinki resulted already in the 1960s in a general awareness within the legal and medical scientific community of the necessity of global regulations for performing clinical research. Also, the regulatory authorities responsible for protecting society from registration of ineffective and unsafe drugs gradually came to understand that more background on the submitted clinical data was needed to guide their decisions.

Unfortunately, it took the EC's CPMP until 1991 to produce its Guidelines on GCP, by which the monopoly of the FDA Regulations was challenged and the discussion on global harmonization funded.

European Good Clinical Practice

The EC's GCP Guidelines were originally issued in July 1991 as a 'Note for Guidance', which means that they should be regarded as recommendations to the EC Member States. Nonetheless all Member States and all pharmaceutical companies recognized its importance and endorsed all principles. Indirectly the Guidelines were promoted to a Directive from 1 January, 1992 onwards. This means that all EC countries agreed on incorporating the GCP Guidelines into their local legislation. Some countries have already done this, some are about to do (Wijnberg, 1993). A solid legal base for GCP does not mean however that the implementation of all GCP procedures in daily research practice can be realized easily.

GCP applies to all clinical studies of medicinal products, including volunteer, pharmacokinetic, bioavailability and bioequivalence studies and clinical trials. The standard, established practice for all these studies should be subject to review in conformity with the GCP principles, and should be adapted if not so. For example, the protection of trial subjects must be in full accordance with the latest revision of the Helsinki Declaration, with the need for informed consent and consulting of an ethics committee. Everybody involved must work according to written Standard Operating Procedures (SOPs). There are requirements on adequate statistical design and analysis, data handling and archiving, Serious Adverse Experience (SAE) reporting, and quality assurance audit.

Clinical research ethics

The current revision of the Declaration of Helsinki is the accepted basis for clinical trial ethics. Protection of the individual is a prime requirement in clinical research (Roscam Abbing, 1993); in the EC's GCP Guidelines this is defined to be the responsibility of the physician conducting the clinical trial (investigator).

Ethics committee

An ethics committee is an independent body, comprising medical professionals and non-medical members, whose responsibility is to verify that the safety, integrity and human rights of the subjects participating in a particular trial are protected, thereby providing public reassurance.

The precise composition of an ethics committee is not defined in most European countries, but the structure given in American regulations for the Institutional Review Board (IRB) is usually the standard. An Institutional Review Board (the American ethics committee) should be comprised of five members with varying background, not all one gender, not all scientists, not all affiliated to the institution, and there should be no conflicts of interest.

The ethics committee must be informed and give its opinion on the suitability of the clinical trial protocol and the way informed consent is obtained from the subjects. The committee must be informed of all protocol amendments and of unexpected and serious adverse events arising during the trial.

Informed consent

According to the current revision of the Declaration of Helsinki informed consent should be implemented in every trial. Informed consent is the voluntary confirmation of a subject's willingness to participate in a particular trial, and the documentation thereof. This confirmation should only be obtained after information has been given about the trial including an explanation of its objectives, potential benefits, risks and inconveniences, and of the subject's rights and responsibilities. Information should be given in oral and written form whenever possible. No subject should be obliged to participate in a clinical trial.

If a patient is unable or incapable of giving consent personally, inclusion in a trial is only permitted if the responsible ethics committee agrees and the investigator is of the opinion that participation is in the best interest of this patient. A legal representative of the patient should agree and preferably sign an informed consent form.

In a life-threatening emergency, where no alternative therapy for saving the life of the patient is available, it is allowed to include a patient in a trial without prior consent. However, as soon as possible thereafter, personal consent should be obtained.

Audit

According to GCP all observations and findings of a clinical trial should be verifiable. This is important to assure the credibility of the data reported and to draw the right conclusions.

An audit is a comparison of raw data and associated records with the interim or final report on the trial results, in order to determine whether these data have been accurately reported, to determine whether testing was carried out in accordance with the protocol, and to establish whether practices were employed in the generation of data that would impair their validity. Audits can be conducted either by an internal, but independent facility from the pharmaceutical company (sponsor), an external contractor, or regulatory authorities.

The investigator's view

At the beginning there was considerable resistance to the introduction of GCP in Europe. In the opinion of investigators, GCP would be a bureaucratic concept and would do little to improve the scientific standards of research.

According to GCP, investigators have to comply with very strict regulations and detailed instructions as set for example in the GCP Guidelines, the SOPs, the protocol and the case report form. They have to complete what they regard as endless documentation. Clinicians are not used to working this way. They are used to make clinical judgements, to diagnose, to do what ever *they* think is best for the patient. That is why it is important that investigators surround themselves with supporting personnel who have the skills essential for organizing, documenting and controlling the trial, such as study coordinators, nurses and secretaries (Rentmeester, 1993).

An investigator who wishes to be involved in a programme of new drug development will now be expected to work in full accordance with the guidelines. Further, the level of excellence required for clinical trials sponsored by the pharmaceutical industry will make it difficult to work to a lesser standard where other clinical trials are concerned.

The pharmaceutical company's view

Certainly, each pharmaceutical company has questioned why they should implement GCP. The following objections could be heard early on.

'It's not necessary!'; 'We will need extra staff!'; 'We already do our own GCP!'; 'We already know the drug is OK!'; 'The clinicians will not like it!'; 'It will cost too much!'.

To understand these reactions it may be helpful to define the GCP concept from another perspective. This definition might be then: 'to obtain and handle data about drugs through a quality control process, which can be validated at any time by the sponsor's own management or regulatory authorities from outside'. This validation, the 'auditing', introduces the aspect of checking the work of the people involved.

In order to have a standard for reference when auditing the process, GCP requires that all functions and activities should be performed according to detailed and written instructions, the so-called Standard Operating Procedures (SOPs).

Due to, for example, the principles of auditing and SOPs it took some effort to convince each and every person in the sponsor's organization, ranging from high to low in the hierarchy, that GCP is a management philosophy that is not based upon mistrust and control but that aims at performing high quality clinical research.

FDA's view on non-US data

In the USA, there is a fully legislated and regulated system, with an adequately funded inspectorate and with established penalties to ensure compliance. In the EC, there is a comprehensive guideline; a number of provisions which will be implemented into the law in the member states and a number of provisions are still in discussion. Inspectorates are not yet set up in the majority of the member states. There is some resistance to the concept of a pan-EC inspectorate (Allen, 1991).

To date the US legislation allows for foreign clinical data to be accepted as valid without on-site FDA inspection, when they are convinced that the quality of the data can be assured sufficiently.

Conclusion

The introduction of GCP has meant for investigators and sponsors that performing clinical trials has become increasingly more time and manpower consuming, and therefore difficult and costly. For society it has meant that clinical trial data carry substantially more credibility which allows regulatory authorities to use these data in the knowledge that all precautions have been taken to ensure their validity and accuracy, and that human rights have been respected. The question remains to be answered whether or not the burden on the former outweighs the blessing for the latter.

References

Allen, M.E. (1991): *Good clinical practice in Europe*. Romford, UK: Rostrum.

Committee for Proprietary Medicinal Products (CPMP) Working Party on Efficacy of Medicinal Products, Note for Guidance (1989): *Good Clinical Practice for Trials on Medicinal Products in the European Community*, vol. 1. Catalogue No. CB–55–89–706-EN-C. Brussels: EC.

Moran, J. (1991): *Good Clinical Practice in Europe*, 3rd ed. PJB Publications Ltd.

Rentmeester, Th. (1993): Guidelines in the European Community. Good Clinical Practice for trials on medicinal products in the European Community. (Original title: Richtlijnen in de Europese Gemeenschap. Good Clinical Practice voor trials met medicinale produkten in de Europese Gemeenschap). *Epilepsie Bull.* **21**, 9–12.

Roscam Abbing, H.D.C. (1993): Directive 'Good Clinical Practice' and the position of the research subject. (Original title: Richtsnoer 'Good Clinical Practice' en de positie van de proefpersoon). *Medisch Contact* **39**, 1189–1191.

Wijnberg, B. (1993): The impact of Good Clinical Practice on public authorities and the Ministry of Health (Original title: De betekenis van Good Clinical Practice voor overheid en WVC). *Medisch Contact* **39**, 1181–1182.

World Medical Association (1989): *Declaration of Helsinki: Recommendations guiding physicians in biomedical research involving human subjects.*

The ethics of animal and human experimentation, edited by P.P. De Deyn.
©1994 John Libbey & Company Ltd., pp. 193–205.

18

Review procedures and review committees for research protocols involving humans

Peter P. De Deyn and Herman Verhaegen

Committee for Medical Ethics, OCMW Antwerp, Jan Palfijn Hospital, Merksem, University of Antwerp and General Hospital Middelheim, Lindendreef 1, 2020 Antwerp, Belgium

Summary

This paper aims to describe the tasks and functions of the committees responsible for reviews of proposals on human experimentation. A brief review is given of these committees world-wide and special emphasis is put on the Belgian Committees for Medical Ethics (CME). The tasks of the CME as imposed by the National Order of Physicians will be described and as an illustration, the authors discuss the procedures and activities of the Committee for Medical Ethics of the Community Hospitals of the City of Antwerp (CME OCMW Antwerp).

The CME OCMW Antwerp was founded in 1985 on the initiative of the General Medical Consultation Committee which consists of medical directors and presidents of medical boards of the different public hospitals. The CME OCMW Antwerp consists of representatives of each hospital (elected by the medical board), two legal experts, and a hospital pharmacist. The CME OCMW Antwerp's major task is to give advice and formulate guidelines concerning medical–ethical issues raised within the Antwerp community hospitals. Guidelines concerning privacy and professional secrecy have been formulated, and a work group on the rights of the child has been formed. These and other advices and guidelines have been published in regional and national journals. One of the major activities of the CME OCMW Antwerp is the review of study protocols. Between 1985 and December 1993, 565 proposals were reviewed by our committee. This paper discusses the nature of the protocols submitted as well as assessment criteria applied by the CME. In the assessment procedure, an attempt is always made to evaluate the scientific value of the proposed study as well as its ethical acceptability.

The majority of the protocols considered are clinical drug trials sponsored by the pharmaceutical industry. These protocols concern phase I to IV trials as well as pre-marketing studies. The guidelines for 'Good Clinical Practice for Trials' stimulated the pharmaceutical industry to prepare the protocols more thoroughly. This, on the other hand, probably resulted in increased bureaucracy (for example, non-relevant amendments are often brought to the attention of the CME). Looking back over the past 9 years the authors clearly note a positive evolution. In the early phases, several trials were undoubtedly never submitted to the CME. In this context it remains important to maintain a good relationship with the investigators, to keep the lines of communication open and not to fall into a judge–accused relationship. The number of submitted protocols is still increasing. Remarkably, the quality of protocols has continued to improve which may have resulted from education provided by the regulatory systems.

Introduction

Institutional Ethics Committees (Australia), Hospital Ethics Committees, Institutional or Non-institutional Review Boards (USA), Medical Ethics Committees (Belgium, The Netherlands) and Research Ethics Committees (Britain) are all names of committees involved with the evaluation of the ethical acceptability of research involving humans.

These committees should primarily be distinguished from (hospital) ethics committees which concentrate on ethical reflection and individual case-oriented health care advice. Robertson (1984) defined the hospital ethics committees as follows: 'A hospital ethics committee is an institutionally authorized or designated group of persons that, on an optional or required basis, will advise, discuss, or consult with a physician, patient, or family about ethical issues that arise in clinical care'. According to Jaffe (1989) four major functions for these committees grew out of governmental actions endorsing their formation. These functions are education, policy-making (for example with regard to do-not-resuscitate orders, *in vitro* fertilization and living wills), retrospective review in order to support the growth of good ethical decision-making and finally, probably most importantly, consultation for specific cases.

Depending on local and national peculiarities, these committees have a different composition and developed quite different working procedures and cover a variety of activities. From what follows, it will become evident that several Committees for Medical Ethics handle problems of ethical reflection as well as specific research-oriented ethical issues.

As early as 1803, Percival wrote that, before proceeding with therapeutic innovations, a physician ought to consult with peers. Some 150 years later however, the Nuremberg Code and the original Declaration of Helsinki did not mention this principle. The first US federal document requiring committee review dated from 1953 and consisted of a set of guidelines entitled 'Group Consideration for Clinical Research Procedures Deviating from Accepted Medical Practice or Involving Unusual Hazard.' As a result of ethical reflection with regard to the first large-scale trial ever mounted, testing the efficacy of the Salk vaccine in a placebo-controlled design, the concept of the Institutional Review Board (IRB) was realized in the 1960s. It is only in the revised version of the Declaration of Helsinki at the World Medical Assembly in Tokyo in 1975 that the principle of committee review is mentioned with following sentence: 'The design and performance of each experimental procedure involving human subjects should be clearly formulated in an experimental protocol which should be transmitted to a specially independent committee for consideration, comment and guidance'.

Institutional review boards or local research committees: an overview

In 1968, 73 per cent of the US IRBs consisted exclusively of scientists and physicians while only a minority had in addition representatives of other professions or lay persons.

In 1974, policies and guidelines related to IRBs were revised and issued as Department of Health, Education and Welfare regulations (45 CFR 46). These guidelines stipulate that the committees must be composed of not fewer than five persons and must include the capacity to judge the research proposals in terms of community attitudes. 'The committee must therefore include persons whose primary concerns lie in these areas of legal, professional, and community acceptability rather than in conduct of research, development, and service programs of the type supported by the Department of Health, Education and Welfare'. In 1981, the Department of Health and Human Services and the Food and Drug Administration (FDA) refined and extended their regulations governing the protection of human experimental subjects. The 1981 revisions also supported the position that all FDA-regulated research required review irrespective of where it was to be performed resulting in the founding of the so-called Non-institutional Review Boards.

However, despite all regulations and guidelines, our US colleagues Rosnow *et al.* (1993) point out that the task of IRBs and the procedures to be applied still remain poorly defined. Historically, the role of review boards was to ensure that informed consent was obtained, the privacy of the participating subjects was guaranteed, and the inclusion process permitted equal access to all relevant potential participants. While a central responsibility of IRBs still consists of ensuring that the potential benefits to the individual research participants and also to society will be greater than any risks linked to participation in research, additional issues have been introduced in IRB discussions. The scientific validity of the proposed protocols, and hence their design and the methods applied became an increasing concern of the IRBs since failure to meet given standards of control and sample size could result in a waste of resources and lead to false conclusions which could eventually even jeopardize general well-being. As pointed out by Rosnow *et al.* (1993) and in other chapters of this volume (e.g. Ch. 20, *Placebo: some scientific and ethical considerations*), the IRB should function as a mirror of scientific and ethical standards. This of course renders its task extremely difficult and inconsistencies in decision making may ensue. According to Williams (1984), IRBs are relatively successful in ensuring privacy and overseeing consent while they are less effective in weighing risks and benefits. These inconsistencies may result among many other factors from different standards applied in the assessment of protocols and the composition of review boards. We all are aware of identical protocols that were approved without amendments by one IRB while amended or even disapproved by another. Although one might regret this phenomenon, we believe it can only be partially prevented.

Some investigators take issue with the activities of the local IRBs which they consider to act as police forces rather than protectors of experimental subjects' rights. Researchers conducting low-risk interventions or epidemiological surveys have particularly felt unduly constrained by IRB processes or advice. In the USA however, protocols of low risk are actually not required to undergo full IRB review if they fulfil some criteria such as anonymity of responses and absence of criminal or civil liability (Department of Health and Human Services, 1981). Similarly, most epidemiological studies are exempt from review by IRBs. On the other hand, International Guidelines urging for Ethical Review of Epidemiological studies have been provided by the Council for International Organizations of Medical Sciences (CIOMS, 1991).

In 1991, the UK's Department of Health issued its guidelines on Local Research Ethics

Committees (Department of Health, 1991). The district health authority appoints the committee whose responsibility has been extended to reviewing research on humans undertaken by any NHS body (including family health service authorities, special health authorities, or trusts), as well as NHS patients treated elsewhere. The committee's role however is an advisory one; the NHS body itself decides whether the research should proceed. Introducing a second level of decision-making will certainly cause inevitable delays in the review procedures. Moreover, the new guidelines recommend that the committee should have two or more lay members as well as medical staff, nursing staff and general practitioners. Further, it is stipulated that both sexes and a wide range of age groups should be represented. However, the new guidelines do not mention the inclusion of a lawyer as member of the committee.

The boundaries of research that need approval by the Research Ethics Committees have been considerably extended in the UK. As an example, epidemiological research using existing records must be submitted to the committee. Similarly, research using questionnaires requires committee approval. Moodie & Marshall (1992) argue that this is completely justified since some of the questions might cause anxiety or distress to patients. In addition, the committee is required to bring to the attention of its appointing body any indication that research is being carried out which it had not been asked to consider. The latter might pose some problems since it is not always evident whether innovative therapies should be considered as research or as therapy. The guidelines with regard to recruitment are not very restrictive. On the other hand, they seem to offer a clear policy concerning subject information in order to permit a choice about whether to participate by stating that participating subjects must be informed in advance of all known risks. Another aspect dealt with in the guidelines is provision of compensation to research subjects who may suffer as a result of their participation. The monitoring function of the committees with regard to ongoing research is not a real requirement. There is only a mention of the fact that investigators should notify the committee if there would be a significant deviation from the original protocol or when there are unusual or unexpected results which might raise questions about the safety of the research. Finally, the guidelines with regard to multicentre trials read as follows: 'Each Local Ethics Committee is free to arrive at its own decision when considering a proposal which is planned to take place in more than one area'. On the other hand, according to the same guidelines, one local ethics committee could consider protocols on behalf of all of them. Nevertheless, a National Ethics Committee has not been formed. In a paper on ethical approval from 28 local research ethics committees, Benster & Pollock (1993) illustrated the absence of clear guidelines for multicentre research applications and the failure to distinguish between patient and population research. The latter usually does not involve patient interventions, neither does it intrude upon the doctor–patient relationship, nor does it have any direct application for the individual subject. Despite all aspects of the presented guidelines, Moodie & Marshall questioned whether these guidelines serve the proposed aims of local ethics committees: protecting the public from harm and enhancing the conduct of good scientific research?

McNeill *et al.* (1990) presented a comprehensive, questionnaire-based survey on 89 out of 101 Australian Institutional Ethics Committees functioning in 1988. The majority of committees complied with national requirements in terms of their membership. With a mean membership of 11, the committees had an average of eight male and three female members. The average age was 40–54 years. On average, committees were composed of four medical graduates, including administrators, clinicians and researchers; the required two lay persons; one lawyer; one minister of religion; and the representatives of two or three other professions, ranging from nurses and psychologists to non-medical researchers and statisticians. Although medical graduates still comprise the largest group on Australian institutional ethics committees, the proportion of non-medical members is greater than that in ethics committees in the United States, the UK, The Netherlands and Belgium (McNeill, 1989). In Denmark and New Zealand it is even required that half of the members are lay persons, and New Zealand committees are required to be chaired by one of the lay members (McNeill, 1989; Gillet, 1989). Sixty-seven per cent of respondents to McNeill *et al.*'s Australian study considered that the ethics committee's role was to consider the scientific validity of the projects, while 65 per cent acknowledged that the committee's role was also to consider the level of competence of the researchers. Thirty-nine per cent of the local committees considered the ethics of treatment at a policy level, and 29 per cent of respondents stated that their committee considered the ethics of treatment of individuals. The mean number of protocols submitted to a committee for review during one year (from July 1987 to June 1988) was 40.5 with 10 per cent of committees considering over 100 protocols. In other countries the number of protocols submitted to committees is often smaller; e.g. the number of protocols submitted to Dutch committees was approximately half the number submitted to their Australian counterparts (Bergkamp, 1988). The following types of research protocols were submitted to Australian Institutional Ethics Committees: medical sciences (65 per cent), behavioural sciences (15 per cent), health services (8 per cent), population and epidemiology (6.3 per cent), social sciences (4.6 per cent) and other (1 per cent). In several other countries, Canada is one, non-medical protocols are subject to separate systems of review (McNeill, 1989).

Less than half of the Australian committees monitored research projects in progress as a general practice. Most of the monitoring that was conducted was based on a report from the researchers on the progress of the study. At present, the surveillance of research projects until completion has been limited world-wide. The major reason is the time-consuming nature of such activity while the lack of resources available to the committees may be important as well. The Canadian system has presented a partial solution to this problem by giving research ethics committees the power to require that surveillance be provided by independent monitors at the expense of the research programme (McNeill, 1989). Of the submitted protocols in Australia, 63 per cent were approved after first consideration, approximately 15 per cent were approved after clarification and further consideration by the committee, 17 per cent approved after modification by the researcher and 2.7 per cent were rejected.

Bai (1992) reported on the ethics committees that have been founded in the past 10 years in the Japanese medical colleges and medical faculties on a voluntary basis. Each of the approximately 80 ethics committees is composed of eight to 12 members among whom an average of seven are professors of medical faculties of university hospitals; a mean of only 1.3 members are persons from other faculties and 1.2 members are from outside the university. The average number of female members is 0.3 and 60 committees contain exclusively men. The Japanese Ethics Committees tackled issues related to organ transplantation and the application of new medical technology without really being involved with cases of daily medical practice. Moreover, although the committees were originally founded, as is still stipulated in their regulations, with the aim of giving ethical advice to research involving human subjects, few research proposals involving new drugs or instruments were submitted in 1990.

Institutional review boards or committees for medical ethics in Belgium

In Belgium, self-regulation plays an important role in the regulation of research involving humans. The Belgian Order of Physicians requires that researchers transmit their experimental protocols to an ethics committee licensed by the Order. Committees are licensed based on criteria that mainly deal with its composition and some formal aspects. While most committees follow the Declaration of Helsinki and the Good Clinical Practice for Trials on Medicinal Products in the EC, no substantial rules or procedures are applied uniformly.

The National Council of the Order of Physicians distinguishes two kind of committees involved with bio-ethics. The first are the so-called Committees for Medical Ethics (CME) while the second are committees for ethical reflection. Since the former ones are comparable with the Research Ethics Committees, they will be discussed in what follows. The latter ones mainly focus on philosophical, religious, sociological and economic aspects related to medical practice in all its perspectives without emphasis on biomedical experimentation. The National Council of the Order of Physicians formulated some requirements with regard to medical research (Articles 89 to 94 and an advisory note of 14 April 1984 replaced by a note of 15 February 1992). The last advisory note (National Council, Order of Physicians, 1992) describes new rules on experiments with human beings and contains directives which are here partially reproduced after free translation:

– Biomedical research involving humans requires that a protocol of the anticipated experiment be made and submitted to a CME. The physicians and investigators are obliged to answer the questions raised by the Ethics Committee and to submit the full text of the advice to the experimental subjects. Any later alteration to the research protocol requires submission to the Ethics Committee. The involved CME has to be informed about the course and results of the study.

– The CMEs need to be composed in such a way that its members can understand biomedical as well as ethical problems. The Committees have permission to call upon experts whenever considered necessary. Persons who are directly responsible for management or financing of a health care institution may be consulted but must not be a member of the CME of their institute.

– Every CME consists of at least eight persons, among whom are non-physician members and members independent of the institute. The latter group consists of at least of one physician. The Committee contains members of both genders; physicians form the majority.

– A member who is directly or indirectly involved with any given research project abstains during the formulation of the Committee's advice.

– A favourable advice requires the approval of at least two-thirds of the members. Secrecy

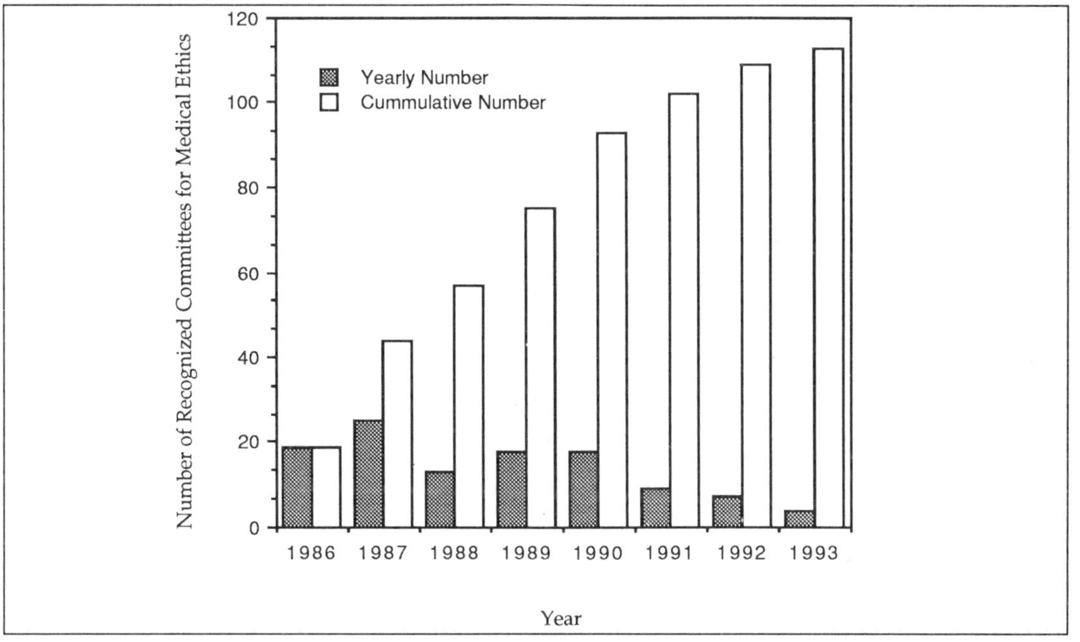

Fig. 1. Committees for Medical Ethics Belgium

applies to all members and people consulted.

– A physician participating in biomedical research on human subjects has to ascertain whether the project has been submitted to a Committee recognized by the National Order of Physicians and whether positive advice has been given. The protocol has to describe the proposed aims, the project and risks of the experiment, the detailed content of the information given to the experimental subject and whether the latter is provided orally or in writing. Moreover, it is required that the participating subjects give oral or written informed consent. Mention of insurance covering the risks related to the experiment is required as well.

– If the investigators publish or publicly report on the results of experiments, the CME involved should be mentioned.

– The Committees deliver a report of activity to the National Council of the Order of Physicians on a yearly basis.

– Any physician participating in biomedical research involving humans that has not been previously submitted to a recognized CME can be prosecuted and sanctioned.

The rules with regard to human experimentations listed above aim at protecting experimental subjects and at stimulating scientifically sound research. However, as outlined by Nys (Ch. 6, *Legislation in Belgium concerning animal and human experimentation*), these rules are more of a formal nature and do not contain substantial requirements in the presence of a relative lack of legislation concerning experiments involving humans in Belgium. Nys concludes that the lack of control mechanisms and real sanctions mean that the Declaration of Helsinki and the 'Good Clinical Practice' which have been im-

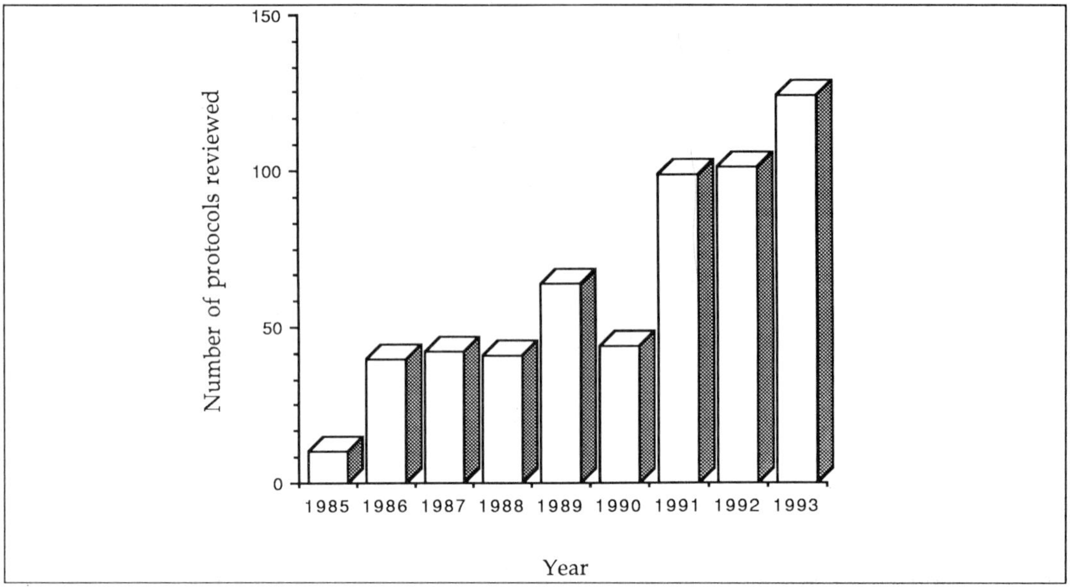

Fig. 2. Number of new protocols reviewed yearly by the CME OCMW Antwerp.

plemented in Belgium by royal decree cannot be considered as an effective tool for the protection of the subjects' rights.

Since 1986 a total of 113 Committees have been recognized in Belgium as shown in Fig. 1. During the first 5 years an average of more than 18 Committees was approved yearly. Fortunately, the number of new Committees has declined since then with only four new Committees in 1993. Of the 113 approved Committees, 42 are localized in the Flemish part of Belgium (approximately 6 million inhabitants) and 71 in Brussels and the Walloon part (4.5 million inhabitants). The abundancy of CMEs that are often responsible for small institutions with a possible lack of sufficient experts and dealing with a limited number of submitted protocols is not very reassuring. Moreover, the independence of members and investigators may not be guaranteed in small institutions. A limited number of CMEs would contribute to a more uniform approach and decision making and would undoubtedly improve the accessibility to experts. On the other hand, a too restricted number of committees would have disadvantages as well. The bureaucratic load would increase and the members would by definition be less well informed about the qualities of submitting centres and investigators. According to the authors, CMEs should be confronted with a minimal number of protocols on a yearly basis, and in addition they should have easy access to experts (e.g. in specific biomedical fields or statistics).

The committee for medical ethics of the community hospitals of Antwerp (CME OCMW Antwerp)

The CME OCMW Antwerp is the Institutional Review Board of all Community Hospitals of Antwerp covering activities in seven hospitals accounting for 2500 acute beds, 3000 nursing-home beds and more than 500 physicians. In addition, our CME is responsible for reviews of research conducted within three large relatively independent clinical research units. The Committee was formally recognized in 1987 but started its advisory functions in 1985 on the initiative of the General Medical Consultation Committee which consists of medical directors and presidents of medical boards of the different public hospitals. The CME OCMW Antwerp consists of physician representatives of each hospital (elected by the medical board), two (external) legal experts, an external physician member and a hospital pharmacist. The committee consists of 10 male and one female member. The major task of the CME OCMW Antwerp is to give advice and provide guidelines concerning medical–ethical issues raised within the Antwerp community hospitals. The activities conducted were primarily those assigned to the CMEs but in addition work has been done with regard to ethical reflection which is not the focus of this volume. Ethical reflection considered the following topics: privacy, attestations, AIDS-related issues, *in vitro* fertilization, children's rights and determination of evaluation criteria for clinical research protocols. Needless to say that our external members with juridical background were of major importance in this regard. Nevertheless, more than 80 per cent of the activities of the CME OCMW Antwerp involves the evaluation of ethical acceptability of research protocols.

The number of submitted protocols has been steadily increasing over the 8 years of functioning. In what follows we will describe the nature and origin of the more than 100 protocols which we receive yearly since 1991 (see Fig. 2). Of a total of 565 studies submitted between 1985 and December 1993, 34 (6 per cent) did not consider medicines. As an example, one of these proposals aimed at investigating the influence of sport activities and physical training on the outcome of dialysis. Among medication-related protocols (94 per cent), 53 (9.4 per cent) were proposals made by the European Organisation for Research and Trials on Cancer (often also inspired or sponsored by the pharmaceutical industry), 41 (7.3 per cent) were not industry sponsored and finally, the majority, 437 (77.3 per cent) were prepared and sponsored by the pharmaceutical industry.

As stated above, the objectives of the CME OCMW Antwerp comply with the guidelines and rules formulated by the National Council of the Order of Physicians. The following basic assumptions were made and continuously influence our decision making: (1) performing experiments are principally and morally acceptable; without biomedical experimentation no progress can be made in medicine; (2) the balance between risks and benefit needs to be positive (for the patient and for scientific research); (3) discomfort or risks are sometimes unavoidable but need to remain acceptable. The deontological obligation 'nil nocere' needs to be weighed against the public health benefit; (4) ethical approval can only be granted to scientifically sound protocols; on the other hand, a scientifically well-designed study project is not necessarily ethically acceptable; (5) the right to self-determination of the individual is essential; and, (6) scientifically sound and ethically acceptable research needs to be protected against fallacy.

Some IRBs develop policies about certain methodologies (e.g. placebo controls are never allowed if there is a standard treatment available, or placebo controls are permissible only for standard treatment non-responders). Set or strict policies like these do not truly permit a weighing of all relevant ethical and methodological concerns in each protocol. As outlined in Ch. 20 (*Placebo: some scientific and ethical considerations*), we believe that every protocol requires individual consideration and well-founded decisions can only be made based upon sufficient scientific knowledge of the disease and studied medication and/or procedure weighing scientific versus deontological obligations of all involved investigators without jeopardizing the well-being of experimental subjects. As a Committee we experienced a learning process: we gradually developed a more methodological approach and set up minimum criteria and guidelines in the evaluation of submitted protocols. After 8 years of functioning, our procedures are still evolving. In what follows, the major general points evaluated by the CME OCMW Antwerp will briefly be discussed. First of all, the aim, the purpose and the rationale of the submitted protocol are considered. Are the goals proposed reachable by the presented design? Which phase of clinical research is proposed if it concerns protocols studying medications? In phase I trials, special attention is given to the animal toxicology data and the information for the subject volunteering in the non-therapeutic experiment. It is obvious that as far as concerns toxicity, some broader criteria are acceptable in, for example, oncological indications. In addition the design of the study is evaluated (e.g. placebo-controlled double-blind trial versus active control double-blind with or without cross-over design) as well as the inclusion and exclusion criteria. Some of the questions raised are of course whether a placebo arm is ethically justified, whether rescue medication is provided when indicated and whether the study is of sufficient scientific relevance (e.g. 'me-too' compounds and premarketing trials). The information provided to the experimental subject (healthy volunteer or patient) is scrutinized in order to assure that the candidate participants are able to give or deny consent after adequate and accessible information. Special attention is also given to informed consent or alternatives in studies involving so-called vulnerable subject populations (see examples given in Chapters 21 (*Dissent on informed consent*), 26 (*Psychiatric patients as research subjects*) and 27 (*Research involving children: scientific and ethical aspects*)). However, some investigators question whether participating volunteers are capable for example of understanding the design, rationale and aim of placebo-controlled trials. Stanley (1987) reviewed the literature and concluded that irrespective of their condition, most patients were fairly able to understand the risks and benefits of a proposed treatment and the purpose of a particular treatment or procedure including placebo. We believe that investigators probably should focus on trying to convey to patients information on important aspects of the study design instead of providing a lot of detailed information on, for example, every possible minor risk of a procedure such as a venapuncture. Often advice is given to investigators or sponsors in order to render the patient information sheet in agreement with the philosophy mentioned above. The research subject information needs to be written in an understandable language, and should not be a mere enumeration of unintelligible terminology. The subject information clearly needs to depict the aims of the study. When it concerns a pharmacodynamic study on volunteers, it needs to be stated that the subject should not anticipate any personal benefit, but that only scientific benefit is to be expected. The patient information also needs to stress the possibility of withdrawal from the study without any influence upon subsequent treatment. Another concern in the evaluation of the protocol is whether adequate insurance has been provided by the sponsor or investigator. Also, the knowledge, reputation and infrastructure of the investigators involved needs to be evaluated in order to reassure that the trial can be successfully conducted in the centre in question by the participating investigators. As far as concerns the 'me-too' protocols, we believe that it is not primarily the task of the local ethics committee to reduce those to a minimum. We believe this should rather be a concern of drug regulatory authorities. With regard to the pre-marketing studies, we judge them acceptable provided that the protocol gives additional benefit to the participating subjects (earlier access to the medication, better information on the compound taken, etc.).

We now will briefly discuss our practical functioning and advices given related to the first 565 protocols submitted for evaluation to the CME OCMW Antwerp (before 1994). If obvious flaws were discovered (such as lacking a Dutch language patient-information sheet), the investigator involved was requested to make the necessary corrections or additions before discussing it with all Committee members. The president (H. Verhaegen) and secretary (P.P. De Deyn) of our Committee carefully examine each protocol and prepare a summary containing all relevant information as outlined above. In the case of a relative emergency the president and secretary can give an expedited though provisional or interim approval if they have no doubt about the ethical acceptability of the protocol. This kind of approval needs to be ratified later by the Committee. In what follows we will describe the number of protocols that were rejected by the committee as a whole. In total 112 protocols did not receive approval after a first evaluation. This is quite comparable with the average situation in Australia and the UK where approximately 75 per cent of proposals are approved after first consideration (Nicholson 1986; McNeill *et al.*, 1992). Of a total of 168 new protocols reviewed in 1982–1983 by the IRB of the UCLA School of Medicine 28 per cent were approved at first review 'without comment', 64 per cent 'with comment', 8 per cent 'deferred' and one 'disapproved' (Chlebowski, 1984). In most of the 112 originally not-approved proposals reviewed by the CME OCMW Antwerp, approval was given later on. Approval was granted after required documents were provided such as elaborate toxicity data, safety profiles of the studied compounds, patient information sheet and patient informed-consent page, or when privacy of experimental subjects were guaranteed or proof of adequate insurance was provided. In certain cases alterations had to be made to the design of the trial or the content of the patient information sheet. Finally, 20 (3.5 per cent) remained rejected because investigators or sponsors were unable or unwilling to comply with our requests.

The regulatory system may have effectively educated researchers and raised the ethical standard of the research protocols presented to the committees. The implementation of 'Good Clinical Practice' guidelines certainly had a beneficial influence upon the lay-out and overall quality of the submitted protocols. On the other hand, bureaucratic aspects have tremendously increased. An illustrative example is the obligatory submission of virtually every amendment, even if it involves only minor items such as extension of the recruitment period or minor changes in inclusion criteria such as a non-significant change in allowable age of an adult study population. In case of merely administrative or minor amendments as judged by the president and secretary, they are not individually discussed within the committee. The same goes for so-called serious adverse events which are often not medication related and which do not warrant interruption of the study protocol. The monitoring of ongoing research protocols by our committee is limited to the reading of annual study update reports of ongoing studies. Our committee does not require the submission of these annual study update reports.

Conclusion

The ethical committees should function as a mirror of scientific and ethical standards. Indeed, research ethics committees implement certain rules and guidelines which aim at protecting experimental subjects and at stimulating scientifically sound research. If a review committee is satisfied that a proposal is scientifically sound, it will then consider whether any risk to the subject is justified by the expected benefit, and whether the proposal is satisfactory with regard to informed consent and other ethical requirements. Nevertheless, research ethics committees worldwide differ in terms of specific aims, guidelines, procedures and sometimes advice given. Often, their function is only an advisory one and in many countries, research protocols involving humans remain unreviewed by independent research ethics committees. Belgium, with a population of 10.5 million inhabitants, has 113 CMEs. While most committees perform a function comparable to the IRBs or Research Ethics Committees, some also fulfil the role of Committees of Ethical Reflection. While it is considered critical that a minimal of protocols be considered per year per ethics committee in order to guarantee sufficient experience, one should realize that too many submitted protocols (e.g. 272 per year in one of the Australian committees) on the other hand might jeopardize the possibility of research monitoring by the committees. Some monitoring of committees may be necessary as is illustrated by McNeill *et al.* (1992) who found evidence that some researchers do not present their research proposals for review by committees and that in addition some deviate from approved proposals without seeking approval for these deviations from a research ethics committee.

Acknowledgements

The authors wish to thank all members of the CME OCMW Antwerp with whom they have on a regular basis very fruitful interactive discussions.

References

Bai, K. (1992): Characteristics of ethics committees of Japanese medical schools. *Med. Law* **11**, 337–343.

Benster, R. & Pollock, A.M. (1993): Guidelines for local research ethics committees: distinguishing between patient and population research in the multicentre research project. *Public Health* **107**, 3–7.

Bergkamp, L. (1988): American IRBs and Dutch research ethics committees: how they compare. *IRB: Rev. Hum. Subjects Res.* **10**, 1–6.

Chlebowski, R.T. (1984): How many protocols are deferred? One IRB's experience. *IRB: Rev. Hum. Subjects Res.* **6**, 9–10.

CIOMS (1991): International guidelines for ethical review of epidemiological studies. *Law, Medicine & Health Care* **19**, 247–258.

Department of Health (1991): *Local research ethics committees.* (HSG(91)5.) London: Department of Health.

Department of Health and Human Services (1981): Final recommendation amending basic HHS policy for the protection of human research subjects (45 CFR, Pt. 46). *Federale Register* **46**, 8366–8392, 19195.

Gillet, G. (1989): The new ethical committee: their nature and role. *N.Z. Med. J.* **102,** 314–315.

Jaffe, G.A. (1989): Institutional Ethics Committees. Legitimate and impartial review of ethical health care decisions. *J. Legal Med.* **10,** 393–431.

McNeill, P.M. (1989): Research ethics review in Australia, Europe and North America. *IRB: Rev. Hum. Subjects Res.* **11,** 4–7.

McNeill, P.M., Berglund, C.A. & Webster, I.A. (1990): Reviewing the reviewers: a survey of institutional ethics committees in Australia. *Med. J. Aust.* **152,** 289–296.

McNeill, P.M., Berglund, C.A. & Webster, I.W. (1992): Do Australian researchers accept committee review and conduct ethical research? *Soc. Sci. Med.* **35,** 317–322.

Moodie, P.C.E. & Marshall, T. (1992): Guidelines for local research ethics committees. *Br. Med. J.* **304,** 1293–1295.

Mukerjee, A.K. (1993): Relation between patent foramen ovale and stroke. *Am. J. Cardiol.* **72,** 863.

National Council of the Order of Physicians (1992): *Official Bulletin* **55,** 35–38.

Nicholson, R.H. (1986): *Medical research with children: ethics, law and practice.* Oxford: Oxford University Press.

Percival, T. (1803): *Medical ethics.* London: Russell.

Robertson (1984): Committees as decision makers: alternative structures and responsibilities. In: *Institutional ethics committees and health care decision making 85.*

Rosnow, R.L., Rotheram-Borus, M.J., Ceci, S.J., Blanck, P.D. & Koocher, G.P. (1993): The institutional review board as a mirror of scientific and ethical standards. *Am. Psychol.* **48,** 821–826.

Stanley, B. (1987): Informed consent in treatment and research. In: *Handbook of forensic psychology,* eds. J.B. Weiner & A.K. Hess, pp. 63–85. New York: John Wiley & Sons.

Williams, P.C. (1984): Success in spite of failure: Why IRBs falter in reviewing risks and benefits. *IRB: Rev. Hum. Subjects Res.* **6(3),** 1–4.

The ethics of animal and human experimentation, edited by P.P. De Deyn.

19

Alzheimer's disease: necessary elements in the review of research protocols

Rob J.M. Dillmann

Royal Dutch Medical Association, Utrecht Free University Amsterdam, Lomanlaan 103, Postbus 20051, NL–3502 LB Utrecht, The Netherlands

Summary

Since 1977 the cholinergic hypothesis of Alzheimer's disease has invoked a large number of clinical trials, involving a large number of patients. Unfortunately cholinergic drugs have not proved to be very successful so far. Nevertheless, the cholinergic hypothesis served for almost two decades as an important scientific lead.

Since clinical research has not shown clinically significant results, the question is justified whether the cholinergic hypothesis is sufficient scientific support for randomized clinical trials with demented elderly.

On the basis of the epistemological characteristics of this line of Alzheimer's disease research, and taking into account the content of international guidelines concerning research with human subjects, it is discussed whether there is a situation of genuine scientific or clinical equipoise with regard to the choice between cholinergic treatment or placebotreatment. In the review of research protocols an overall estimate of the viability of the underlying scientific framework should be included. Methodological aspects should be taken into account as well. Clearly the scope of the ethical review should not be limited to the direct interests of the research subjects. The analysis concludes with three rules of thumb for an epistemological evaluation of the overall strength of a particular theoretical framework.

Introduction

Since 1977 the cholinergic hypothesis of cognitive dysfunction in Alzheimer's disease (AD) has invoked a large number of clinical trials. Unfortunately however cholinergic drugs – a family of drugs which would correct cholinergic deficits in AD patients – have not proved to be very succesful so far. The cholinergic hypothesis is nevertheless supported and upheld by a large body of scientific literature, and served for almost two decades as an important scientific lead. Participation of subjects in clinical research is based on the presumption that there is a reasonable and justified scientific belief that the therapy in question indeed might be better than existing therapies (which in the case of Alzheimer's disease are virtually absent), i.e. that there is an 'honest null hypothesis' (Freedman, 1987). Since clinical trials have not shown clinically significant results so far, the question whether or not the scientific belief that the cholinergic hypothesis is sufficient support for randomized clinical trials with demented elderly is justified. In the ethical review of randomized clinical trials (RCTs) the question whether or not the investigator is in a state of true uncertainty regarding the comparative merits of treatment A and B for a particular population (i.e. is in equipoise), has received substantial attention. These discussions focused especially on the interests of the subjects enrolled in RCTs, paying much attention to the treatment preference of the physician of those subjects, and the question whether or not these subjects received the best possible treatment. The question of equipoise has also been raised in the sense that subjects might receive less than the best treatment when evidence accrued during the trial that the alternative treatment yielded better results. Research into AD on the basis of the cholinergic hypothesis indicates that the question of equipoise should include the question on what basis a particular scientific hypothesis is judged to be a potential success. A researcher should not only be in equipoise as far as the comparative merits of the treatments in the two arms of an RCT, but he should also have indication that the tested treatment indeed has potential, although nobody knows for sure whether this potential will be realized.

International guidelines

In many international guidelines, research involving human subjects has been addressed, in particular by the Declaration of Helsinki, and the recently published CIOMS-WHO guidelines (1993). CIOMS guideline 14 reads as follows: 'All proposals to conduct research involving human subjects must be submitted to review and approval to one or more independent ethical and scientific review committees.' (p. 37). Normally – according to the commentary on guideline 14 – ethical review committees consider both the scientific and the ethical aspects of proposed research, since scientific review and ethical review cannot be clearly separated. Scientific review should imply a judgment whether or not a research proposal conforms '. . . to generally accepted scientific principles and should be based on adequately performed laboratory and animal experimentation and on a thorough knowledge of the scientific literature' (Declaration of Helsinki, Article I.1). If a research protocol is judged to be scientifically sound, then the ethical review committee should address the risk/benefit ratio for the subjects, and the procedures for informed consent and the selection of subjects (CIOMS-WHO Guidelines, 1993). As far as the risk/benefit ratio is concerned, the Declaration of Helsinki gives the following picture: (a) the importance of the objective must be in proportion to the inherent risk to the subject (I.4), (b) there should be a careful assessment of predictable risks in comparison with foreseeable benefits (to the subject or others) (I.5), (c) the hazards involved are believed to be predictable (I.7). Hence, the Declaration of Helsinki seems to reject the imposition of any risk to a subject which is (1) unpredictable, and (2) not in proportion with the foreseeable benefits. We may conclude therefore that any risk imposed in the absence of a reasonable expectation of any benefit cannot be legitimate.

These general statements, however, are not practical guidelines for ethical review committees. They do not indicate how it can be decided that a research proposal – and the scientific theories, principles and opinions on which it is based – gives a reasonable expectation of benefit for the patient, a benefit which is moreover in proportion to the risks for the patient. In view of the difficulties which surround this part of scientific and ethical reviews it is to be expected that the review focuses on such matters as the methodology and statistical analysis of the trial, informed consent procedures and inclusion and exclusion criteria. The viability of the scientific framework on which the research proposal is based is likely to remain outside the scope of the ethical review committee, and possibly also outside the scientific review committee. It is of course far from obvious in what way the potential success of a scientific theoretical framework might be estimated. In order to shed some light on this problem the clinical research into cholinergic drugs for AD patients will be used as an example. In this respect it is of course particularly relevant to review the evidence whereupon it was decided that clinical research was (and still is) scientifically and ethically justified. An analysis of this evidence and of the difficulties of this area of research can offer us two things at once: (1) a conclusion regarding the legitimation of current clinical AD research into cholinergic drugs, and (2) an indication of additional analytic tools for scientific and ethical review committees.

The cholinergic hypothesis of Alzheimer's disease

Alzheimer's disease is the primary cause (60 per cent) of dementia. In the Netherlands, the number of patients is about 50 000, in the United States about 2 million. Above the age of 70 years, 3.2 per cent of the population has AD, whereas in the age-category from 80 to 89, about 10.8 per cent of the population has AD (Rocca *et al.*, 1991). The clinical picture of AD is characterized by a progressive and irreversible dementia, with disturbances in perception, cognition, language and memory, with motor disturbances and emotional changes. AD is neuropathologically signified by the presence of extensive plaques and tangles in the brain, especially in the frontal and temporal cortex and hippocampus, with concomitant neuronal cell death and atrophy (Katzman *et al.*, 1978; Reisberg, 1983; Iqbal *et al.*, 1991). The disease has been associated with chromosome 21 (early-onset familial AD) and chromosome 19 (the sporadic late-onset type of AD) (Corder *et al.*, 1993).

In the early 1980s the somewhat pessimistic atmosphere which had pervaded AD research for a long time seemed to have changed into cheerful optimism. The reason for this optimism was the (re)discovery of a certain area in the brain, the nucleus basalis of Meynert (NBM). This area, localized in the substantia innominata in the basal forebrain, just above the optic chiasm, was hypothesized to be one of the predilection sites of cell loss and neuropathological changes in AD. If true, this would imply that an anatomical background and a therapeutic possibility for AD might have been found.

The attention of researchers was directed to this group of cells because at the end of the

1970s a reduced level of choline acetyltransferase (ChAT) activity, an enzyme necessary for the synthesis of acetylcholine* in presynaptic neurons, had been found in the brains of patients with AD (Davies & Maloney, 1976; Perry *et al.*, 1977a). Furthermore, reduced levels of ChAT activity had been found in animals with lesions in their basal forebrain (Coyle *et al.*, 1983). These findings made researchers suppose that this particular region in the brain could be the cause of decreased levels of ChAT activity in AD.

In general the 'cholinergic hypothesis' is that cognitive changes (particularly memory deficits) in elderly people and especially in patients with AD, are caused by disturbances in a (cholinergic) neural circuit from the NBM, via the hippocampus to the frontal and temporal cortical areas. The disturbances in this circuit are explained both by loss of neurons and by impaired function of the remaining neurons. Other symptoms of AD and the possible causes thereof do not belong to the domain of the hypothesis.

Development of the cholinergic hypothesis

The first findings relevant to the development of the cholinergic hypothesis were reported by Gauss in 1906 (Gauss, 1906; Bartus *et al.*, 1986). Gauss's publication reviewed the facilitation of childbirth by administering light anaesthesia. The women appeared to have difficulties in remembering the events preceding and during the delivery. The provision of anaesthesia during delivery was common practice during the 1950s in the United States and many other countries, and stimulated the search for effects on learning and memory of these anaesthetics which also had anticholinergic properties (Lambrechts & Parkhouse, 1961; Pandit & Dundee, 1970). During the 1960s much attention was directed to the presence of the enzyme acetylcholinesterase (AChE) in the central nervous system. Lewis & Shute (1967), for instance, used the detection of AChE to construct a map of the cholinergic areas and the connections between them in the diencephalon of the rat brain.

The functional importance of these connections was initially understood in the context of the Reticular Activating System (RAS), a system possibly involved in the regulation of the cortical activity, and therefore linked to vigilance, attention and concentration. Cholinergic neurons were thus initially not considered as important for memory, but for the processes of activation of the cortex. Lewis & Shute (1967) mentioned their importance

* Acetylcholine is a neurotransmitter and as such is produced by particular neurons, using acetylcholine-precurs- ors (choline, lecithine) and the enzyme choline acetyltransferase (ChAT). It is released in the synaptic cleft following an impulse-train in the presynaptic neuron. After passing this cleft it stimulates cholinergic receptors in the membrane of the post-synaptic neuron. There it is broken down by the enzyme acetylcholinesterase. Enhancing cholinergic transmission can in principle be accomplished by stimulating acetylcholine production, and by blocking acetylcholine breakdown. Anticholinesterase drugs are substances capable of inhibiting the activity of the enzyme acetylcholinesterase (AChE) in the membrane of postsynaptic neurons. Inhibition of AChE increases the concentration of acetylcholine in the synaptic cleft, stimulating postsynaptic impulse generation up to a certain level. When the concentration of acetylcholine increases beyond this level, impulse generation is blocked. Several pharmaceuticals, some insecticides and substances for chemical warfare belong to the group of anticholinesterases. Pharmaceuticals usually belong to a subgroup of reversible anticholinesterases; insecticides and substances for chemical warfare exert, as a rule, an irreversible effect. One of the best known pharmaceuticals is physostigmine, isolated in 1864, and used in 1877 for the first time in the treatment of glaucoma. Its chemical structure was elucidated in 1923, which induced the development of many synthetic analogues (Witter *et al.*, 1978).

for memory but they considered them only secondary to the effects concerning arousal.

In 1971 Deutsch reintroduced the (19th century) hypothesis that learning and memory are due to changes in synapses, and specifically, cholinergic synapses. Changes in synaptic transmission – depending on the amount of neurotransmitter (acetylcholine) synthesized and released, as well as on the sensitivity of the post-synaptic membrane – could explain the processes of learning and forgetting. Deutsch's approach of the problem can be recognized clearly in the first study which related cholinergic impulse transmission to the memory changes in elderly people, the study of Drachman & Leavitt (1974). Young people receiving scopolamine (an anticholinergic agent wich competes with acetylcholine for the post-synaptic receptors) showed memory disturbances wich were quite similar to changes in elderly people. In particular, the 'storage' of new information was compromised during scopolamine administration. Drachman & Leavitt pointed out the similarity between their findings and those in patients with severe hippocampal lesions.* Moreover, they suggested that the preference of 'ageing changes' (neurofibrillary plaques and tangles) for the hippocampus indicates that cholinergic impulse transmission, hippocampus and plaques and tangles are related to each other.

The research of Deutsch (1971) and Drachman & Leavitt (1974) concerning anticholinergic drugs and their effect on human memory, shifted the attention from arousal and attention towards memory. The functional effects of 'anticholinergic drugs' (on memory) were ascribed, via the demonstration of 'cholinergic neurons' in the brain by AChE and ChAT assays, to particular brain regions. Four important links – memory, ageing, cholinergic neurons and anticholinergic drugs – were combined in their work.

The model provided an important rationale to investigate the importance of cholinergic neurons in AD. By the end of 1976 and in the beginning of 1977 the occurence of cholinergic deficits in AD was reported (Davies & Maloney, 1976; Perry *et al.*, 1977b; Perry *et al.*, 1978). The expression 'cholinergic hypothesis' was suggested by Perry *et al.* (1978) and the subject extensively discussed by Bartus *et al.* (1982). Bartus *et al.* reported some 40 investigations directed to the distribution of ChAT activity in several brain regions (such as hippocampus, cortex and striatum), in animals and humans, both elderly people and patients with AD (Bartus *et al.*, 1982). In general it was assumed that ChAT activity is consistently lowered in AD, whereas the findings regarding elderly people are equivocal.†

* Earlier Scoville and Milner (1957) had conjectured from the effects of partial frontal lobotomy (in which two-thirds of the hippocampus is removed) that the anterior hippocampus and the hippocampal gyrus were of particular importance for the retention of new knowledge, i.e. the recent memory. One patient in particular became quite famous because of the dramatic effects of the procedure on his memory (Milner *et al.*, 1968; Milner, 1970). Thus the hippocampus and gyrus hippocampus became known as an important structure for memory processes, especially the 'storage' of recently acquired information. The relationship between hippocampus, nucleus basalis and cholinergic neurons was not revealed by these findings of course. Lewis & Shute (1967) provided the link between hippocampus and cholinergic neurons, and the link between the nucleus of the diagonal band of Broca (continuous with the nucleus basalis of Meynert) and the hippocampus.

† The results of these studies are difficult to appreciate. Clinical criteria for AD or senile dementia of the Alzheimer type yielded at the time false-positive results ranging from 10 to 50 per cent (Gurland & Toner, 1983). The neuropathological criteria were based on criteria like those of Blessed *et al.*, (1968) but these did not appreciate the considerable variation of changes according to brain region. This is of course also

In the early 80s the decrease in cholinergic activity in the cortex was associated with the loss of neurons in the NBM (Whitehouse *et al.*, 1981). Earlier, the nucleus basalis had been identified as a cholinergic structure projecting to the neocortex (Kievit & Kuypers, 1971). A considerable loss of ChAT activity in this group of neurons (90 per cent) preceded a decrease of the number of neurons (by 35 per cent) (McKinney *et al.*, 1982; Nakano & Hirano, 1984). Additionally, cholinergic neuron endings were found in the senile plaques in the cortex.* This was taken as a suggestion that a functional loss of cholinergic activity in the neurons of the NBM was responsible for the decrease in cholinergic activity in the cortex (Perry & Perry, 1985).

In general, the NBM was referred to as the primary cause of the decrease of cholinergic activity (Sagar, 1985). One particular analogy seems to be in function here: the function of the NBM – assumed to be the source of input for the cortex – suggests a direction from NBM to cortex. This functional direction is subsequently used to infer – by analogy – a pathological direction, of course also from NBM to cortex. Anatomically speaking, however, there are two possible explanations: anterograde and retrograde degeneration. In the anterograde explanation the changes in the NBM are presumed to be the origin. Via transaxonal transport (or a lack of it) they are guided to the cortex and possibly to the post-synaptic neurons too (Whitehouse *et al.*, 1985). In the case of retrograde degeneration, the process starts in the neuron-endings and is transferred to the NBM (Harrison, 1986; Winblad *et al.*, 1986). Then one has to infer another cause for the cortical lesions, such as an infectious agent, or perhaps aluminium (Crapper *et al.*, 1973; Wisniewski *et al.*, 1975; Wisniewski, 1978).

Gradually, Meynert's nucleus started to emerge as the central element in the cholinergic hypothesis, although the consistency and severity of the degeneration of basal forebrain cholinergic neurons in AD was questioned and significant loss of cells in the NBM in several other clinical diseases was reported in the period 1982–83 (Bartus *et al.*, 1986). Knowledge concerning Parkinson's disease particularly favoured the central position of the nucleus basalis. Parkinson's disease is generally acknowledged as due to the loss of neurons and neuronal function in the substantia nigra, a complex of cells which provides the brain with dopamine. The analogy is tempting: while the motor disturbances in Parkinson's disease are related to the lack of input to the cortex from a particular subcortical group of neurons, the memory and cognitive changes in AD are related to the subcortical nucleus basalis. Moreover, AChE activity appeared to be strong in immature and mature plaques.

These observations changed the modest 'hypothesis' which was suggested in 1978 by Perry *et al.* into the firm statement of Coyle *et al.* (1983): 'The delineation of cholinergic deficits in AD along with the selective degeneration of nerve cells in the Diagonal Band of Broca and NBM provides the first example of a major disorder of higher cognitive

a problem in determining the level of ChAT and AChE activity in neuropathological specimens. Furthermore, the brains investigated were usually obtained after autopsy. The cases coming to autopsy are as a rule highly biased (more severe cases, selected from a hospital population), which is a problem in all forms of retrospective research.

* The search for cholinergic activity in plaques was stimulated by the observation that the plaques contained neural endings. Fischer had reported this in 1910 and it was revived by Wisniewski & Terry (1973).

functions in which transmitter-defined neuronal pathways responsible for dementia have been identified.'

It seems as if AD had been successfully reconceptualized as 'a disorder of central cholinergic innervation.' What needed to happen to turn this reconceptualization into a descriptive success? The first association between 'cholinergity' and AD was made by Drachman & Leavitt (1974), who conflated the pharmacological and the anatomical fields of knowledge. In the subsequent years this gap seemed to have been filled, that is, a relationship of cholinergity between AD (plaques) and the NBM had been found. But how could cholinergic neurons become responsible for the whole of dementia, as Coyle *et al.* (1983) suggested? On which grounds was it decided that the changes in the cholinergic circuits were pivotal and the cortical changes merely a consequence? How did researchers deal with the conflicting findings regarding the important role of the NBM?

Some epistemological observations

To answer these questions we must analyze thoroughly how researchers develop strategies to deal with conflicting evidence. Bartus and his co-authors (1982; 1986) discussed some of the problems which are associated with the cholinergic hypothesis. One of the deductive requirements ('hypotheses') they propose is this:

> '. . . (i) specific dysfunctions in cholinergic markers should be found in the brains of subjects suffering from age-related memory loss . . .' (Bartus, 1993).

The cholinergic hypothesis (which is in fact a theory) gives an explanation for the relation between 'age-related central nervous system disorders' (i.e. dementia caused by AD) and the 'cognitive loss' which accompanies them. The disruption in 'the cholinergic neurotransmitter system' is considered to be a major factor in this relation.

Close inspection reveals that this 'deductive requirement' involves more than simple 'deduction'. Three shifts appear to have taken place. Firstly, there is a shift from 'cholinergic system' to 'cholinergic markers', secondly, there is a shift from 'cognitive loss' to 'memory loss', and thirdly, 'age-related memory loss' is used instead of dementia. The first shift brings the ontological claim – 'there are cholinergic neurotransmitter systems' – back to: 'we need to show changes considered to be *markers* of those systems'. The question whether or not 'cholinergic systems' can be identified as such, or should be identified as such, is thus glossed over.* The second shift introduces some specification, i.e. from the clinical picture of dementia to cognition and especially to memory, and narrows down the domain in which the theory is considered to be relevant. The third shift identifies age-related memory loss with the clinical picture (and neuropathological findings) of dementia. These shifts are necessary strategies to keep the scientific work going. The first strategy infers from knowledge (markers) the being of theories as objects

* This point is of direct interest. Thal *et al.* (1989) for instance stated: 'Of all the neurotransmitter changes reported, however, decreases in choline acetyltransferase (ChAT) are the only neurotransmitter changes that have been strongly correlated with changes in memory'. This sentence serves as the crucial legitimation of the clinical trial which the authors report. It is quite clear from the quotation how the probe 'ChAT' is equated with 'neurotransmitter', which in its turn is assumed to be the cause of the clinical deficits. Thus it is rational to try to influence the amount of neurotransmitter by blocking its breakdown. The shift from a particular probe to something which is pointed out by it, is overtly in use to legitimize particular clinical studies. That is an important consequence of this epistemological shift.

(cholinergic systems), the second and third limit the complexity of the domain to be investigated, at the same time trying to yield knowledge which is assumed to be valid for a much larger domain than the one which is investigated.

These shifts are supported by particular ways of reasoning when dealing with research results. This can be illustrated by the next quotation: 'There is no apparent explanation for the success of some authors in finding reliable changes in this enzyme marker (ChAt) with normal aging and the failure of many others' (Bartus *et al.*, 1986). Several explanations for these differences are offered: assay techniques, difference between animal and human studies, age of the patients, the extent of the changes (so small that they are difficult to detect), and regional variations in the brain.

There are some important points here. (1) Senile dementia of the Alzheimer type was not mentioned in the cholinergic hypothesis (theory). The theory dealt with ageing, not with AD, and yet, the changes in AD are used as an argument for the theory. Somehow the theory shifted from ageing to AD. (2) The changes in the NBM are anatomical, not 'cholinergical', and yet, they are used as supportive evidence. (3) Conflicting findings are dealt with in a particular way: the (sources of) variation are reasoned away, and are neutralized by pointing out that the number of studies finding a difference is larger than the number of those finding no difference.

The conclusion is that AD as a disorder of cortical cholinergic innervation was literally carved from the given correlations. These were moulded according to a functional hypothesis which linked the cholinergic system and the NBM to memory performance, supported by the example of Parkinson's disease. Correlations constitute a network of associations, and analogies borrowed somewhere else (Parkinson's disease) were used to give the associations a particular direction. But it was not merely a matter of directing the associations, it also implied that somewhere on the road dementia was restricted to memory disturbances. The story of the cholinergic hypothesis is a story of directing the correlations, of selecting the relevant facts, and identifying markers of reality as reality itself.

Clinical picture: 'bridging the brain–behaviour barrier'

In what sense were cholinergic neurons assumed to be of importance for the clinical picture? The first study which related AD to the cholinergic hypothesis was published by Perry *et al.* (1978). Subjects were rated according to Blessed's Dementia Scale, and post-mortem the number of plaques and ChAT/AChE levels in the brain were assessed. Cortical ChAT activity appeared to be correlated with the average number of plaques and the score on the Dementia Scale. The authors suggested that a 'cholinergic hypothesis' was compatible with the functional abnormalities. The neuropsychological function of the cholinergic system (including NBM, the diagonal band of Broca and the hippocampus, as well as several cortical areas), remained, however, unclear, except for the prevailing opinion that these nuclei and circuits played a functional role in mediating recent memory.

The precise importance of cholinergic abnormalities for the clinical phenomena AD patients display, appeared to be difficult to assess. These rating scales were badly suited for the assessment of the changes in patients with AD (Crook, 1983). They were constructed on the basis of particular theoretical viewpoints concerning memory processes, such as the distinction between short-term, recent and long-term memory. The operationalization inherent to these rating scales thus failed to verify the changes as present in AD patients. Furthermore, AD patients showed disturbances in such measures that it was in fact impossible to test them. Their results were located in that part of the test range where the tests had a very low discriminatory power. Crook therefore defended the use of psychometric instruments which reflect the actual behavioural impairments, rather than an 'abstract psychological construct' (Crook, 1983). The development of testing procedures which were better adjusted to the abilities of AD patients, improved the possibilities for neuropsychological assessment. It introduced a shift from test procedures particularly directed to memory performance, to procedures directed to the abilities of daily life, like dressing and eating (the so-called ADL scales – assessment of daily life), the recognition of faces and pictures, the ability to remember short lists of items, like grocery shopping lists, etc.

The 'memory model' of AD, as measured by psychometric procedures based on theoretical memory models and adapted to people with less serious changes than AD patients show, thus shifted towards assessment procedures which were closely linked to the phenomena which can be encountered in the daily life of an AD patient. This implied at the same time that the possibilities of linking the cholinergic hypothesis, which was understood to be paralleled by memory changes on the clinical level, to the clinical picture of dementia in AD, decreased to almost zero.

It becomes hard to understand in what sense the cholinergic hypothesis indeed offered a bridge which linked brain and behaviour. So far what had been linked was brain (as perceived by some neurochemical procedures) and behaviour as assessed by rating scales which emphasized memory as an important element of AD. The link between the neuropathological, the neurochemical and the clinical fields of knowledge was, however, not provided.

Therapeutic endeavour: a cholinergic disease?

Nevertheless, the therapeutic possibilities suggested by the cholinergic hypothesis, generated great enthusiasm among neurobiologists (Rosenberg *et al.*, 1983). The post-mortem findings in AD patients, the effects of cholinomimetic drugs in enhancing learning and the provoking of memory deficits by anticholinergic drugs in normal subjects were considered to provide a 'sound rationale' for the investigation of therapeutic effects of cholinomimetic drugs. The form and character of the cholinergic hypothesis was in fact inspired by therapeutic possibilities. Rossor (1982), for instance stated that: '. . . it provides a useful theoretical basis for therapy, but it does not assume any relation between the cholinergic deficit and pathological abnormalities within the cortex such as the senile plaques and neurofibrillary tangles'.

Soon after the first publications concerning decreases in AChE in AD, oral choline treatment was administered to patients with AD, during experiments in 1977 and 1978

(Perry *et al.*, 1978; Bartus *et al.*, 1982). At that time most of the elements of the 'cholinergic hypothesis' still had to be formulated. Apparently, the cholinergic hypothesis did not inspire therapeutic trials as mere application of the hypothesis or theory. The therapeutic trials of course followed from it, but at the same time the presumed therapeutic possibilities were a major argument for developing the hypothesis.

The cholinergic hypothesis indicates several therapeutic possibilities: (1) stimulating the function of intact neurons, and (2) replacing the function of neurons which have disappeared.* The first possibility implies the stimulation of the synthesis and/or release of acetylcholine, or the blockade of the breakdown of acetylcholine by acetylcholinesterases. The second possibility implies the stimulation of the cholinergic post-synaptic membrane by substances similar to acetylcholine.

The stimulation of the synthesis of acetylcholine has been tried to achieve with cholinergic precursors like lecithin and choline. In this case, however, the presynaptic neuron needs to be intact. In attempting to enhance the release of acetylcholine, piracetam, a derivative of GABA (γ-amino-butyric-acid) which increases ATP synthesis, has been used. Enhancing acetylcholine release is also based on the assumption that the presynaptic neuron is intact. The blockade of acetylcholinesterase by physostigmine or tetrahydro-aminoacridine (tacrine or THA), both anticholinesterases has also been attempted.†‡ Although in this case the existing neurons are not forced to increase their production, it still is assumed that acetylcholine production does take place. The direct stimulation of the postsynaptic membrane has been attempted using arecoline. Combinations of these drugs, such as the combination of lecithin and physostigmine or THA have been used too (Bartus *et al.*, 1982; 1986; Reisberg, 1983; Summers *et al.*, 1986).

The results obtained in these studies are, however, not very promising. Bartus *et al.* (1982) reviewed 17 precursor studies, and none of them showed significant effects, neither clinically, nor in psychometric performance. Studies with physostigmine were hampered by the fast turnover of physostigmine and the necessity to administer the drug intravenously; furthermore there appeared to be large variations in dose-response (if any). Kumar & Calache (1991) reviewed 22 clinical trials with acetylcholine precursors, 32 trials with physostigmine with different modes of administration, 12 trials with THA, and eight with muscarinic agonists (four with betanechol§ and four with RS–86). These

* Recently a new development came into being: the possibility of neuronal grafts of embryonic neurons restoring neurotransmitter production (Gage *et al.*, 1988). So far, the results have been obtained in animal studies and a small number of studies concerning Parkinson's disease. The theoretical pivot of this approach is similar to the other cholinergic therapeutic strategies. In other words: embryonic neurons serve as an envelope and production unit for a locally administered drug.

† Especially THA gained popularity in this field, induced by a positive report by Summers *et al.* (1986). The design of this study has, however, been criticized. In various countries the efficacy of THA has been investigated since. The advantage of THA above physostigimine is the possibility of administering the drug orally. More than one drug had a turbulent history, as did THA. It was developed at the turn of the century as a potential antihelminthic. Diaminoacridines were found to have an antiseptic effect. Monoaminoacridines were investigated during World War II for their antibacterial effects. Tetraaminoacridine was one of the compounds investigated, but showed no bacterial effects, and instead it appeared to be analeptic (Summers *et al.*, 1988).

‡ It has been reported that the mechanisms of action of THA might involve irreversible inhibition of AChE, and reversible binding with muscarinic acetylcholine receptors (Adem *et al.*, 1990).

authors concluded that 'The cholinergic deficit in AD patients was reported more than a decade ago and several attempts have been made to correct this deficit with disappointing results. The severe side-effects associated with various drugs in this group have hampered the progress in correcting cholinergic deficits . . . To achieve a clinical improvement in AD patients by cholinergic drugs alone is somewhat unrealistic' (Kumar & Kalache, 1991).

Recently two large studies have been published by Farlow *et al.* (1992) and Davis *et al.* (1992), enrolling respectively 468 and 632 patients. Davis *et al.* concluded that tacrine showed a statistically significant effect as compared with placebo on cognitive performance, although the difference was too small to be detected clinically. This study used a so-called enrichment design, using only patients showing a clear response to tacrine. Farlow *et al.* found significant effects, both on psychometric performance and clinically, but this study was hampered by the withdrawal of around 200 patients, including 100 because of the side-effects of tacrine. Therefore the authors conclude that tacrine might be efficient and safe in some patients with AD.

Difficulties in cholinergic AD research

It is important to indicate some of the background to the failure to produce clinically significant results in the framework of the cholinergic hypothesis so far.

(1) AD is probably not a homogeneous disorder, and in combination with difficulties in clinical diagnosis, it is not to be expected that homogeneous patient groups can be obtained (Boller *et al.*, 1992; Dillmann & Stam, 1992).

(2) The 'cholinergic hypothesis' as such came about on the basis of an analogy with Parkinson's disease, and is based on a clear selection of information, a necessary but risky step in all scientific enterprises. How this worked in the case of the cholinergic hypothesis has been presented in the section entitled *Some epistemological observations.*

(3) There is no known animal model of AD. Biochemical explanations and theories can therefore not be tested *in vivo* in animals before starting clinical research.

(4) Drugs are not particularly suited to replace neuronal function which is time- and place specific: '. . . NBM neurons discharge at higher rates and are phasically active with rapid alterations in firing in relation to behaviour. The loss of a neuronal system that exerts tonic modulatory influences, like the dopaminergic system, may be more amenable to pharmacologic correction, than the loss of a neuronal system, like the NBM, which conveys spatially and temporally coded information' (Coyle *et al.*, 1983).

(5) The choice of outcome parameters in AD research is particularly difficult. Sometimes positive effects have been reported in THA trials concerning particular psychometric procedures, like word recognition, recall and long-term memory. But these effects are hardly significant when the whole clinical situation is taken into consideration. Moreover one must be aware that patients might improve their performance in psychometric

§ In three out of four trials with betanechol it was administered into the cerebral ventricles. One might sincerely wonder whether this is justified in view of the low probabilities of success, and the substantial side-effects.

assessment because of learning-effects. Effects upon ADL or the global clinical impression should also be included as outcome parameters. The use of enrichment procedures – i.e. selecting a subpopulation of AD patients who appear to be particularly responsive to treatment with THA – makes it also difficult to generalize results over the whole population of AD patients.

(6) Other neurotransmitter systems are compromised in AD such as serotonergic (5-hydroxytryptamine) and noradrenergic systems.* Concentrations of somatostatin (a neuropeptide) and GABA (a cortical neurotransmitter) are also lowered in the brains of AD patients.

(7) Assessment of the clinical effects of pharmacological treatment must take into account the natural progression of the disease. This implies among other things that cross-over designs have an important disadvantage. Moreover, the efficacy of drug therapy is probably strongly dependent on the stage of the disease.

(8) Side-effects of tacrine – the most commonly investigated drug at the moment – are quite serious, although reversible and not life threatening. In the studies of Davis *et al.* (1992) and Farlow *et al.* (1992) many patients were withdrawn because of side-effects (respectively 18 and 23 per cent). In general the side-effects are nausea or vomiting, headache, diarrhoea, abdominal pain, and a rise in serum levels of liver enzymes (ALAT). Dizziness, sweating, hypotension, bradycardia, and agitation have also been reported.

Equipoise

The general principles and guidelines such as the Declaration of Helsinki and the CIOMS-WHO (1993) guidelines clearly indicate that any risk imposed in the absence of a reasonable expectation of any benefit cannot be legitimate.

In randomized clinical trials (RCTs) the interventions to be compared must be equally advantageous to the prospective subjects, and there should be no scientific evidence to establish the superiority of one over another (CIOMS-WHO, 1993). When this evidence is lacking, the physician can argue that there is no professional judgment possible on the basis of which he could prefer one therapy over the other. So there is no reason to advise his patient to take one particular therapy, which makes it ethically justified to ask (or to accept) that his patient be enrolled in a clinical trial. This condition of professional uncertainty on the basis of insufficient scientific evidence has been coined 'equipoise' by Fried (1974). Although equipoise is often presented as an important prerequisite in RCTs to prevent the patient unjustifiably receiving placebo instead of 'real' treatment, or

* The potential involvement of noradrenergic systems in the intellectual deterioration in Alzheimer's disease has evolved into something which might be designated with the term 'noradrenergic hypothesis'. Clinical trials with centrally acting adrenergic agonists, such as clonidine and guanfacine, have been performed although with negative results. The similarity with the cholinergic hypothesis is striking: the noradrenergic system was associated with 'certain aspects of learning and memory'. Lesions in – and pharmacological blockage of – adrenergic projection systems (such as those of the locus ceruleus) produced learning impairments in rodents, which could be reversed by intraventricular administration of noradrenaline. These findings entailed clinical trials with the adrenergic agonists mentioned. (Mohr *et al.*, 1989; Schlegel *et al.*, 1989).

'standard' treatment instead of 'better' treatment, the state of AD research clearly shows that the opposite problem could also be present.

The problem of equipoise was framed by Schafer (1982) as a problem of providing 'completely individualized treatment' versus a standardized treatment assigned by chance in one of the arms of an RCT. Schafer argued that – even if a physician does not know whether one treatment should be preferred over the other – he or she often has a personal or intuitive preference for one rather than the other. Withholding such information would be to violate the right of the patient to the best possible care. One of the cases Schafer had in mind was an RCT for radical versus partial mastectomy for breast cancer, a trial which had failed because participating physicians hesitated to enroll their patients, since they had strong opinions about the efficacy and safety of the treatment options (Taylor *et al.*, 1984). It is, however, difficult to understand in what way intuitive judgments of physicians really contribute to the choice for the best treatment option. Marquis (1983) used another definition also following the presumption that the role of the physician as an individual healer is primary. He stated that a physician has a 'therapeutic obligation' to recommend a patient therapy such that, given present medical knowledge, the hypothesis that the particular therapy is superior to some other therapy is more probable than the opposite hypothesis. Hence, using the same point of departure, Marquis ended up with a definition quite different from Schafer's.

Freedman (1987), however, rejected this approach of 'equipoise' as theoretical, because it presents equipoise as an exact balance of all the available evidence for each of two options. Freedman suggested the concept of 'clinical equipoise', in which there is a current or imminent conflict in the clinical community over what treatment is preferred for particular patients, or when there is a split in the community with some clinicians favouring A and some favouring treatment B. Hence, there is '. . . no consensus within the expert clinical community about the comparative merits of the alternatives to be tested' (Freedman, 1987). When evidence has accumulated to the point that any well-informed physician would have a treatment preference, then equipoise would have been disturbed, and a trial would not be justified. This definition is more consistent with Fried's original proposal (1974), in which professional judgment – i.e. the judgment based on the body of established medical knowledge – is central. Personal intuition and the like are – by definition – not part of professional knowledge, but are personal opinions of a particular physician. It is not likely that patients seek advice on the basis thereof. Presumably they do so because of his of her professional expert opinion. Such a professional attitude could imply a '. . . decided treatment preference on the part of the investigators. They simply must recognize that their less-favored treatment is preferred by colleagues whom they consider to be responsible and competent' (1983).

We can characterize four different ways of defining 'equipoise': (1) on the basis of personal intuitions (Schafer), (2) on the basis of professional judgment (Fried), (3) on the basis of controversies in the scientific community (Freedman), and (4) on the basis of all available scientific evidence (Marquis). Freedman's definition indicates that the weighing of scientific evidence might be a difficult task, and that in performing this task we should take into account that scientific belief is influenced by the scientific community, and in addition, that scientific community is influenced by political and economical factors. The pivotal role of the scientific controversy in his definition makes one aware of the underlying dynamics of scientific work. In this sense we should also modify his definition: scientific controversies are relatively rare. That, however, does not imply that there are no difficulties in evaluating research proposals in the absence of a clear controversy, nor that a condition of equipoise could exist in the absence of a controversy. In this sense perhaps Freedman's definition is a little bit too practical, and might perhaps best be used in combination with an evaluation of the scientific evidence so far accrued, such as in Marquis' definition.

A particular point of interest is the situation such as in AD research when there is no 'standard' therapy available, implying that cholinergic treatments, such as tacrine, are tested against placebo. The situation of equipoise does then not come down to a controversy or a lack of consensus regarding treatment A versus treatment B, but to a general evaluation whether or not this new type of treatment might have a relevant (clinical) effect. The situation of placebo-controlled therapy is therefore difficult to evaluate in terms of Freedman's 'clinical equipoise', since we all would tend to try whether the new treatment is successful provided that we can safely assume that no harm will be done to the patients. In this case we should use a wider scope, and assess the dynamics of the scientific work. This is especially important when we are discussing a particular line of research into a very common disease, with devastating consequences, when this disease cannot be treated such as AD.

Equipoise in AD research

So far more than 7000 patients have been treated with tacrine in the clinical trials of only one pharmaceutical company (Gage *et al.*,1988). The total number must therefore be even higher than that. Dosages were used from 20 to 150 mg a day, often in combination with various dosages of lecithine. A range of research designs has been used such as uncontrolled trials, randomized intervention studies, with and without cross-over. Many different outcome parameters have been used, including psychometric assessments, ADL scales and clinical observation scales. More than 100 trials have been done, often with a relatively small number of subjects enrolled (sometimes about 10 patients). The two largest trials enrolled 468 and 632 patients (in collaboration with the previously mentioned pharmaceutical company), whereas the third largest trial enrolled 89 patients. The general picture is that around 25 per cent of the patients are withdrawn from these studies because of the side-effects.

What conclusions can be drawn regarding a situation of equipoise, i.e. general scientific legitimation concerning THA-trials in AD? Here a real scientific controversy seems to exist. In an editorial in the *New England Journal of Medicine* (*NEJM*) – the same issue as the report of Davis *et al.* (1992) – Growdon (1992) concluded that '. . . despite 15 years of intensive study and trials of cholinergic precursors, agonists and cholinesterase inhibitors, the expectation of benefit still exceeds the reality . . . From a scientific point of view, the very modest effects of short-term tacrine administration that enhancement of acteylcholine transmission is inadequate to reverse the signs and symptoms of AD. Pending discovery of another neurotransmitter deficit that fully accounts for the dementia, it is now time to abandon simple replacement therapy and to develop treatments that can affect the fundamental mechanisms of neuronal degeneration'. This viewpoint is consistent with previous publications by Kumar & Calache (1991), and Fibiger (1991), and was supported by several authors in letters to the Editor in the *NEJM* issue of 18 March, 1993. Lachs (1993) for instance wrote that more evidence was needed before approving a marginally efficacious drug entailing considerable expense.

An opposite point of view was defended by Davis and Thal in their response to the comments on their publication and the editorial of Growdon. Researchers from other study groups stated that 'The call to abandon neurotransmitter based therapy is both premature and one-sided. In the short-term there is no other option'(Levy, 1993). Davis and Thal suggested that continuing research might be important in order to identify subgroups of responsive patients. In these defences the devastating effects of AD, and the lack of alternatives, are usually mentioned as important reasons to continue this line of research.

Must we conclude at this point that there is a situation of 'clinical equipoise'? It is obvious that there exists a controversy with regard to the effectiveness of cholinergic replacement therapy in general and tacrine specifically. It is also obvious that the results of the two largest clinical trials so far yield small, and clinically marginal, yet statistically significant results with tacrine. It is also obvious that any study with a design of lower quality, and generally speaking with a fewer number of subjects, does not add anything to the outcome of this controversy. It is also possible that the findings so far will not be replicated in forthcoming studies. It is clear that the side-effects are considerable, causing 20 to 25 per cent of the subjects to be withdrawn from clinical trials. It is clear that the methodological problems in AD trials are large, and that the theoretical framework ('the cholinergic hypothesis') shows some obvious weaknesses.

It can therefore be defended that the condition of equipoise is met: there is a situation of genuine scientific uncertainty whether or not cholinergic treatment is better than placebo. When two effective treatments had been compared, then we might easily have accepted that clinical trials might be justified, provided they have a proper design, and provided that the side-effects are found to be acceptable. In this case however, there seems to be genuine scientific uncertainty whether cholinergic therapy is better than placebo therapy. From that point two alternative conclusions can be drawn: (1) cholinergic treatment does not clearly work better than placebo, and since the cholinergic framework has a low *a priori* probability of success, further cholinergic RCTs should not be started, especially with regard to the side-effects, or (2) cholinergic treatment might be working better than placebo, and since AD has such devastating effects, there is in fact no other option.

At this point we clearly need an evaluation of the scientific merits and viability of the cholinergic hypothesis as a whole in order to decide whether or not RCTs are justified, and this evaluation must be confronted with the interest of patients with AD and society in general to find a treatment for the disease. It should also be noted that the 'interests' of society could take the form of commercial interests in marketing AD drugs after their registration has been completed. In the previous sections such an evaluation of the cholinergic hypothesis has been attempted, and many other authors have done so. In view of this evaluation the conclusion is warranted that further cholinergic trials should not be started, thus following the first of two alternative conclusions. The fact that AD patients in general are not fully competent because of their disease is an additional reason to be cautious. On this general rule an exception could be made if the quality of the research proposal is at least equal to the best reported study so far, and if the research proposal is directed towards subgroups which are particularly susceptible to cholinergic therapy.*

This conclusion is supported by the general rules and principles as outlined in the section entitled *International guidelines*. There the conclusion was drawn that the imposition of any risk in the absence of a reasonable expectation of any benefit cannot be legitimate. It seems to be the case that cholinergic research involving demented elderly subjects does not warrant a reasonable expectation of benefit for the patients themselves, or for society in general. The imposition of risks as in trials with tacrine can therefore not easily be legitimized.

Ethical review of research proposals

The example of the cholinergic hypothesis of AD enables us to draw several conclusions with regard to ethical and scientific review of research proposals. The first conclusion concerns the scope of ethical review, the second the methodological aspects of research proposals, and the third concerns the relevance of epistemological analysis for scientific and ethical review.

The scope of ethical review is often limited to the interests of the subject: the risks imposed, the possible benefits and the contents and procedures of informed consent. A proper analysis of the concept of equipoise (which can be deduced from the Declaration of Helsinki as a condition for starting an RCT) shows that the scientific viability needs to be an integral part of the process of review. In order to have the best estimates of the risk–benefit ratio for the subjects involved, we obviously need good estimates of the benefits, and to have those we need an overall judgment of the theoretical framework of the research proposal.

This overall judgment also points the way to several methodological aspects which need to be taken into account somewhere in the review process. In AD research several methodological issues are relevant: the heterogeneity of patients meeting the criteria for a diagnosis of AD, the choice of clinically relevant outcome parameters, the natural progression of the disease, and the absence of an adequate animal model which complicates the step from theoretical assumptions and laboratory findings to relevant clinical findings. Apart from these all the general methodological issues are relevant, such as those of randomization, inclusion and exclusion criteria, dosage, report of side-effects, sample size, data analysis etc.

From an epistemological viewpoint several other observations can be made. The theoretical foundation of many findings and observations in biology and biochemistry is often incomplete. This is even more so in human neurobiology, and also in AD research. Moreover, scientists have the same tendency as other people to try to make an under-

* 'The results of adequately large and well-designed multicentre studies will allow reasonable inferences to be made about the clinical importance and usefulness of THA. In the interim, while these results are being awaited, what emerges are a series of uncoordinated, small-scale efforts, none of which are adequate or could have been adequate to address the relevant issue.' (Schneider, 1990).

standable and plausible explanation for the enormous amount of observations. In doing this they also tend to mix description with theoretical elements, thus moulding the observed phenomena. The cholinergic hypothesis is a clear example of this process. Some processes have been pointed out, such as selection of the data, giving causal direction to statistical relationships, conflating different areas of knowledge with each other, and presuming real phenomena on the basis of presumed indicators thereof. With these processes understandable theoretical frameworks are constructed which serve as the a priori legitimation for doing clinical research. The overall strength of these frameworks is an important feature in ethical review of a research proposal, since this strength is probably correlated with the chances of success of research conducted on the basis of that particular theoretical framework. Measuring this overall strength is a difficult task, and to date no guidelines and procedures exist by which this task might be accomplished. As a first indication thereof some rules of thumb can be formulated: The strength of a theoretical explanation decreases if (1) more fields or domains of knowledge must be used simultaneously (e.g. microscopic anatomy, neurohistochemistry, neuropharmacology, neuropsychology, clinical observation, regular activities of daily living), (2) if processes of selecting the data, of directing the causal relationships, and of taking indicators for reality take place more often, and (3) if the theoretical explanation is based on an analogy with another scientific problem, without addressing the observations which make such an analogy less plausible.

Of course the question can be raised whether ethical review committees should be able to perform review procedures taking all these issues into account. At this point, however, it seems irrelevant where these judgments are formed, provided they come about. Close collaboration between scientific and ethical review committees would of course be preferred from this point of view. In general this would improve scientific efficacy, and this is in itself an attainable ethical goal.

References

Adem, A., Mohammed, A.K. & Winblad, B. (1990): Multiple effects of tetrahydroaminoacridine on the cholinergic system: biochemical and behavioural aspects. *J. Neural Transm.* **2**, 113–128.

Ahmad, S.R. (1993): Tacrine approved. *Lancet* **342**, 736.

Bartus, R.T., Dean, R.L., Beer, B. & Lippa, A.S. (1982): The cholinergic hypothesis of geriatric memory dysfunction. *Science* **217**, 408–417.

Bartus, R.T., Dean, R.L., Pontecorvo, M.J. & Flicker, C. (1986): The cholinergic hypothesis: a historical overview, current perspective and future directions. *Ann. NY Acad. Sci.* **44**, 332–358.

Blessed, G., Tomlinson, G. & Roth, M. (1968): The association between quantitative measures of dementia and of senile changes in the cerebral grey matter of elderly subjects. *Br. J. Psychiatr.* **114**, 797–811.

Boller, F., Forette, F., Khachaturian, Z. *et al.* (1992): *Heterogeneity of Alzheimer's Disease.*. Heidelberg: SpringerVerlag.

CIOMS-WHO (1993): *Guidelines for medical research with human subjects*. Geneva: WHO.

Corder, E.H., Saunders, A.M., Strittmatter, W.J. *et al.* (1993): Gene dose of Apoliprotein E Type 4 allele and the risk of Alzheimer's disease in late onset families. *Science* **261**, 921–923.

Coyle, J.T., Price, D.L. & Delong, M.R. (1983): Alzheimer's Disease: a disorder of Cholinergic innervation. *Science* **219**, 1184–1190.

Crapper, R.D., Krishnan, S.S., & Dalton, A.J. (1973): Brain aluminium distribution in Alzheimer's disease and experimental neurofibrillary degeneration. *Science* **180**, 511–513.

Crook, T. (1983): Psychometric assessment in Alzheimer's disease. In: *Alzheimer's disease*, ed. B. Reisberg, pp. 211–213. New York/London: The Free Press.

Davies, P. & Maloney, A.J.F. (1976): Selective loss of cholinergic neurons in Alzheimer's disease. *Lancet* ii, 1403.

Davis, K.L., Thal, L.J., Gamzu, E.R. *et al.* (1992): A double-blind, placebo-controlled multicenter study of tacrine for Alzheimer's disease. *N. Engl. J. Med.* **327**, 1253–1259.

Deutsch, J.E. (1971): The cholinergic synapse and the site of memory. *Science* **174**, 788–794.

Dillmann, R.J.M. (1990): *Alzheimer's disease. The concept of disease and the construction of medical knowledge.* Amsterdam: Thesis Publishers.

Dillmann, R.J.M. & Stam, F.C. (1992): De ziekte van Alzheimer: verscheidenheid zonder eenheid. *Tijdschr. Gerontol. Geriatr.* **23**, 41–47.

Drachman, D.A. & Leavitt, J. (1974): Human memory and the cholinergic system: a relationship to aging? *Arch. Neurol.* **30**, 113–121.

Farlow, M., Stephen, I., Gracon, D.V.M. *et al.* (1992): A controlled trial of tacrine in Alzheimer's disease. *JAMA* **268**, 2523–2529.

Fibiger, H.C. (1991): Cholinergic mechanisms in learning, memory and dementia: a review of recent evidence. *TINS* **14**, 220–223.

Freedman, B. (1987): Equipoise and the ethics of clinical research. *N. Engl. J. Med.* 317, 141–145.

Fried, C. (1974): *Medical experimentation. Personal integrity and social policy.* Amsterdam: North Holland Publishing Company/Elsevier.

Gage, F., Privat, A. & Christen, Y. (eds.). (1988): Neuronal grafting and Alzheimer's disease. Berlin: Springer.

Gauss, C.J. (1906): Gebürten im Künstlichen Dammerschlaf. *Arch. Gynaek.* **78**, 579–631.

Growdon, J.H. (1992): Treatment for Alzheimer's Disease? *N. Engl. J. Med.* **327**, 1306–1309.

Gurland, B. & Toner, J. (1983): Differentiating dementia from non-dementing conditions. In: *The Dementias*, eds R. Mayeux, W.G. Rosen, pp. 1–17. New York: Raven Press.

Harrison, P.J. (1986): Pathogenesis of Alzheimer's disease – beyond the cholinergic hypothesis: discussion paper. *J. Roy. Soc. Med.* **79**, 347–352.

Iqbal, K., McLachlan, D.R.C., Winbald, B. & Wisniewski, H.M. (1991): *Alzheimer's disease: Basic mechanisms, diagnosis and therapeutic strategies.* Chichester: Wiley.

Katzman, R., Terry, R.D. & Bick, K.L. (1978): Recommendations of the nosology, epidemiology, and etiology and pathophysiology of the workshop-conference on Alzheimer's disease-senile dementia and related disorders. In: *Alzheimer's disease: senile dementia and related disorders* (*Aging*, Vol. 7) eds. R. Katzman, R.D. Terry & K.L. Bick, pp. 579–585. New York: Raven Press.

Kievit, J. & Kuypers, H.G.J.M. (1971): Basal forebrain and hypothalamic connections to frontal and parietal cortex in the Rhesus monkey. *Science* **187**, 660–662.

Kumar, V. & Calache, M. (1991): Treatment of Alzheimer's disease with cholinergic drugs. *Int. J. Clin. Pharmacol. Ther. Toxicol.* **29**, 23–37.

Lachs, M. (1993): Tacrine in Alzheimer's disease. Letter to the editor. *N. Engl. J. Med.* **328**, 809.

Lambrechts, W. & Parkhouse, J. (1961): Postoperative amnesia. *Br. J. Anaesth.* **33**, 397–404.

Levy, R. (1993): Tacrine in Alzheimer's disease. Letter to the editor. *N. Engl. J. Med.* **328**, 808.

Lewis, P.R. & Shute, C.C.D. (1967): The cholinergic limbic system: projections to hippocampal formation, medial cortex, nuclei of the ascending cholinergic system, and the subfornical organ and supra-optic crest. *Brain* **90**, 521–540.

Marquis, D. (1983): Leaving therapy to chance. *Hastings Center Report* **8**, 40–47.

McKinney, M., Stuble, R.G., Coyle, J.T. & Price, D.L. (1982): Monkey nucleus basalis is enriched with choline acetyltransferase. *Neuroscience* **7**, 2363.

Milner, B., Corkin, S. & Teuber, H.L. (1968): Further analysis of the hippocampal amnesic syndrome: 14-year follow-up study of H.M. *Neuropsychologia* **6**, 215–34.

Milner, B. (1970): Memory and the medial temporal regions of the brain. In: *Biology of memory*, eds. K.H. Pribram & E. Broadbent, pp. 29–50. New York: Academic Press.

Mohr, E., Schlegel, J., Fabbrini, G. *et al.*(1989): Clonidine treatment of Alzheimer's disease. *Arch. Neurol.* **46**, 376–378.

Nakano, I. & Hirano, A. (1984): Parkinson's disease: neuron loss in the nucleus basalis without concomitant Alzheimer's disease. *Ann. Neurol.* **15**, 415–418.

Pandit, S.K. & Dundee, J.W. (1970): Preoperative amnesia: the indicence following the intramuscular injection of commonly used premedicants. *Anesthesia* **25**, 493–499.

Perry, E.K., Perry, R.H., Blessed, G. & Tomlinson, B.E. (1977a): Necropsy evidence of central Cholinergic deficits in senile dementia. Letter to the editor. *Lancet* i, 189.

Perry, E.K., Gibson, P.H., Blessed, G., Perry, R.H. & Tomlinson, B.E.(1977b): Neurotransmitter enzyme abnormalities in necropsy brain tissue. *J. Neurol. Sci.* **34**, 247–265.

Perry, E.K., Tomlinson, B.E., Blessed, G., Bergmann, K., Gibson, H. & Perry, R.H. (1978): Correlation of Cholinergic abnormalities with senile plaques and mental test scores in senile dementia. *B.M.J.* **2**, 1457–59.

Perry, E.K. & Perry, R.H. (1985): A review of neuropathological and neurochemical correlates of Alzheimer's Disease. *Dan. Med. Bull.* **32**, 27–34.

Reisberg, B. (ed.) (1983): *Alzheimer's Disease.* New York, London: The Free Press.

Rocca, W.A., Hofman, A., Brayne, C. *et al.* (1991): Frequency and distribution of Alzheimer's disease in Europe: A collaborative study of 1980–1990 prevalence findings. *Ann. Neurol.* **30**, 380–90.

Rosenberg, G.S., Greenwald, B. & Davis, K.L. (1983): Pharmacologic treatment of Alzheimer's Disease: an overview. In: *Alzheimer's Disease*, ed. B. Reisberg, pp. 329–339. New York, London: The Free Press.

Rossor, M.N. (1982): Neurotransmitters and CNS Disease: Dementia. *Lancet* ii, 1200–1204.

Sagar, H.J. (1985): Brain behaviour relationships in amnesia and dementia. In: *Senile Dementia of the Alzheimer Type. Neurology and Neurobiology* Vol. 18, eds. J.T. Hutton & A.D. Kenny, pp. 205–218. New York: Alan Liss Inc.

Schafer, A. (1982): The ethics of the randomized clinical trial. *N. Engl. J. Med.* **307**, 719–724.

Schlegel, J., Mohr, E., Williams, J. *et al.* (1989): Guanfacine treatment of Alzheimer's Disease. *Clin. Neuropharmacol.* **12** (2), 124–128.

Schneider, L.S. (1990): Letter to the editor. *N. Engl. J. Med.* **323**, 919–920.

Scoville, W.B. & Milner, B. (1957): Loss of recent memory after bilateral hippocampal lesion. *J. Neurol. Neurosurg. Psychiatry* **20**, 11–21.

Summers, W.K., Majowski, L.V., Marsh, G.M., Tachiki, K. & Kling, M.D. (1986): Oral tetrahydroaminoacridine in long term treatment of senile dementia, Alzheimer type. *N. Engl. J. Med.* **315**, 1241–1245.

Summers, W.K., Majovski, L.V., Marsh, G.M., Tachiki, K. & Kling, A. (1988): Tacrine, back to the future? (Abstract) In: *Advances in Alzheimer therapy: cholinesterase inhibitors*, p. 21. Springfield, IL: Southern Illinois University.

Thal, L.J., Masur, D.M., Blau, A.D., Fuld, P.A. & Klauber, M.R. (1989): Chronic oral. Physostigmine without lecithin improves memory in Alzheimer's disease. *Am. J. Geriatr. Soc.* **37**, 42–48.

Taylor, K.M., Margolese, R.G. & Soskoline, C.L. (1984) Physicians' reasons for not entering eligible patients in a randomized clinical trial of surgery for breast cancer. *N. Engl. J. Med.* **310**, 1363–1367.

Whitehouse, P.J., Price, D.L., Clark, A.W., Coyle, J.T. & DeLong, M.R. (1981): Alzheimer's disease: evidence for selective loss of cholinergic neurons in the nucleus basalis. *Ann. Neurol.* **10**, 122–126.

Whitehouse, P.J., Price, D.L., Struble, R.G., Clark, A.W., Coyle, J.T. & Delong, M.R. (1982): Alzheimer's disease: loss of neurons in the basal forebrain. *Science* **215**, 1237–1239.

Whitehouse, P.J., Struble, R.G., Uhl, G. & Price, D.L. (1985): Dementia: bridging the brain–behavior barrier. In: *Senile dementia of the Alzheimer type (neurology and neurobiology)* Vol. 18, eds. J.T. Hutton & A.D. Kenny, pp. 221–229. New York: Alan Liss Inc.

Winblad, B., Bucht, G., Fowler, C.J. & Wallace, W.C. (1986): Beyond the transmitter-based approach to Alzheimer's Disease. In: *Treatment development strategies for Alzheimer's disease*, ed. T. Crook. New Canaan: Mark Powers Associates Inc.

Wisniewski, H.M. & Terry, R.D. (1973) Reexamination of the pathogenesis of the senile plaque. In: *Progress in neuropathology*, ed. H.M. Zimmerman, pp. 1–26. New York: Grune & Stratton.

Wisniewski, H.M., Bruce, M.E. & Fraser, H. (1975): Infectious etiology of neuritic (senile) plaques in mice. *Science* **190**, 1108–1110.

Wisniewski, H.M. (1978): Possible viral etiology of neurofibrillary changes and neuritic plaques. In: *Alzheimer's disease, senile dementia and related disorders* (*Aging* Vol. 7), eds. R. Katzman, R.D. Terry & K.L. Bick, pp. 555–557. New York: Raven Press.

Witter, A., van Ree, J.M. & Versteeg, D.H.G. (1978): *Farmacologie I: Algemene Farmacologie van het autonome zenuwstelsel.* Utrecht: Wetenschappelijke Uitgeverij Bunge.

The ethics of animal and human experimentation, edited by P.P. De Deyn.
©1994 John Libbey & Company Ltd., pp. 227–247.

20

Placebo: some scientific and ethical considerations

Peter P. De Deyn[*†], Rudi D'Hooge[†] and Barbara A. Pickut[*]

[*]Department of Neurology, General Hospital Middelheim and [†]Department of Neurochemistry and Behaviour, Born-Bunge Foundation, University of Antwerp, Universiteitsplein 1, 2610 Wilrijk-Antwerp, Belgium

Summary

The authors give a historical introduction with regard to placebo. While placebo was originally, until approximately 1940, mostly used as a therapeutic tool, its main application is currently situated in clinical scientific research. The definition of placebo as being an inert substance without (specific) pharmacological effects contrasts with the multitude of effects associated with its prescription and administration. Since the 1940s the placebo effect, a term that refers to diverse non-specific, desired or non-desired effects of substances or procedures and interactions between, e.g., patient and physician, and patient and paramedic, has been described. The placebo effect can be positive as well as negative. In medical practice placebo can be administered intentionally or non-intentionally. The effect of every treatment, irrespective of its nature, is a summation of placebo effect and specific therapeutic effect. The unpredictability of the impact and nature of the placebo effect in any individual or patient population necessitates the placebo-controlled design in most clinical trials.

While prescription or administration of the intentionally therapeutically applied placebo almost necessarily implies deception from the care-giver, this is certainly not the case when placebo is used in scientific research. The consenting subject in the placebo-controlled randomized clinical trial is fully informed about the possible chances of being 'treated' with placebo, thereby excluding deception. In contrast to our opinion, some authors perceive an incompatibility between conducting placebo-controlled clinical trials and obtaining informed consent.

There is however a genuine possibility of conflict that might exist between the care-giving physician and the physician investigator. The treating physician's first obligation is to provide the best available standard therapy in order to help his patient, while the physician-scientist's obligation is to generate objective, valid and patient-oriented applicable scientific data.

The authors argue that objective clinical scientific data and well-considered guidelines allow sensible decision making solving the ethical dilemma mentioned above. Different experimental designs with specific limitations and advantages (or possibilities) are discussed in the light of some case studies. A double-blind placebo-controlled design is considered ethically acceptable provided that: (1) no adequate standard therapy exists for the studied disease; or (2) the possibly active standard therapy has serious side effects; (3) the placebo treatment period is sufficiently short; (4) the administration of placebo or withholding active treatment does not inflict unacceptable risks to the patient and finally; (5) when the patient is informed about his/her possible randomization to the placebo arm and has given consent.

Introduction

History and definitions of placebo

Placebo is the first person singular of the future indicative of the Latin verb *placere* and means: 'I shall please' or 'I shall serve'. To our knowledge, the first written document about placebo dates from 1386 when Chaucer defines placebo as a sycophant or servile flatterer. The power of positive expectation in medical practice was frequently described in literature, throughout the 17th and 18th centuries while the word placebo first entered the medical vocabulary late in the 18th century: Motherby's *New Medical Dictionary* and Quincy's *Lexicon* again defined placebo quite negatively, this time as 'a commonplace method in medicine'. In the early 19th century emphasis was put on the importance of merely pleasing the patient besides curing him. The concept of placebo at that time was the deceptive prescription or administration of an inert medicine with deception in order to please. The negative connotation of placebo persisted into the early 20th century when Richard Cabot still defined placebos as inert medicines, given intentionally by physicians to unsuspecting patients.

The so-called modern concepts and applications of placebo and placebo effects however are more bona fide. To our knowledge, the first rather isolated placebo-controlled clinical trial took place in 1916 and was conducted by Macht who injected physiological saline as a control to check the analgesic action of morphine (Delay & Pichot, 1973). In his note on placebo however, Pepper (1945) still did not refer to this use but enthusiastically defended its therapeutic use. It was only later, in the 1940s and 1950s, that the new usage of placebo in clinical research developed on a larger scale simultaneously with the concept of the placebo effect. In the placebo-controlled clinical trial, for the first time patients were given placebos, not for their own immediate benefit but for the benefit of biomedical sciences. Rather surprising observations on the clinical consequences of administering placebos in the research setting entailed a new term, the 'placebo effect'. Although placebos were still defined as inert medicines or treatments, both inert and active therapies were observed to produce effects beyond their predicted physiological properties. The total of unexplained consequences of administering placebos and active treatments became loosely known as 'the placebo effect'. In 1955, Modell even defined the placebo reaction as 'the only single action which all drugs have in common'

Shapiro (1961) defined placebo as 'any therapeutic procedure (or that component of any therapeutic procedure) which is given deliberately to have an effect, or unknowingly has an effect on a patient, symptom, syndrome, or disease, but which is objectively without specific activity for the condition being treated. The therapeutic procedure may be given with or without conscious knowledge that the procedure is a placebo, may be an active (noninert) or inactive (inert) procedure, and includes, therefore, all medical procedures – no matter how specific, oral and parenteral medications, topical preparations, inhal-ants, and mechanical, surgical and psychotherapeutic procedures. The placebo must be differentiated from the placebo effect which may occur or may not occur and which may be favourable or unfavourable. The placebo effect is defined as the changes produced by placebos'. Some authors even assign a placebo effect to the mere act of diagnosis itself (Brody & Waters, 1980). Finally, Lyerly *et al.* (1964) illustrated that placebo instructions, such as telling the subject that he/she received a drug with such and such activity, influences the perception of the drug's effects.

According to Shapiro & Morris (1978), 'A placebo is defined as any therapy or component of a therapy that is deliberately used for its non-specific, psychological or psychophysiological effect, or that is used for its presumed specific effect, but is without specific activity for the condition being treated'. Other authors referred to the latter as pseudo-placebos, also called unclean placebos, which are active substances without specific effect on the treated condition as for example, vitamin preparations in certain conditions and antibiotics in viral diseases. Also subtherapeutic dosages or administration in homoeopathic dosages of active substances can be seen as (pseudo)placebo treatment.

While, in a historical context, placebo applications were originally exclusively therapeutic, their present day scientific application is the focus of this chapter. Since the earliest days of medical science, and certainly since the advent of clinical drug trials, the placebo effect has been considered a nuisance rather than a therapeutic tool. Given the unpredictability of placebo effects in individual patients and patient groups, the placebo became an irreplacable tool as 'inactive' control in randomized clinical trials. On the other hand, it has to be stressed that placebos have no diagnostic value. The conclusion that a positive reaction to placebos points to the fact that the disease treated or the symptoms are of psychogenic origin is just as incorrect as the assumption that a negative placebo response would be an indication for the existence of an organic disease.

Placebo effects

The placebo effect has been responsible for the efficacy of a majority of therapies throughout the history of medicine, but only in the past 40 to 50 years, along with the introduction of medications with proven specific efficacy, have the effects of placebo treatment been systematically studied. A substantial group of papers discussed the possible mechanisms of placebogenesis which will not be dealt with extensively in this chapter. Lundh (1987) presented a cognitive-emotional model of the mechanisms involved in placebogenesis. Conditioning has been suggested as contributing to the placebo effect, as illustrated by the fact that the order of administration of placebo versus active drug has a definite influence on the frequency of positive responses, those patients treated initially with placebo having a lower response rate than those who are exposed to placebo after taking one or more pharmacologically active agents. Moreover, the placebo effect is exclusively a characteristic of the alert, conscious human being. Levine *et al.* (1978) have presented evidence that naloxone may block placebo analgesia, which may indicate that endorphins play a role in this kind of placebo analgesia, a conclusion that was later disputed by other authors (Gracely *et al.*, 1983).

The placebo (and 'nocebo') effect

Rather surprising observations on the clinical consequences of administering placebos in research setting entailed a new term, 'the placebo effect'. It is important to stress that the placebo effect may be expressed both in the form of subjective clinical variations and in the form of evident objective anatomical and functional variations. Although placebos were still defined as inert medicines or treatments, both inert and active therapies were observed to produce effects beyond their predicted pharmacological properties. The total of unexplained consequences of administering placebos and active treatments became known as the placebo effect.

Placebo effects are known to contribute to the power of many therapeutic interventions and in some cases they might be the most important or even only factor involved. There is still much debate about the effectiveness of psychotherapy (Smith *et al.*, 1980). Research seems to indicate that nonspecific aspects of therapy (placebo effects) determine much of the outcome of psychotherapeutic intervention. Some researchers (e.g. Fish, 1973) have even argued that patient's beliefs about the effectiveness of therapy and the ability of the therapist to influence these beliefs are the key factors that determine the success of therapy.

Certain symptoms, syndromes or diseases are known to be responsive in varying degrees to placebo effects. In 1946, Jellinek studied 199 subjects with headache and found that approximately 60 per cent obtained relief when given placebo while 85 per cent responded to active analgesics. Jellinek, however, as many others, was not aware of the power of placebo and mistakenly dismissed placebo reactors as those having 'imagined pain, psychological headaches'. Lasagna *et al.* (1954) found that 72 per cent of patients with postoperative pain responded to morphine injections, but 40 per cent of these same patients responded to placebo as well. In an analysis of 15 studies involving 1082 patients with various diseases, Beecher (1955) demonstrated placebos to have an average significant effectiveness of 35.2 ± 2.2 per cent. In this review, reported percentages of placebo response ranged from 21 to 58 in the following conditions: postoperative wound pain, cough, drug-induced mood changes, pain from angina pectoris, headache, seasickness, anxiety and tension and common cold. Evans (1974) demonstrated that an average of 36 per cent of patients had at least 50 per cent pain relief under placebo administration. Endogenous-type depressions have placebo response rates around 30 per cent, while those of lesser severity have rates approaching 70 per cent. Also surgical procedures have been demonstrated to induce placebo responses. The earlier discussed relief of angina pectoris by sham operations consisting of a parasternal incision is a clear example of the placebo effect related to surgery (for review see Beecher, 1961). Placebo responses in different studies considering the same symptoms, varied from 0 to 100 per cent indicating the importance of differences in populations, the relationship patient–physician–healer and many other factors (Meyer & Kindli, 1989).

It remains important however to note the distinction between placebo effects and spontaneous remission. Therefore, some placebo effects reported in the literature may instead represent the natural course of the disease or symptoms. Spontaneous remission may be defined as that kind of improvement which occurs independently of contact with a caregiver, as part of the natural course of the disease. Consequently, in the evaluation of the efficacy of any therapeutic procedure, one has always to take three factors into account, namely the nature or natural evolution of the disease, the specific effect of the therapy and finally the placebo effect.

In addition to the beneficial effect of placebo, Beecher (1955) also reported toxic effects associated with placebo use. Warm glow was reported in 8 per cent, dry mouth in 9 per cent, nausea in 10 per cent, sensation of heaviness in 18 per cent, headache in 25 per cent, difficulty concentrating in 15 per cent, drowsiness in 50 per cent, relaxation in 9 per cent, fatigue in 18 per cent and sleep in 10 per cent. Reidenberg & Lowenthal (1968) however, suggested a more cautious interpretation of these findings and introduced a new concept: the 'adverse nondrug reaction'. These authors performed a questionnaire survey, involving students and hospital staff taking no medications, on the occurrence of many symptoms often listed as side-effects of drugs. Their astonishing results indicated that only 19 per cent of the 414 respondents (healthy persons who did not take any medication at all) stated that they had not experienced during the previous 72 hours any of 25 often reported drug side-effects.

Factors that influence the placebo effect

While it remains difficult to determine what causes these placebo effects, it seems more feasible to discuss the elements that appear to contribute to them. These can be categorized into elements in the doctor–patient relationship, the physician, the patient, the treatment situation and the placebo preparation or procedure itself. As those different factors will be dealt with systematically in what follows, it will appear that irrespective of numerous studies, it remains impossible to predict a placebo effect or placebo response in any given subject or patient population.

The therapist–patient relationship

The patient's transference relationship with the therapist, and the countertransference relationship with the patient, are important elements in the placebo reactions and are supposed to contribute to the direction of placebo reactions (positive, negative or absent) and therefore to influence outcome of all treatment. While the concept of transference is difficult to demonstrate experimentally, the term physician–patient relationship refers to it.

The personality of the physician

The friendly, interested, empathic and reassuring physician who thoroughly examines his patients and is not anxious or conflicted is likely to elicit positive placebo effects. On the other hand, negative placebo effects are more likely when the physician appears angry, rejecting, reproaching or contemptuous. Moreover, the therapist's attitude (positive, enthusiastic, negative or doubtful) towards the prescribed or given treatment is also believed to contribute importantly to the treatment outcome. For example, several studies demonstrated that the effectiveness of tranquillizers increased or decreased depending on the attitude of the therapist (Feldman, 1956; Uhlenruth *et al.*, 1959).

The personality of the patient: placebo responders?

Beecher *et al.* (1953) found that persons obtaining relief from placebos got increased relief from some studied oral analgesics as compared to the whole population and concluded that the placebo reactor merited further study. In 1954, Lasagna *et al.* attempted a study of the profile of the so-called placebo reactor and found no differences in sex ratios or in intelligence between reactors and nonreactors. However, they concluded that 'there are significant differences in attitudes, habits, educational background and personality structure between consistent reactors and nonreactors'. Most placebo responders displayed placebo effects inconsistently, that is to say, sometimes the placebo produced relief and sometimes not. Several investigators have attempted to relate the placebo effect to personality and characterized placebo reactors as compliant, religious, hypochondriac, anxious, depressed, neurotic, dependent and so on. However, many of the personality clusters found in some studies could not be duplicated in others. Although there does not seem to exist a placebo type or a global personality type that responds to placebo under all conditions, placebo response may still correlate with more limited personality characteristics. For example, Steinbook *et al.* (1965) were able to relate primary suggestibility to placebo response.

Moertel *et al.* (1976) studied several possible characteristics of placebo responders in a population consisting of 288 cancer patients undergoing controlled trials of oral analgesics. Among those, 112 received 50 per cent or greater pain relief from placebo formulations. Patients who responded to placebo had a greater response rate to active drugs. They also had a higher incidence of central nervous system side effects to placebo. Patient groups showing an increased placebo response included those with a high level of education, those with a professional occupation, farmers, women working outside the home, and patients who were widowed, separated, or divorced. Those resistant to placebo were patients with a low educational level, unskilled workers, housewives, married women without children, and smokers. Also according to this study, gender, age, number of siblings, alcohol consumption and pain severity did not influence the placebo responsiveness. Surprisingly, smokers were clearly less susceptible to placebo than non-smokers. The higher placebo response rate as found by Moertel *et al.* for highly educated people was in contradiction with the findings of Lasagna *et al.* (1954) who suggested the opposite correlation.

Since the awareness of the existence of the placebo effect, numerous other studies further aimed at characterizing the placebo responders. However, their attempt to identify 'placebo reactors' with the objective of eliminating individuals so identified from inclusion in experimental trials, obviating the need for controls, remained unsuccessful.

The therapeutic setting

An important variability of placebo effect between different centres has been documented. The nature and degree of placebo effect may be influenced by staff attitudes, expectations and biases. Moreover, importance has rightly been attached to the healing context of the medical visit (e.g. diplomas displayed, physician wearing a white coat).

Factors of the preparation or procedure

Characteristics of the administered placebo influence its effect. For example, reactions to the taste, smell, size, colour, shape and price of tablets or capsules may vary considerably. Blue medications are experienced as more sedative, red ones as more stimulating, white ones as analgesic and lavender ones as hallucinogenic. As an example, 'sleep-inducing' placebo administered as a tablet was active in 49 per cent of subjects while when administered as 'sleepdrink' it was efficient in 71 per cent and finally, when administered as as gelatine capsule, it was active in 81 per cent (Kuschinsky, 1975). In a study of 48 patients with anxiety states, green oxazepam tablets were more active than red and yellow ones whereas depressive symptoms appeared to respond best to yellow tablets

(Schapira *et al.*, 1970). Buckalew & Coffield's (1982) data showed non-random distributions for nine capsule colours in anticipated action, with specific effects of four colours. There was a clear agreement between Jacobs & Nordan's data (1979), Schapira *et al.*'s data (1970) and this study in the perception of a yellow capsule as stimulant–antidepressant. Moreover, a significant difference between capsule and tablet for perceived strength was found in favour of the capsule, as was a trend relating capsule size to preceived drug strength. Greater placebo effects can be expected with injections, various complicated procedures and impressive machines. As an example of the latter, medical students often remember the patients they adequately 'cured' from angina pectoris by performing an electrocardiography.

Placebo-controlled RCTs

It is precisely the variability of the placebo effect which emphasizes the need for controlled clinical trials. Essential in this application is that the placebo is not meant to please but to provide a good control, denominated 'dummy' by certain authors. The inclusion of a placebo arm in randomized clinical trials (RCTs) permits adequate evaluation of the efficacy, safety and toxicity of new potential pharmacologically active agents.

Several stories with regard to the development of originally presumed therapeutic procedures illustrate the tremendous need of placebo-controlled clinical trials. An example is a surgical technique (ligation of the internal mammary artery) once proclaimed to be efficacious for the treatment of angina pectoris which turned out to be a mere placebo. In the 1950s, considerable relief of symptoms was reported for patients with angina pectoris subjected to bilateral ligation of the internal mammary artery. It was postulated that increased coronary flow was facilitated through collateral channels proximal to the site of ligation. An Italian clinician, Battezzati and his colleagues (1955) were the first to apply this technique in the early 1950s. An enthusiastic report written by Ratcliff (1957) was published in *Reader's Digest*. As early as one year later, promising results were also reported by several American researchers who communicated their enthusiasm based upon data provided by non-controlled trials (Brill *et al.*, 1958; Harken, 1958; Kitchell *et al.*, 1958). Placebo-controlled trials however disproved the presumed efficacy of this 'popular' surgical treatment for angina pectoris. It took two double-blind studies involving a total of 35 subjects. Fourteen of them were placebo-treated or sham-operated and 21 underwent a ligation of the internal mammary arteries demonstrating the lack of efficacy of the procedure which was performed under local anesthesia (Dimond *et al.* 1958; Cobb *et al.*, 1959). The 'placebo' procedure consisted of parasternal skin incisions without ligation while the 'active' treatment consisted of parasternal skin incisions followed by ligation of the internal mammary artery. Later, it was demonstrated that internal mammary artery ligation did not result in an increased perfusion of the cardiac muscle and had no effect on the pathophysiology of coronary-artery disease. Although deception was obvious in these two placebo-controlled trials, patients not being informed about the possibility of a sham operation, the double-blind evaluation of the procedure's effect in 35 patients prevented the wide-spread introduction of this not efficacious surgical procedure.

The demonstration that a new drug is safe and effective for its intended use is a legal requirement for marketing a new drug in the United States of America (USA) and in many other countries. Evidence submitted to the USA Food and Drug Administration (FDA) to satisfy this requirement must include 'adequate and well-controlled investigations' characterized in regulations as clinical studies capable of distinguishing 'the effect of a drug from other influences, such as spontaneous change in the course of the disease, placebo effect, or biased observation'. According to the FDA regulation this usually necessitates standard clinical trial features such as (inactive) control groups, randomized assignment to treatment, and blinded assessment outcome.

In a recent paper Leber from the USA FDA (1991) stresses the necessity of performing randomized controlled clinical trials and strengthens his point by a couple of case reports in the field of psychiatry. Although Leber, an FDA division director making recommendations on the marketing of drug products used in psychiatry and neurology, states that 'There is no alternative to the randomized controlled design – no ifs, ands, or buts!' he certainly does not claim the infallibility of the RCT device. The authors agree with him that in the absence of fraud and/or break of blinding, a difference in outcome among patients concurrently randomized to therapy cannot be attributed to personal beliefs, secondary interests, or prejudgements of patients, investigators or sponsors. Open studies, case series and studies relying on external or historical controls do not allow sound conclusions. Usually, it is highly unreliable to draw conclusions based on historical controls, even more so when they are applied for evaluating efficacy against diseases with poorly known natural history or when the history is known but characteristically highly variable, such as, e.g., insomnia, anxiety, depression and pain syndromes (Lasagna, 1961; Leber, 1983, 1989).

As Leber (1991) illustrates, even RCTs that fail to find differences between treatment groups often cannot be interpreted without danger. Indeed, a study failing to demonstrate a difference between a new drug and a standard drug does not necessarily indicate the efficacy of the new drug because the assumption that the outcome of the experiment is merely a function of the drugs administered is treacherous. In his 1989 paper, Leber describes the results of six placebo-controlled clinical trials on the treatment of depression with an imipramine and a new drug arm. Statistical analysis of the results in all six studies indicated that the patients treated with imipramine and the new drug improved to the same extent, implying that the new drug was not only effective but equipotent to imipramine. However, taking the response in the placebo-treated group into account, only one out of six studies was indicative of an antidepressant effect of the new agent. Without the inclusion of a placebo arm, it would have been impossible to show that the improvement was probably not related to pharmacological effects of the administered agents. Another example, provided by the same author (Leber, 1989), regards the difficulties that a pharmaceutical company encounters in documenting the efficacy of an antidepressive agent already widely marketed outside the USA. Here again, the new drug was as 'efficacious' as the standard controls, desipramine and imipramine, but did not induce a significantly different change on the Hamilton scale than did placebo. While according to some authors, (placebo)-controlled RCTs lack sufficient sensitivity in identifying active agents, the authors refer to the above examples on antidepressants and internal mammary artery ligation and stress that the RCT certainly will keep the number of ineffective drugs marketed and widely introduced nontherapeutic surgical and other procedures to a minimum.

Possible ethical problems related to the use of placebo

The two major ethical problems in the use of placebo involve deception when used therapeutically or used in research without adequate patient information and informed consent, and the potential conflict between the deontological and scientific obligations of the physician-researcher. The ethical issues related to the therapeutic applications of placebo will be addressed only briefly since this volume mainly focuses on experimentation and therefore also on placebo's application in this context.

Deceipt related to placebo application

While it is general practice to apply placebo in a deceptive way in a therapeutic setting, this is certainly unacceptable when applying placebo as a scientific tool, as an inactive control in clinical research. Even in the former case, some reports demonstrated the possible disclosure of the placebo nature of the treatment. Indeed, studying a neurotic population, Park & Covi (1965) disproved the view that unawareness of the real nature of the placebo is a necessity for the placebo effect. These authors demonstrated that placebo could be applied successfully as a therapeutic agent in an open manner in a neurotic population presenting signs of anxiety. The patient information consisted in part of the following statement: 'Many different kinds of tranquilizers and similar pills have been used for conditions such as yours, and many of them have helped. Many people with your kind of condition have also been helped by what are sometimes called "sugar pills", and we feel that a so-called sugar pill may help you, too. Do you know what a sugar pill is? A sugar pill is a pill with no medicine in it at all. I think this pill will help you as it has helped so many others. Are you willing to try this pill'? Virtually all patients accepted the placebo 'treatment' and improved over 1 week. However, Park & Covi (1965) also found that a number of patients refused to believe they received placebo.

However, many other authors, including Elander (1991) still quite vividly defend the therapeutic use of placebo and suggest that the principle of autonomy or self-determination may be violated provided that one adopts a consequentialistic or utilitarian strategy towards the individual patient and/or the patient population as a whole. Goodwin *et al.* (1979), on the other hand, point to the important unethical and non-scientific use of placebo in so-called therapeutic and diagnostic contexts. These investigators surveyed 60 house officers and 39 registered nurses to ascertain their knowledge of placebo action and their patterns of placebo use. Obviously, most respondents underestimated or were unaware of the power of placebo. Moreover, and unfortunately, the following patterns of placebo use emerged: (1) use of placebo to prove the patient 'wrong', that is, to diagnose psychogenic symptoms in a patient who is thought to be exaggerating, imagining or faking his symptoms; (2) use of placebos in disliked or 'undeserving' patients such as alcoholic, psychotic or manipulative and demanding patients; (3) use of placebos in situations in which standard treatments are either failing or making the patient worse; and (4) use of placebo as a group activity to release staff frustration towards 'difficult' patients.

We believe that deception in the therapeutic use of placebo still might be ethically acceptable in certain well-defined limited cases, when the physician is for example dealing with subjects with a tendency to substance abuse or when subjects have to be withdrawn from certain addictive agents. The other therapeutic usages of placebo in non-informed patients as described above are regrettable, ethically unacceptable and illustrative of ignorance and prejudice. With regard to the first use as described by Goodwin *et al.* (1979), we insist upon informing the reader that malingerers or drug addicts do not have a greater likelihood of being relieved by a placebo. On the contrary, the impression given by most of the studies is that such patients are less likely to be placebo responders. Moreover, there is also no evidence that a complaining or 'manipulative' patient is more likely to respond to placebo than a patient who is well liked by the hospital staff (Lasagna *et al.*, 1954).

In the scientific application of placebo, however, informed consent should be mandatory, implying that complete information with regard to the rationale, the design, the eventual standard therapeutic procedures for the given disease, the randomization procedure, and the chance of being randomized to placebo should be communicated and discussed. Moreover, the informed consent procedure as dealt with extensively in Ch. 21 (*Dissent on informed consent*), requires the patient to be informed about all risks and benefits associated with the trial and the patient's right to withdraw at any time. Some authors disagree here and as an example we would like to cite from Brewin (1982): 'But in certain situations – especially if we describe every treatment hazard (likely, unlikely, remote) or spell out every unpleasant possibility [. . .] – the very same informed consent that is helpful to one patient may turn out to be a disaster for the peace of mind of another'. In the same paper, Brewin, who opposes compulsory informed consent, furthermore states that, 'Part of the trouble, as with communication of diagnosis and prognosis, is that our present age – hating secrecy, despising paternalism, and reluctant to take anything on trust – finds it especially difficult to accept that too much information may be as bad as too little'. The author goes even further by suggesting that some doctors, once in possession of written informed consent, might become less concerned than they should be about their ethical responsibilities. The authors of this chapter do not share this fear.

Still other authors perceive an incompatibility between informed consent and placebo control or treatment yielding a conflict between deontological obligation and scientific rigor (Levine, 1987). Levine (1987) warrants for the fact that in subjects who are informed of the expected therapeutic and adverse effects of pharmacologically active agents in placebo-controlled trials, types of behaviour are likely to be influenced by having been so informed. In some cases these behavioural changes may introduce serious biases in the results of the study. For example, in several clinical trials, providing such information, the subjects have been able to correctly 'guess' their treatment assignments. Such unblinding is, of course, detrimental to the purposes of using a double-blind design in the first place. Therefore, Levine (1987) proposes a modification of the process of informed consent to placebo-controlled clinical trials in a way that would eliminate or at least reduce its tendency to undermine the results of these studies without defeating the ethical purpose of informed consent. The author suggests that disclosure be presented in the following form: 'If you participate in this study, there is a possibility that you may develop some side effects of the drugs. These include some but not all of the following: gastro-intestinal distress, headache, ringing in the ears, skin rashes, dizziness, joint pain, and blurred vision. If in the course of this study, you have any of these problems, please report them to the investigator.' In other words, Levine proposes giving a list containing in addition to the eventually well-known side effects, irrelevant ones that are of the same order of importance as the actual expected side effects. This proposal is consistent with the ethical purposes of informed consent in that it entails disclosure of material risks. It will also reduce the probability of correct 'guesses' about treatment group assignment and otherwise reduce the introduction by informed consent of bias into the results of the study.

An ethical issue to be discussed concerns what patients are capable of understanding about placebo-controlled trials. Do the patients really know what placebo means, do they realize that they have a certain chance of receiving placebo, and why they will? Stanley (1987) reviewed the literature and concluded that irrespective of their condition and whether or not they were psychiatric patients, patients were fairly able to understand the risks and benefits of a proposed treatment and the purpose of a particular treatment or procedure.

Potential ethical conflict between deontological and scientific obligations related to placebo application in RCTs

The physician is subject to two fundamental ethical obligations, a deontological one and a scientific one. The clinician's deontological obligation obliges him to apply all existing knowledge for the best possible treatment of each individual patient. On the other hand, in agreement with the physician's scientific obligations it is unethical not to produce sound scientific data. According to the latter obligation, it is the duty of the physician to acquire new knowledge so that, by such advance, future patients might benefit, and, having acquired new knowledge, to communicate it accurately to the scientific community in order to contribute to the collective benefit. However, these two obligations may at certain occasions be in contradiction in the execution and design of placebo-controlled RCTs. According to certain people, randomization by itself means that the patient is no longer being treated purely for his own good. It is feared he is being 'used' – at best for the benefit of future sufferers from his condition, at worst merely to satisfy scientific curiosity – and that, in terms of hazard, benefit, or both, he risks being treated in a way that would not normally be considered appropriate for him. It is thought that some kind of sacrifice is being demanded of him and that he should either be given a full explanation or else not randomized. A physician in his normal practice, giving treatment without randomization however, is trusted to choose from several options, even though there may be no way that he can be sure which is best. The authors prefer to term the physician's treatment choice for a given individual the 'individual trial'. This individual trial is practiced daily by every physician world-wide and often does not apply the safeguards of well-designed controlled clinical trials.

The primary question is whether it can be ethically justified to deprive a certain percentage of patients in placebo-controlled trials of their 'right to receive' a drug of acknowledged efficacy merely in order to verify whether other active drugs exist. Although withholding a treatment of proved efficacy potentially violates the physician's commitment to individual patient welfare, it does not imply that allocating patients to the standard therapy control group, or to the placebo standard group when no standard therapy exists, or when doing so in developing new drugs for treatment of an already (partially) treatable disease does not inflict unnecessary danger to the subject, is a violation of the deontological commitment. Basically speaking, the choice in the latter case is between adopting a form of treatment known to be efficacious and attempting to come up with an alternative, more beneficial and safer form of therapy.

The conflict between physician and physician–investigator is often less founded on scientific than on emotional basis. Some physicians tend to stress the pragmatic viewpoint of the RCT: only the application of an accepted treatment as the control arm can answer the question whether the new treatment improves a standard method. According to these clinicians, explanation that a new drug is better than no treatment may interest drug regulatory agencies, but has no practical implication for the treatment of patients. We believe this is a weak and short-sighted reasoning. Indeed, the use of placebo-controlled clinical trial designs is the only way to keep the number of ineffective drugs marketed and widely introduced nontherapeutic surgical and other procedures to a minimum, as is also illustrated above by the internal mammary artery ligation case and the examples given by Leber. The conviction that ignorance may cause patients harm may not only be used as a justification for research but in addition renders research an ethical obligation. The important ethical difficulties associated with the widespread application of a new treatment without a trial and consequently potentially without specific effects but with varying degrees of side-effects, is far greater than those associated with the trial itself. The optimal and therefore often placebo-controlled and ethically founded clinical trial meets the duties of benefiting society and increasing knowledge without jeopardizing the well-being of the experimental subjects.

There are many examples of marketed compounds without proven efficacy and, in addition, several companies marketed so-called alternative medicines such as homoeopathic and anthroposophic compounds, herbs and 'pseudovitamins' evading or disregarding drug regulatory requirements. Recently, Pope (1992) correctly stated that 40 different compounds for treatment of Alzheimer's disease are available in Europe without any proven efficacy. An example where the pharmaceutical industry deliberately disregards high scientific standard placebo-controlled clinical trials and continues to actively market a placebo or at best a (pseudo)placebo is provided by the *Ginkgo biloba* case (Schönhöfer *et al.*, 1989). In 1988, 5.24 million prescriptions for *Ginkgo biloba* extract involved a cost of DM 370 million to former West German sickness insurance. In 1992 sales were comparable with total costs of approximately DM 368 million. The drug, licensed under the drug law of 1986 which does not require scientific evidence from controlled trials but merely positive therapeutic 'experiences', is promoted for treatment of peripheral arterial disease, memory impairment, vertigo, impotence and so on. Although the company sponsors a lot of clinical studies testing their preparation, they seem to carefully avoid using clinically relevant items as efficacy parameters. Scientists publishing scientifically sound negative information with regard to this preparation were threatened with legal action, were unsuccessfully sued and subjected to personal attacks (Schönhöfer, 1990). In 1992, Kleijnen & Knipschild, published a review paper that was more in favour of *Ginkgo biloba*. Unfortunately, this review was based on a rather small selection of studies conducted with this extract (most trials 'have shortcomings in the methods, including small numbers of patients, inadequate descriptions of randomization, patient characteristics, and effect measurements, and poor data presentation'). Moreover, as Kimbel (1992) also pointed out, most studies were not really conclusive and referred to papers not published in peer-reviewed journals. Kimbel (1992), moreover, writes that 'The obvious discrepancy that *Ginkgo biloba* extracts are among the most prescribed medicines in France and Germany but not licensed in Anglo-American and Scandinavian countries suggests widely differing standards of acceptance. Would it not be advisable to base any therapeutic conclusions on the criteria of leading regulatory agencies i.e. evaluation of all published and unpublished studies and use of established standards for clinically relevant efficacy?' We fully agree and conclude that the presented case illustrates that well-controlled RCTs are an ethical obligation and that drug-approval authorities should base their decisions exclusively on high standard data disregarding 'anecdotal' clinical 'experiences'.

Another, although less extreme, example concerns an agent with presumed efficacy in the treatment of diabetic and alcoholic polyneuropathy. The compound is being marketed in Germany without extremely convincing evidence of its activity, and the manufacturing and marketing company prefers not to take the option of distributing their compound throughout Europe since this would entail a registration procedure necessitating additional placebo-controlled RCTs. If their compound has does indeed have specific efficacy against these forms of polyneuropathy, it would be unethical not to provide it to all patients world-wide. As a matter of fact, this specific company prefers to keep a significant market for a possible placebo or pseudoplacebo instead of developing a potential panacea for patients suffering from diabetic and alcoholic neuropathy world-wide.

Methodologically well-designed trials may be unethical

A methodologically bad trial is always unethical but a methodologically good one is not in itself ethical. Beecher (1966) discusses an impressive series of examples of unethical studies in an attempt to prevent repetition of such practices. His examples date from the 1940s to the 1960s and involve studies in which patients were denied active antibiotic treatment, leading to death in many of them, and research protocols in which mentally handicapped subjects and juvenile delinquents were subjected to toxic agents. In other studies, the toxicity of certain substances inducing lethal effects was studied and non-therapeutic invasive surgical procedures were performed without informed consent. In still other studies, cerebral ischaemia was induced and alcoholic patients were subjected to certain toxins inducing hepatic encephalopathy. Artificial induction of hepatitis was carried out in a vulnerable patient population of mentally defective children. Finally, cancer cells were injected into 22 human subjects and a highly malignant melanoma was transplanted from a daughter to her volunteering and informed mother. While most of these studies were scientifically sound, they were ethically unacceptable since informed consent was not obtained in most cases and/or experimental subjects were subjected to unacceptable risks.

As another example, already discussed above, well-designed placebo controlled trials that disproved the presumed efficacy of the internal mammary artery ligation for angina pectoris involved deception, patients not being informed about the possibility of a sham operation (Dimond *et al.*, 1958; Cobb *et al.*, 1959).

Still another remarkable case of unethical research was the well-known Tuskegee syphilis study. This study was designed to determine the natural course of untreated latent syphilis. The studies started in 1932, an era when syphilis still was treated with various drugs containing heavy metals. Although it was supposed that such treatment reduced mortality and morbidity, it was suspected that some of the complications attributed to syphilis were actually iatrogenic. The recruited subjects (black men) were not informed about the withholding of treatment and were even deceived by being told that some of the investigational procedures were actually therapies. Already in 1936 it was evident that the control group developed many more complications than the treated group, leading to increased death rates. Even in the 1940s, when an adequate treatment, namely penicillin, became available, the men were not informed of this. Although there was evidence that withholding treatment shortened life expectancy by approximately 20 per cent, the study was continued until approximately 1972 (Brandt, 1978).

The 'San Antonio Contraceptive Study' was designed to determine which of the alleged side effects of an oral contraceptive were due to the drug and which 'reflect the symptomatology of every day life'. Although the study was well designed in order to obtain the requested information, some ethical considerations were disregarded. Most of the enrolled subjects were impoverished Mexican-American women who had previously had multiple pregnancies and came to the clinic seeking contraceptive treatment. The study had a placebo-controlled double-blind cross-over design in which one-half of the women received placebo first and the other half received the active contraceptive with a switch of medications midway through the study. None of the women were told that a placebo was used as part of the study. However, all women were advised to use a vaginal cream as a contraceptive for the duration of the study. Of the 76 subjects, 11 became pregnant during the course of the study, 10 while taking placebo and one while receiving the active contraceptive.

At present, as discussed amply in several other chapters of this book, practices as outlined above no longer take place. Sufficient ethical safeguards have been introduced to prevent this, through activities of Institutional Review Boards, increased awareness of patients of their rights to self-determination and rather well defined publication policies; scientific journals requiring ethical approval for performed studies and editors and referees judging the ethical acceptability of the presented research.

A couple of case studies on the acceptability of placebo-controlled RCTs

One is often surprised by the prejudices that exist in evaluating the ethical acceptability of certain clinical trial protocols. It is essential to be fully informed about the current state of the biomedical knowledge with regard to the disease being considered in order to be able to give advice correctly. A couple of case studies will illustrate this necessity. An example will be given with regard to the development of new agents against gastroduodenal ulcers, depression and schizophrenia. Ethical concern is also related to the development of many other medications among which are new antiepileptic agents as will be dealt with elsewhere in this volume (Ch. 24, *Clinical evaluation of antiepileptic drugs: guidelines of the International League Against Epilepsy*). Determining factors for the rejection of placebo- controlled non add-on trials in most cases in epileptology, are the nature of the disease with the well known possibility of immediate damage resulting from epileptic seizures and the possibility that certain types of seizures may cause remote permanent neurological injury.

Gastroduodenal ulcers

An intriguing example is the development of new agents with therapeutic efficacy against gastroduodenal ulcers. With the advent of potent agents such as cimetidine, ranitidine and omeprazol one could prematurely conclude that any placebo-controlled trial is to be considered ethically unacceptable. Indeed, Institutional Review Boards or Commissions on Medical Ethics are sometimes reluctant to approve placebo-controlled therapeutic trials for peptic ulcer or inflammatory bowel disease on the grounds that placebo treatment for these potentially serious conditions might not be ethically justifiable. However, several studies yield data consistent with Sircus's (1980) assumption that 40 per cent of ulcers heal with placebo in 4 weeks, 60 per cent in 6 weeks and 80 per cent by week 8. Scheurer *et al.* (1977) reported that in the third week of placebo treatment the original ulcer size reduced by 71 per cent in gastric ulcer and by 83 per cent in duodenal ulcer, and these percentages increased to 82 per cent and 83 per cent respectively by week 6. This is of course a substantial placebo effect which may even have justified the provocative paper of Blum (1982) entitled 'Is placebo the ideal anti-ulcer drug?'. Isenberg *et al.* (1983), however, demonstrated that compared with placebo, cimetidine significantly expedited the healing of benign gastric ulcers, shifting the time-response curve to the left. The time for healing of ulcers in 50 per cent of patients was 3.8 weeks in the cimetidine group and 7.0 weeks in the placebo group. By 12 weeks, the total proportion of patients whose ulcers had healed was 90 per cent in the cimetidine group and 70 per cent in the placebo group. By 12 weeks, the results with low-dose antacid were similar to those with cimetidine, suggesting that the maximum incidence of healing was comparable. Neither cimetidine nor antacid was more effective than placebo in relieving symptoms. The potential advantages of faster healing include a lower overall cost of therapy and perhaps a lower incidence of ulcer complications.

The important placebo response in gastroduodenal ulcers necessitates the placebo-controlled arm, as outlined above by Leber for depression, in order to avoid the erroneous conclusion that both agents are effective if equivalence is shown in active control trials. Adequate statistical information may be obtained in placebo-controlled trials (even in single centres) with only a relatively limited number of patients and the exposure of important numbers of patients to ineffective and toxic compounds may be prevented. Trials in this area should consider a placebo arm, an investigational drug group and a standard drug group. A new efficacious drug should be equally potent to the other standard therapy and display fewer side-effects or have a higher efficacy with equal side-effects or have a decreased dose frequency and additionally be significantly better than placebo (in relieving pain, accelerating ulcer healing or preventing ulcer complications). In order to achieve this in an ethically acceptable manner, several guidelines and safeguards in the experimental designs have been introduced in order to produce scientifically sound data without inflicting suffering or unnecessary damage to experimental subjects. Proposals in this regard were made by several authors among whom are Dobrilla (1983), Sachar *et al.* (1984), Freston (1986), Schiller & Fordtran (1986), Lauritsen & Rask-Madsen (1987) and Smith (1989, on behalf of the American College of Gastroenterology (ACG) Committee on FDA-related Matters).

In 1986 Schiller & Fordtran stated that the low incidence of serious ulcer complications (bleeding, obstruction and perforation) with placebo makes it reasonable and ethical to continue to do placebo-controlled trials on patients with uncomplicated duodenal ulcer disease, provided that: (1) specific entry and exclusion criteria are applied (e.g. are excluded patients with preexisting ulcer complications, elderly patients, and those with large ulcers); (2) the treatment period is sufficiently short; (3) patients understand the risks and give informed consent; and (4) patients in such trials are observed carefully. Moreover, the AGC's Committee on FDA-related Matters concludes that placebo-controlled trials remain the least ambiguous method of evaluating drug efficacy for peptic ulcer disease; that short-term trials with strict entrance criteria are associated with low risk for participants; that the inclusion of escape clauses (antacid use or withdrawal from the study) is an important protective mechanism; that comparison of a new drug against a standard drug is the least convincing method to assessing drug efficacy; and finally, that dose-ranging studies, to demonstrate dose-related efficacy of the new drugs might offer an alternative to simple placebo-controlled trials (Smith, 1989; on behalf of ACG Committee on FDA-related Matters). On the other hand, one might at present entertain doubts about how far there is still potential for yet another therapeutic gain in gastroduodenal ulcer healing.

Depression and schizophrenia

The acceptability of conducting placebo-controlled RCTs for development of new antidepressants is another topic of ethical concern. Endogenous-type depressions have placebo response rates around 30 per cent, while neurotic or reactive depressions have rates approaching 70 per cent (see Brown, 1988, for review). The more severe depressions, for example those with Hamilton Psychiatric Rating Scale for Depression scores greater than 20, have placebo responses between 30 and 40 per cent while those with less severe illness (Hamilton score below 14) have placebo-response rates greater than 50 per cent. Brown (1988) also found no difference between baseline clinical and demographic characteristics of placebo responders and non-placebo responders in a rather large group of patients with major depression, illustrating the limited predictability of placebo response in any patient subgroup. Quitkin *et al.* (1991) analysed the heterogeneity of clinical response during placebo treatment in 144 patients who met the DSM-III criteria for depressive illness and who were randomly assigned to placebo medication in four double-blind antidepressant drug trials. Half of the patients were rated as improved for at least 1 week, whereas 23 per cent had abrupt improvements and 27 per cent had gradual improvements. Abrupt improvements were observed early and were less likely to persist while gradual improvements occurred evenly throughout the first 6 weeks of treatment and tended to persist. The gradual improvements resembled the true drug response since 70 per cent occurred after a 2 week delay. The authors attributed the gradual improvement to spontaneous remission. The difference in improvement rates between drug-treated and placebo-treated non-endogenous patients is probably not great enough to make placebo control unethical. Moreover, in psychiatry, the case in favour of placebos is perhaps stronger than in other fields of medicine because there is a heavy reliance on self-reporting to evaluate improvement and the greater possibility of subjective response to treatment. While the previously described problems in testing the efficacy of antidepressants in active control studies are clearly illustrated above by the examples given by Leber, we believe that caution is warranted. Indeed, in certain cases placebo use may not be advisable; for instance, with depressed patients at significant risk of suicide, with psychotic features, or with severe functional impairment.

Several authors have questioned the ethical acceptability of short-term placebo treatment of chronic schizophrenics (Curson *et al.*, 1986). Again an equilibrium between our scientific and deontological obligations should be sought. It is obvious that double-blind placebo-controlled trials are here also the most reliable methods of assessing potential new antipsychotic agents. Nevertheless, some clinicians fear that relapse contributes to long-term deterioration and therefore that subjects exposed to placebo or inactive new agents might be put at a long-term disadvantage when the trial leads to an additional relapse. Although 66 per cent of patients given placebo and only 8 per cent of those given the active drug fluphenzine decanoate relapsed during their original trial, Curson *et al.* (1986) were unable to demonstrate differences between the groups in any clinical or social variable measured at the end of 7 years of follow up. Moreover, there was no difference in the number of relapses after the end of the trial between patients who received placebo and those who received the active drug. Nevertheless, one should not overlook the suffering experienced by the placebo-treated persons who suffered relapses during the placebo-controlled trial. The authors of this chapter are of the opinion that placebo-controlled clinical trials are acceptable in this patient population on condition that escape antipsychotic treatments are provided by well thought-through exit criteria applicable a within reasonable time after relapse.

Proposed possibilities for ethically inspired modifications of placebo-controlled RCTs

While the placebo-controlled RCT is the gold standard for development of new pharmaceutical compounds, some alternatives have been proposed with varying degrees of success and scientific validity. Positive control studies, comparing the new drug with a previously proven effective one, have several pitfalls as demonstrated by several antidepressive trials (type II errors). Placebo-controlled add-on designs may be valid but drug interactions and other difficulties for the study of side effects are frequently encountered. Equally active new compounds with fewer side effects may not be identified. Still an alternative is randomizing to active drug *vs* placebo but allowing access to standard therapy (e.g. antacid for peptic ulcer on a p.r.n. basis, with utilization thereof being one of the criteria of therapeutic response). Here, the use of the rescue medication may serve both as protection for the placebo group and a measure of efficacy of the treatment under study. Introducing an open active treatment extension may render the placebo-controlled design more acceptable or attractive to the participating subjects. In a sometimes rather deceptive way, some protocols do not consider a placebo arm but include a low-dosage arm of which the lack of efficacy has already been proven in earlier trials. Dose-dependency of the observed effects however would be indicative of the specific nature of the observed effects. Double-blind RCTs with a cross-over design as opposed to a parallel design deserve to be mentioned as well. These designs may allow all patients to receive active medication during at least part of the trial. One of the major flaws however, is the fact that carry-over effects may cloud the obtained results. Finally, we would like to mention our view that reduction of the proportion of patients randomized in the placebo arm does not render the trial design more ethically acceptable. Indeed, if a placebo control is unethical in any given study, it remains unethical, whether applied to 50 per cent or 1 per cent of patients.

Conclusions

Since it is ethically unacceptable to perform clinical trials that are not scientifically well designed and to market active compounds without specific effect, that is with efficacy not exceeding that of placebo in a given disease and with side effects potentially more important than those of placebo, the authors argue that well-designed optimally controlled randomized clinical trials form the only valid tool for improvement of biomedical sciences. The placebo control group represents a control for a 'package' of effects which potentially could obscure and confound the demonstration of drug efficacy. These include: (1) the passage of time, particularly for patients with disorders with an inherent tendency to remit; (2) the increased attention and encouragement given to the patient; (3) the patient's expectations and hope for improvement; and (4) the psychosocial consequences of being legitimized in the sick role. Placebo controls are not always mandatory but neither are they always dangerous. The need for placebos as controls has to be evaluated in a case-by-case manner. Discussing placebo issues involves discussing both scientific issues and ethical issues.

The nature of the disease process being treated, the duration of the study period, the probable therapeutic–toxic ratio of the agent being tested, the availability and appropriateness of alternative therapy, and many other considerations must all play their roles in the design of any clinical trial. The placebo-controlled RCT is the domain in which deontological and scientific obligations can be reconciled. A placebo-controlled experimental design is not only ethically acceptable but often an ethical obligation provided some of the following criteria are applied: (1) there is no adequate standard therapy for the studied disease; or (2) the (presumed) active therapy has important side-effects; (3) placebo 'treatment' period is not too long; (4) giving a placebo treatment does not inflict unacceptable risks to the patient; and (5) the experimental subject is fully informed and informed consent given. These principles and guidelines help the physician in achieving equilibrium between not jeopardizing patients' welfare and not compromising high standards of scientific investigation.

References

Battezzati, M., Tagliaferro, A. & de Marchi, G. (1955): La legatura delle due arterie mammalie interne nei disturbi di vascolarizzazione del miocardio: nota preventiva relativa de primi dati sperimentali e clinici. *Minerva Med.* **46,** 1178–1188.

Beecher, H.K., Keats, A.S., Mosteller, F. & Lasagna, L. (1953): The effectiveness of oral analgesics (morphine, codeine, acetylsalicylic acid) and the problem of placebo 'reactors' and 'non-reactors'. *J. Pharmacol. Exp. Ther.* **109,** 393–400.

Beecher, H.K. (1955): The powerful placebo. *J.A.M.A.* **159,** 1602–1606.

Beecher, H.K. (1961): Surgery as placebo. A quantitative study of bias. *J.A.M.A.* **176,** 1102–1107.

Beecher, H.K. (1966): Ethics and clinical research. *N. Engl. J. Med.* **274 (24),** 1354–1360.

Blum, A.L. (1982): Is placebo the ideal antiulcer drug? In: *Peptic ulcer disease. advances in pathogenesis and treatment*, eds. P.G. Bianchi & K.D. Bardhan, pp. 57–61. Verona: Cortina International.

Brandt, A.M. (1978): Racism and research. The case of the Tuskegee syphilis study. *Hastings Center Report* **8,** 21–29.

Brewin, T.B. (1982): Consent to randomized treatment. *Lancet* **ii** 919–921.

Brill, I.C., Rosenbaum, W.M., Rosenbaum, E.E. & Flanery, J.R. (1958): Internal mammary artery ligation. *Northwest Med.* **57,** 483–486.

Brody, H. & Waters, D.B. (1980): Diagnosis is treatment. *J. Fam. Practice* **10,** 445–449.

Brown, W.A. (1988): Predictors of placebo response in depression. *Psychopharmacol. Bulletin* **24,** 14–17.

Buckalew, L.W. & Coffield, K.E. (1982): An investigation of drug expectancy as a function of capsule color and size and preparation form. *J. Clin. Psychopharmacol.* **2,** 245–248.

Cobb, L.A., Thomas, G.I., Dillard, D.H., Merendino, K.A. & Bruce, R.A. (1959): An evaluation of internal-mammary-artery ligation by a double-blind technique. *N. Engl. J. Med.* **260,** 1115–1118.

Curson, D.A., Hirsch, S.R., Platt, S.D., Bamber, R.W. & Barnes, T.R.E. (1986): Does short term placebo treatment of chronic schizophrenia produce long term harm? *Br. Med. J.* **293,** 726–728.

Delay, J. & Pichot, P. (1973): *Medizinische Psychologie*. Stuttgart: Thieme.

Dimond, E.G., Kittle, C.F. & Crockett, J.E. (1958): Evaluation of internal mammary artery ligation and sham procedure in angina pectoris. *Circulation* **18,** 712–713.

Dobrilla, G. (1983): Placebo in the evaluation of antiulcer drugs. *Int. J. Tiss. React.* **4,** 329–337.

Elander, G. (1991): Ethical conflicts in placebo treatment. *J. Adv. Nurs.* **16,** 947–951.

Evans, F.J. (1974): The placebo response in pain reduction. *Adv. Neurol.* **4,** 289–296.

Feldman, P.E. (1956): The personal element in psychiatric research. *Am. J. Psychiatry* **113,** 52–57.

Fish, J.M. (1973): *Placebo therapy*. San Francisco: Jossey-Bass.

Freston, J.W. (1986): Dose-ranging in clinical trials: rationale and proposed use with placebo or positive controls. *Am. J. Gastroenterol.* **81,5,** 307–311.

Goodwin, J.S., Goodwin, J.M. & Vogel, A.V. (1979): Knowledge and use of placebos by house officers and nurses. *Ann. Intern. Med.* **91,** 106–110.

Gracely, R.H., Dubner, R., Wolskee, P.J. & Deeter, W.R. (1983): Placebo and naloxone can alter post-surgical pain by separate mechanisms. *Nature* **306,** 264–265.

Harken, D.E. (1958): Clinical conference: long-term management of patients with coronary artery disease. *Circulation* **17,** 945–952.

Isenberg, J.I., Peterson, W.L., Elashoff, J.D., Sandersfeld, M.A., Reedy, T.J., Ippoliti, A.F., Van Deventer, G.M., Frankl, H., Longstreth, G.F. & Andersen, D.S. (1983): Healing of benign gastric ulcer with low-dose antacid or cimetidine. A double-blind, randomized, placebo-controlled trial. *N. Engl. J. Med.* **308,** 1319–1324.

Jacobs, K.W. & Nordan, F.M. (1979): Classification of placebo drugs: effect of color. *Percept. Mot. Skills* **49,** 367–372.

Jellinek, E.M. (1946): Clinical tests on comparative effectiveness of analgesic drugs. *Biometrics Bull.* **2,** 87–91.

Kimbel, K.H. (1992): *Ginkgo biloba. Lancet* **340,** 1474.

Kitchell, J.R., Glover, R.P. & Kyle, R.H. (1958): Bilateral internal mammary artery ligation for angina pectoris. *Am. J. Cardiol.* **1**, 46–50.

Kleijnen, J. & Knipschild, P. (1992): *Ginkgo biloba. Lancet* **340**, 1136–1139.

Kuschinsky, G. (1975): Wirkungell un Indikationen von Plazebo. *Deutsches Ärzteblatt* 663–667.

Lundh, L.-G. (1987): Placebo, belief, and health. A cognitive-emotional model. *Scand. J. Psychol.* **28**, 128–143.

Lasagna, L., Masteller, F., von Felsinger, J.M. & Beecher, H.K. (1954): A study of the placebo response. *Am. J. Med.* **16**, 770–779.

Lasagna, L. (1961): Testimony given at Hearings before the Subcommittee on Antitrust and Monopoly of the Committee on the Judiciary, United States Senate, 87th Congress, 1st Session S. Res. 52 on S. 1552: Part 1: 282–283.

Lauritsen, K. & Rask-Madsen, J. (1987): Review: clinical trials in peptic ulcer disease – problems of methodology and interpretation. *Aliment. Pharmacol. Therap.* **1**, 91–123.

Leber, P. (1991): Is there an alternative to the randomized controlled trial? *Psychopharmacol. Bull.* **27**, 3–8.

Leber, P.D. (1983): The implicit assumptions of active control trials (a critical examination). *Controlled Clin. Trials* **14**, 133.

Leber, P.D. (1989): Hazards of inference: the active control investigation. *Epilepsia* **30 (S1)**, 57–63.

Levine, J.D., Gordon, N.C. & Fields, H.L. (1978): The mechanism of placebo analgesia. *Lancet*, **ii** 654–657.

Levine, R.J. (1987): The apparent incompatibility between informed consent and placebo-controlled clinical trials. *Clin. Pharmacol. Ther.* **42**, 247–249.

Lyerly, S., Ross, S., Krugman, A. & Clyde, D. (1964): Drugs and placebos: the effects of instructions upon performance and mood under amphetamine sulphate and chloral hydrate. *J. Abnormal Soc. Psychol.* **68**, 321–327.

Meyer, U.A. & Kindli, R. (1989): Plazebos und Nozebos. *Therapeutische Umschau* **46**, 544–554.

Modell, W. (1955): *The relief of symptoms*. Philadelphia: Saunders WB.

Moertel, C.G., Taylor, W.F., Roth, A. & Tyce, F.A.J. (1976): Who responds to sugar pills? *Mayo Clin. Proc.* **51**, 96–100.

Park, L.C. & Covi, L. (1965): Nonblind placebo trial. An exploration of neurotic patient's responses to placebo when its inert content is disclosed. *Arch. Gen. Psychiatry* **12**, 336–345.

Pepper, O.H. P. (1945): A note on the placebo. *Am. J. Pharmacol.* **117**, 409–412.

Pope, K. (1992): FDA chief answers critics. *Acad. Focus* **28**, 28a-d.

Quitkin, F.M., Rabkin, J.G., Stewart, J.W., McGrath, P.J., Harrison, W., Ross, D.C., Tricamo, E., Fleiss, J., Markowitz, J. & Klein, D.F. (1991): Heterogeneity of clinical response during placebo treatment. *Am. J. Psychol.* **148**, 193–196.

Ratcliff, J.D. (1957): 'Internal-mammary-artery ligation probably has no effect on the pathophysiology of coronary-artery disease'. New surgery for ailing hearts. *Reader's Digest* **71**, 70–73.

Reidenberg, M.M. & Lowenthal, D.T. (1968): Adverse nondrug reactions. *N. Engl. J. Med.* **279**, 678–679.

Sachar, D.B. on behalf of the College's Committee on FDA related matters (1984): Placebo-controlled clinical trials in gastroenterology. A position paper of the American College of Gastroenterology. *Am. J. Gastroenterol.* **79**, 913–917.

Schapira, K., McClelland, H.A., Griffiths, N.R. & Newell, D.J. (1970): Study on the effects of tablet colour in the treatment of anxiety states. *Br. Med. J.* **ii**, 446–449.

Scheurer, U., Witzel, L., Halter, F., *et al.* (1977): Gastric and duodenal ulcer healing under placebo treatment. *Gastroenterology* **72**, 838–841.

Schiller, L.R. & Fordtran, J.S. (1986): Ulcer complications during short-term therapy of duodenal ulcer with active agents on placebo. *Gastroenterology* **90**, 478–481.

Schönhöfer, P.S., Schulte-Sasse, H., Manhold, C. & Werner, B. (1989): Sind Extracte aus den Blättern des Ginkgobaumes bei peripheren Durchblutungs-und Hirnleistungsstörungen im Alter wirksam? Beurteilung von Tebonin un Rökan. *Intern. Praxia* **29**, 585–601.

Schönhöfer, P.S. (1990): *Ginkgo biloba* extracts. *Lancet* **i**, 788.

Shapiro, A.K. (1961): Factors contributing to the placebo effect. Their implications for psychotherapy. *Am. J. Psychother.* **18**, 73–88.

Shapiro, A.K., & Morris, L.A. (1978): The placebo effect in medical and psychological therapies. In: *Handbook of psychotherapy and behavior change*, 2nd edn, eds. S.L. Garfield & A.E. Bergin, pp. 369–410. New York: Wiley.

Sircus, N. (1980): Modern management of peptic ulcers with special reference to the placebo phenomenon. *Ital. J. Gastroenterol.* **12**, 315.

Smith, L.J. on behalf of the ACG committee on FDA-related matters (1989): Placebos in clinical trials of peptic ulcer. *Am. J. Gastroenterol.* **84**, 469–474.

Smith, M.L., Glass, G.V. & Miller, T.I. (1980): *The benefits of psychotherapy*. Baltimore: Johns Hopkins University Press.

Stanley, B. (1987): Informed consent in treatment and research. In: *Handbook of forensic psychology*, eds. J.B. Weiner & A.K. Hess, pp. 63–85. New York: John Wiley & Sons.

Steinbook, R.M., Jones, M.B. & Ainslie, J.D. (1965): Suggestibility and the placebo response. *J. Nerv. Ment. Dis.* **140**, 87–91.

Uhlenruth, E.H., Canter, A., Neustadt, J.A. & Payson, H.E. (1959): The symptomatic relief of anxiety with meprobamate, phenobarbital and placebo. *Am. J. Psychiatry* **115**, 905–910.

The ethics of animal and human experimentation, edited by P.P. De Deyn.

21

Dissent on informed consent. Tension between medical, legal and communication science related conceptions on informed consent: an argument to reformulate the role and responsibilities of physicians

Gerrit K. Kimsma

Department of Family- and Nursing Home Medicine, Faculty of Medicine, Free University, Van der Boechorststraat 7, 1081 BT Amsterdam, The Netherlands

Summary

In this contribution it is argued that the legal conception of the informed consent procedure in case of research is one-sided and unnecessarily unreflective of the many sided patient–physician relationship. A case is argued for a more detailed and better understood integration of research and the medical relationship in research as processes of communication. A redefinition of informed consent from this perspective should lead to a redefinition of the roles and responsibilities of physicians in the informed consent procedures, better suited to varieties of patients and diseases.

Introduction

In a celebrated article from 1989, Howard Brody observed that 'it appears that the theory and practice of informed consent are out of joint in some crucial ways' (Brody, 1989).

Essentially, so his article reads, accepted legal standards of informed consent send physicians the wrong message about what is expected from them. In this contribution I will argue that the reason for this 'misreading' on analysis must be found both in the context of medicine as essentially a therapy-directed enterprise and a legalistic one-sided interpretation of the patient–physician relationship (Kimsma, 1987, 1992). I will argue that the legal and ethical safeguards themselves are insufficient to guarantee a non-influenced decision of patients to accept proposed treatment or to participate in medical research, either therapeutic, experimental or basic. I will argue my case for research and draw comparisons with medical practice, because what is being said for medical practice bears deep consequences for research.

Institutional Review Board-experience

During my more than six years' membership of the Institutional Review Board (IRB) of the Academic Hospital of the Free University of Amsterdam, it has occurred only once in about 1200 protocols that the Board advised against participation of the researcher/physician in the informed consent procedure. The Board justified taking this unorthodox decision because it questioned the ability of the enthusiastic physician to perform the procedure in a neutral and objective manner. It is unknown whether the physician has followed-up the board's suggestion or whether the Hospital Administration, which is legally responsible for the practice of medical research, implemented our request. In fact, it is generally unknown how these procedures take place or how the quality of the informed consent *procedure* is protected and promoted. Veatch's recommendation (1976), that it never may be expected or allowed that researchers or their associates request permission themselves, thus creating a sharp distinction between clinical care and research, is not followed anywhere in the Netherlands and probably in few other places. Recently in the Netherlands, Zwart (1992) has suggested the desirability of creating a sharp division between clinical care and research physicians.

What *is* known is that written informed consent is one of the items that almost always forms a source of criticism. In about 70 to 80 per cent of the forms, minor and sometimes major defects are corrected by the Board before a positive recommendation is given. This means that positive recommendation is restrained in about 150 out of 200 yearly protocols because of deficient written information. The shortcomings were of the following nature: inadequate medical information justifying the research protocol; inadequate information on drug toxicity; misleading information; lack of explanation on methodology of randomization (e.g. placebo-controlled designs); lack of information on extra tests and procedures resulting from participation in a study as compared to standard treatments; and absence of the clause pertaining to voluntariness, and the right to end participation at any time without explanation.

This observation on a relatively small number of informed consent forms has been confirmed in a larger sample at the Academic Hospital at Maastricht of the State University Limburg in the Netherlands. In this extensive research the conclusion is that present day written information is deficient in a number of informative items, in style, and in comprehensiyeness (Wittebrood, 1993).

These deficiencies in *written* information certainly do not create confidence with regard to the quality of the *oral* information provided to potential research subjects.

It is generally unknown how informed consent is obtained in the Netherlands. The actual practice for getting patients to consent is unknown territory. The information on scientific research is scanty in general. At the Free University Hospital of Amsterdam this void has been met, with due respect to and recognition of the professional responsibilities and independence of physicians, by introducing a 'convenant', a kind of contract, between Hospital and researcher(s). This convenant describes the rights of patients and researchers, the conditions by which a protocol must be ended, and the events that require a renewed consent from the IRB. However, it is unknown to what extent researchers deviate from the convenant, and because there are no sanctions, its status is reduced to a gentleman's agreement.

Disregarding the conditions spelled out in the 'convenant' is however not entirely without consequences, since the liability insurance policy of the hospital does not cover claims from patients if they incur physical harm or other damages in the course of the execution of these particular unauthorized protocols.

It *is* known that some researchers hold a grudge against the review procedure and the IRB, apparently based on feelings of unwarranted interference with professional activities. Other researchers produce protocols that, in the words of the Leiden University epidemiologist Vandenbroucke (1990), are polished up and contain informed consent forms that are written with the explicit intent to pass the local IRB and to get a positive advice.

This professional ambivalence has been fostered recently by the position health lawyers tend to take on issues that are experienced as clear obstruction to further medical research that is viewed as socially relevant and medically necessary. Maintaining that consent is an absolute condition for research indeed makes it impossible to investigate left-over sera or tissue of deceased patients, since consent as a requirement is impossible to receive unless given in advance. Also research to investigate the prevalence of hepatitis or HIV positivity anonymously does not seem to serve a socially responsible policy but seems no more than legal dogmatism to prevent 'violation of individual rights'. This obstruction, however irritating it may be for medical researchers, in itself does not, however, justify a hands-off policy or passive resistance.

What *is* further known, is reason for concern, and possibly for action by the medical profession. It may even be, if the profession does not take action, reason for legal action and legislation. Informally and through research it is known that physicians differ greatly in their capacity to communicate and in their propensity to talk patients 'into treatment or into a protocol'. Significant in this respect is a claim by one physician to be able to perform any feat on a patient merely by playing the cards right. This polemical expression is the reverse side of the coin of proven observations that, in more neutral language, patients tend to follow their physicians' advice. Especially where the threat of disease is imminent, patients want their physicians to guide them, as Penman (cited by Mark & Shapiro, 1990) has illustrated in the case of patients with a tumour.

It is also known that patients, not surprisingly, 'tend to have bad memory' for risks that do not fit their hopes or that are too devastating to comprehend (Cassileth, 1980).

From the 1970s on, the constant flow of research on informed consent practices and conceptions reveals a host of misunderstandings and partial truths regarding quality and quantity of comprehension between physicians and patients. In research, these observations tend to be exaggerated with patients consenting before having heard the risks of procedures or consenting even before having read the written information. The picture that emerges is that of patient involvement in the process of informed consent depending on factors that usually are not integrated into the chosen procedures. Involvement depends on number of things, such as:

1. location of treatment,
2. nature of medical treatment,
3. nature of the disease,
4. social status of patients,
5. nature of the patient–physician relation,
6. estimation by physicians whether patients wish to participate in the decision-making process,
7. differences in patients in their wish to participate in the decision making (Bolt, 1991).

These studies clearly reveal a sharp discrepancy between the ideal of informed consent as a fundamental part of medicine, and real life. To the analysis of the factors that influence the quality of informed consent, one fundamental factor must be added which illustrates the gravity of the issue: informed consent is not perceived by patients as protection of patients by informing, but as protection of physicians against unwanted law suits (Annas, 1989).

This discrepancy between fact and theory cannot be explained merely by malfunctioning physicians or overenthusiastic researchers. A more plausible explanation must take into account the primacy of the relation between patients and physicians and the consequences of this relation for the secondary process information.

Medicine and information

From the point of view of medicine and medical professionals, information is part and parcel of medicine (Tomlinson, 1986). Informing is an activity that is crucial in the relationship between physician and patient. In this relationship trust plays a vital part. It goes without saying that the interests of patients and physicians run a parallel course. Without some level of trust, no fruitful action is possible except in cases of compromised consciousness or unconsciousness. In this relationship, the patient's interest always comes first. Even when it is granted that there are fundamental differences between patient and physician, as there are in knowledge and often in social status, the exchange of information serves as a means to materialize the durability and effectiveness of the relationship. The exchange of information is part of medical procedures and is guided by reflections on the patient's interest, and on what is potentially harmful or not. The relationship between patient and physician is one of a continuous nature: it starts during the first moments of an encounter, and often long before that, as it can be based on past contacts regarding different medical problems.

Legal conceptions on information in medicine

For the law and lawyers, the medical relationship is not one of trust *per se*. Trust may enter into it, but only after the process of negotiating a contract. From a legal point of view, the medical relationship is *not a continuum*, but a *series of events*, that can lead to a contract, but not necessarily so. The nature of the process of informing is not part of the relationship but a condition that may or may not make a contract possible. Indeed, the interests of physician and patient may not necessarily run a parallel course. Essentially, opposite ideas on the patient's best interests may exist, or the physician-researchers may have interests that differ from or even conflict with the patient's best interests. An even more basic opposition is founded on experiences of both physicians' malpractice and the emergence of multiple medical treatments. This development is influenced further by social changes favouring more autonomy as opposed to institutional inclinations towards paternalism, underlining ideas of opposite interests and the need for patient protection. This protection finds a further expression in the development of patients' rights, ending in the consequential step that only the patient is the final judge of his own situation. In the end, the differences between patient and physician are reconciled through the making of a contract. Only after a contract has been made, can one speak of a formal relationship: everything before this phase is preliminary, and from a legal point of view: reconnoitring the territory.

The differences between the medical and the legal conceptions comprise two points:

1. different view on the patient/physician relationship;
2. different view on the meaning and the flow of information.

Medicine and the law on the medical relationship

Medical experience demonstrates that a trusting relationship is essential for medical success or compliance. A poor relationship means: the patient not following advice or not taking medication. From the 1970s on, a wave of research has revealed that non-compliance is almost as common as compliance. For long-term therapies, compliance does not exceed 50 per cent (Schouten, 1985).

The causes for this phenomenon are not entirely clear. There is no clear-cut relationship between non-compliance and seriousness of the illness, length of treatment, or amount of costs (Sacket & Snow, 1979). Neither does non-compliance relate to personality characteristics (Schretlen & Tillemans, 1979). What is clear, however, is that physicians tend to underestimate the importance of information. Thus, informing patients, discussing risks, advising life-styles, and taking effective precautions become more prominent when enough attention is being paid to this aspect. Even if it is not completely effective, its need is clearly stated. This statement applies to daily medical routine as well as to research. To patients, the line between treatment and investigation is a subtle one, since the word investigation itself carries a double meaning. Patients are investigated: what else would they do in a hospital? This view of patient–physician interaction with an obligatory relationship in order to become effective has a psychological price. The importance of this relationship for therapeutical effectiveness *in the patients' interest* is a prerequisite for getting therapy compliance. It seems impossible, however, for a physician to withdraw from this relationship when the information does not concern therapy but research. It is possible for a physician to tell a patient that the decision to participate in a project would have to be made without considering the existing patient–physician relationship. Nevertheless, the fact that a physician will distance himself in words from his relationship for the sake of a physician-directed (research) interest will carry an emotion that enhances the existing relationship. It is proof itself that one can trust this physician. Trust or a fiduciary relationship is present or absent and anything that is said, is interpreted within this context.

Information within a relationship aimed at healing is supplied with the intention to convince patients that a proposal is made in their interest: a physician is allowed to influence a patient's decision, but not allowed to manipulate. Of fundamental importance is the recognition that one always influences another person and that the extent of this influence is limited by a person's competence to draw limits and the freedom to choose. Within the healing relationship, influencing is justified by the assumption of the patient's interest. But this justification is insufficient if the interest is ambiguous or merely that of the physician. At this point, the problem boils down to this: the difference between asking for participation in medical care, and asking for it for research purposes without unacceptably influencing the patient is highly difficult to discern.

This problem is viewed differently from the position of health law and current medical ethics. The dominant position in this field is the protection of patient's rights and a reluctance to invade these rights in which physical integrity and right of self-determination are crucial. In health law, influencing a patient, if at all unavoidable, must be as limited as possible. A patient is not a passive actor but is supposedly and fundamentally a free agent in possession of adequate capacities to decide whether to participate in actions, be they medical, legal, patient care- or medical research-related. For health-law, and in its wake present day medical ethics, the relationship between physician and patient seems to be rather a threat to decision making. This threat becomes stronger if within a process of general care, some parts of medical research are built in; where a therapeutic interest is mixed up with or even replaced by a related research interest. Participation, from the legal point of view, is acceptable only on condition of all materially relevant information and the ability to decide in freedom without interference.

Information means information that is spoken or written in comprehensive, non-professional, clear language. This information should not be alluring or inviting; it should be emotionally neutral, and as complete as possible. Description of the research must be as extensive as necessary, comparisons with standard treatment must be made, risks and extra interventions must be mentioned, including research methodology (randomized controlled treatment, involving placebo-treatment, and the possibility of receiving no treatment at all).

It is highly questionable whether or not these demands would, if met, prevent unwanted interference. Of course IRBs must rid the patient 'information' of unwanted alluring or obscure elements, and must eliminate references to unproven potential advantages of participation (such as more frequent medical check-ups). But the gist of the matter remains that influencing patients cannot really be prevented. And there is no absolute way of knowing whether a patient has been merely influenced, seduced, manipulated or even forced into participation, because this is an internal process of which the physician only gets a glance.

So, in conclusion, it is not realistic to try to attempt to withdraw from an already existing relationship between physician and patient. Neither is it realistic to state that there is no relationship until the patient has decided to participate in the trial. On the contrary, the relationship is primary and determines, more often than not, whether the patient is going to participate at all, sometimes independent of the information. An alternative however could consist of having patient recruitment to a controlled trial done by an independent party.

A communication-science context

The statement that it is impossible *not to influence* a patient is self-evident in communication science. In this field, concerned with communication and behaviour, a general consensus exists that it is even *impossible not to communicate*, based on the fundamental assumption that it is *impossible not to behave* in ways that signify the attitudes and values of the speaker. Processes of information and advice, such as informed consent procedures, must essentially be viewed as forms of behaviour. The problem of informing patients then becomes one of effectiveness The ideas that have been developed in this field clarify that communication is not equal to a process of 'sending and receiving messages'. On the contrary, based on research by Watzlawick and others (1967), the behaviour involved is subdivided into verbal and non-verbal elements, each of which plays an important part in effective communication. All communication is influenced by content, but also by the relationship between the persons who communicate. The gist of the matter is that for effective communication the relational aspect guides the informative and is thus of primary importance. This relational aspect in itself is differentiated into two categories: a symmetric or a complementary one. Roughly speaking, a symmetric relationship is one in which there exists some degree of equality; a complementary relationship is one in which inequality is expressed by differences in goals of communication, and in roles.

Translated to the information process in the physician–patient relationship in research conditions, it should become clear that an effective information process can be accomplished easier when there is a fiduciary relationship. This aspect of trust is a necessary condition for effective communication (Hoenen, 1988). The use of a perfectly informative written consent form is in itself important, but only to the cognitive aspect of the process. Concentrating on this part while neglecting the relational aspect can make the whole process ineffective. That is one lesson, based on experience in the science of communication.

A second lesson relates what has been said above about the unrealistic assumption that within the therapeutic relationship of healing, one cannot expect a patient to detach from the already existing relationship, and decide on participation in research in freedom as if this relationship did not exist. The distinction between symmetrical and complementary relationships, as important for understanding effective communication, can be used to show the same paradox. Allowing that the usual relationship between physician and patient can be described as a complementary one, the suggestion of the freedom to choose for or against participation in research introduces a symmetric element within the context of complementarity. At the least this is confusing, at worst it is paradoxical, and possibly detrimental to the relationship without further clarification.

Redefining the role and responsibilities of physicians in the informed consent procedure

According to Veatch (1976), those carrying out research should never be allowed to ask their potential 'subjects' for permission. This suggestion seemed at first glance very dogmatic and rigid, and it has not much adherence, as far as I know. Zwart (1992) has suggested, as others before him, that in The Netherlands one should create a sharp demarcation between clinical caretakers and researchers.

These proposals may have some merit, because pitfalls may be avoided. One such pitfall is the prevention of a relationship influencing a patient's decision. In other words: one avoids the suggestion that within a complementary relationship it is realistic to introduce elements of symmetry, and to expect a patient to decide in freedom based on some particular conception of freedom in an equal relationship. However, in most places clinical reality is a mixture of care and research. Even in purely research facilities, patient care has high priority. Given this reality, and the nature of the physician–patient relationship that I outlined above, several conclusions can be drawn.

The first is that a fiduciary relationship can be conducive to the information process; it can be termed a desirable condition. The second is that even excellent written information is in itself no guarantee of quality. In other words, the ethical and legal conditions, which outline acceptable research protocols and written information, are restrained, without the guarantee of an acceptable execution of the process itself. This fact and the intertwining of the information process with the physician-patient relationship, in addition to the mixture of care and research, make a redefinition of physicians' involvement necessary. Exactly because involvement of law and ethics is limited, it means that the medical profession should re-take and integrate its responsibilities in care and research.

'Protecting the right and welfare of patients is a higher goal than medical progress' (Kopelman, 1986). In the context of research this protection means that patients need to be protected against undue interference, such as friendly invitation, manipulation or gentle techniques of force. In broad terms this means that physicians who are incapable of understanding the subleties of these varieties of influence and of acting accordingly, should not be allowed to request permission from patients for research. Their interest in research should not cloud the ability to judge the influence of their relationship on a particular patient. In narrower terms this means also that physicians should be trained to understand the intricacies of the different levels of communication within their relationship with patients in these differently orientated actions.

This does not only mean training of junior physicians in cognition and skill with guidance and evaluation. It also means understanding that the information process is essentially a *medical* affair, encompassing the conditions of ethics and law. The information process is not something delegated *in extenso* to IRBs, ethicists or lawyers. This approach of acknowledging the subleties of the informational process should also take into account the varieties of contexts where informed consent is requested and varieties of psychological inclinations in patients depending on the stages and seriousness of the disease. To the responsibility of senior researchers at least one must be added: to teach, to guide, and to evaluate the quality of the information process on their wards, as a part of their overall responsibility in care and research.

References

Annas, G.J. (1989): The emerging stowaway: patients' rights in the 1980s. In: *Contemporary issues in bioethics*, eds. T.L. Beauchamp & L. Walters, pp. 335–340. California: Wadsworth.

Bolt, I. (1991): *Informed consent*. Wetenschapswinkel Geneeskunde, Free University, Amsterdam.

Brody, H. (1989): Transparency: informed consent in primary care. *Hastings Center Report*, Sept/Oct, 5–9.

Cassileth, B.R. (1980): Informed consent: why are its goals imperfectly realised? *N. Engl. J. Med.* **17**, 896–900.

Hoenen, J.A.H.J. (1988): *Patiëntenvoorlichting stap voor stap*. Rijswijk: uitgeverij voor gezondheidsbevordering.

Kimsma, G.K. (1987): Control of informed consent? *Verslag 6-e Landelijke Bijeenkomst Medische Ethische Toetsingscomissies*, Academisch Ziekenhuis van de Vrije Universiteit te Amsterdam, October, 3–11.

Kimsma, G.K. (1992): Informed consent. In: *Praktische medische ethiek*, eds. R. Dillmann, E. Van Leeuwen & G.K. Kimsma, pp. 94–106. Utrecht: Bunge-KNMG.

Kopelman, L. (1986): Consent and randomized clinical trials: are there moral or design problems? *J. Med. Phil.* **11**, 320.

Mark, J.S. & Spiro, H. (1990): Informed consent for coloscopy. *Arch. Intern. Med.* **150**, 777–780.

Sacket, D.L. & Snow, J.C. (1979): The magnitude of compliance and non-compliance. In: *Compliance in health care*, eds. B. Haynes, D.W. Taylor & D.L. Sacket. Baltimore, London: The Johns Hopkins University Press.

Schouten, J.A.M. (1985): *Anamnese and Advies*. 2nd edn, p. 113. Brussels: Stafleu, Alphen aande Rijn.

Schretlen, I. & Tillemans, J. (1979): Therapietrouw. *Medisch Contact* **51**, 1609–1617.

Tomlinson, T. (1986): The physician's influence on patient's choices. *Theor. Med.* **7**, 105–123.

Vandenbroucke, J.P. (1990): Medische Ethiek en Gezondheidsrecht: hinderpalen voor de verdere toename van kennis in de geneeskunde. *Ned. Tijdschr. Geneeskd.* **1**, 5–6.

Veatch, R.M. (1976): *Three theories of informed consent: philosophical foundations and policy implications*. Prepared for The National Commission for the Protection of Human Subjects of Biomedical and Behavioral Research.

Watzlawick, P., Beavin, J. & Jackson, D. (1967): *Pragmatics of human communication*. New York: W.W. Norton.

Wittebrood, L. (1993): *Kwaliteit van schriftelijke informatie aan proefpersonen*. Maastricht: RUL.

Zwart, H. (1992): De arts als arts in strikte zin en als wetenschappelijk onderzoeker. *Medisch Contact* **9**, 270–272.

The ethics of animal and human experimentation, edited by P.P. De Deyn.

22

Kant's pain: Ethical considerations on medical experiments in the general practice

Alex K. Huibers

Centre for Bio-ethics and Health Law, Heidelberglaan 2, NL–3584 CS Utrecht, The Netherlands

Summary

Medical experiments in general practice may often seem very normal and 'innocent'. Nevertheless it is important to perform a critical ethical evaluation of these experiments. This is necessary because in most experiments people are used as means to an end, as research material. This is in conflict with an important moral principle, formulated by Immanuel Kant. On the other hand, medical research is aiming at the furtherance of human well-being. For this reason medical experiments can be allowed, on the condition that they serve this important and relevant goal. In general practice a number of specific questions concerning medical experiments can rise. These have to do with the special relationship of loyalty and trust between a general practioner (GP) and his patient and with the relevance of research for the general practice. In this article it is argued that a GP should carefully check whether or not a research project yields relevant information for general practice before deciding upon participation. According to the author, GPs should not participate in so called 'seeding trials' which have marketing of a product as their main objective.

Introduction

In order to illustrate that tough and important ethical questions do rise during the reviewing of general practice-bound standard research protocols within an Institutional Review Board (IRB), I describe the following example.

The protocol submitted to our IRB concerned a phase II trial evaluating an analgesic drug in patients with severe acute lower back pain. The effectiveness of the drug administered orally or intramuscularly was to be compared with a placebo. In order to optimize the blindness of the experiment all participants were to receive both an injection and a pill. Consequently, two-thirds of the participants would receive an injection with an ineffective substance. According to the protocol patients were allowed to use paracetamol as emergency medication. Before doing so, however, they had to call the physician to ask for permission.

The review board was confronted with a number of questions. First of all, would this analgesic drug contribute enough to our armamentarium so as to justify the exposure of patients to the burden and possible risks of the experiment. Or was this a so called 'me too' drug for which any added value could hardly be expected ? Another question was the matter of the two ways of administration: was there no possibility to limit the experiment to the less-invasive oral administration?

The availability of the emergency medication posed another problem: according to the protocol quite a number of participants were to receive placebo. This is in spite of the fact that those people went to the physician with a severe lower back pain. They did not go to the doctor to get a placebo, but a pain-killing drug.

Was there no possibility to compare the compound with another analgesic drug instead of placebo? Unfortunately this was no feasible option, since a drastic rise in the number of participants would then be necessary to get statistically relevant results. The review board, however, felt that the administration of placebo is a serious problem when this kind of pain is concerned. Consequently the board decided that emergency medication had to be more easily available. This was the least of demands one had to live by. Furthermore the board judged that the patient should not have to ask the physician for permission for using the emergency medication, and that in the patient's information brochure there had to be a generous and explicit invitation to use this medication if necessary. Placebo-related ethical considerations are more extensively dealt with in Ch. 20 (*Placebo*).

Another striking point was the matter of informed consent. Is it very realistic to suppose that a person who consults his or her GP with a severe lower back pain is really free in deciding whether he or she wants to participate in an experiment or not? This matter was complicated by the fact that there was no time for reflection, because the drug concerned had to be administered immediately. Because of this, the review board took a very close look at the patient's information brochure.

The general conclusion of the review board was that the research could only take place if considerable changes in the protocol were made.

Nevertheless the briefly discussed protocol was of very reasonable quality. Moreover, the drug concerned was 'just' an analgesic, and the complaint concerned appears very frequently in general practice. Thus, there was no question of spectacular research on a possibly life-saving but very risky drug. And yet, as I stated, some rather important questions were raised by the IRB members. Strikingly the sponsor of a protocol is quite often surprised by such a number of questions. Still, these questions have to be asked, even if rather common research is concerned.

Apparently the use of human subjects is a morally very sensitive area. I will explicitate this by referring to the theory of Immanuel Kant. After this philosophical exploration, I will concentrate on a number of specific problems in connection with medical experiments in general practice. Subsequently, I will discuss the role of the physician as a doctor and researcher, the relevance criteria and 'seeding trials'. Finally, I will briefly touch on the method for reviewing general practice experiments which is now being developed in The Netherlands.

Kant's pain

Medical experiments with drugs are – at least since World War II – a morally sensitive area and subject to much regulation, such as the Nuremberg code (De Beaufort, 1985). This moral sensitivity has other reasons besides the crimes in Nazi Germany. In my opinion, it is mainly caused by the fact that performing medical experiments as such is always in conflict with an important ethical principle. The participant becomes a research-object, he is research material. We doubt this statement. This discomfort is well formulated in Kant's principle, known as the practical imperative. Immanuel Kant (1734–1804) states that human beings are never to be used solely as a means, but should always be considered as an end.

> *'Handle so, dass du die Menschheit, sowohl in deiner Person, als in der Person eines jeden andern, jederzeit zugleich als Zweck, niemal bloss als Mittel brauchest.'* (Kant, 1991)

This practical imperative is in close connection to the 'categorical imperative' which states that one should act according to the rule which could just as well be made a principle of law.

> *'Handle nur nach derjenigen Maxime, von der du zugleich wollen kannst, dass sie ein allgemeines Gesetz werde.'* (Kant, 1991)

An example: it is morally wrong to steal. Otherwise, if you are of the opinion that you are allowed to steal, it should be possible to make this rule a principle of law. Others would then be allowed to steal from you. Of course such a principle of law would be irrational. In the same way it is unthinkable that others should be allowed to use you as a mere means to their ends. Consequently one should not use others as a mere means to one's own ends.

An important feature of medical experiments is that human beings are used as a means. In an experiment the main objective is to get information on safety, efficacy and possible side-effects of a drug. Could one say that in an experiment people are used solely as a means? In my opinion the answer to this question should be affirmative, at least for research on healthy volunteers and placebo-controlled trials. In the first case it is evident that these persons have no therapeutic benefit whatsoever from participating. The same goes however to a certain extent for placebo-controlled trials. In most of the cases it is unclear to which group – placebo or active treatment – a patient is randomized. Consequently, we should take as a presupposition that the person involved is without medication. The fact that there is such a chance is the relevant feature from the viewpoint of the practical imperative. As far as therapeutical experiments and experimental therapies are concerned, one could argue whether or not people are used solely as a means. Participants do get medication with posssible efficacy in the studied condition. Unless randomized in a placebo arm – as a baseline – it is not possible to determine whether or not the medication has been effective.

If we state it as a principle that human beings ought not to be used as means to an end, and we realize that in many experiments exactly this is taking place, should our conclusion be that medical experiments are morally unjustified? Superficially this seems to be the case indeed. In the following I will consider three counter-arguments to this conclusion, the first two of which will not prove to be decisive, but the third will.

A first counter-argument that can be made, is that the practical imperative is no argument against medical experiments, as long as participants give their explicit and free consent. This counter-argument is not decisive. If an act is morally wrong, its wrongness is not waived solely because someone has given his permission for this act. An example – perhaps somewhat extreme – might clarify this point. Imagine a situation in which the life of three seriously ill people could be saved by offering the life of one person. For example the situation may occur that there are three patients in desperate need of a kidney, a liver and a heart transplant. Suppose someone was to be found with the correct tissue-match who is prepared to give his life for these three patients. I think no surgeon would be willing to cooperate in such an initiative. Indeed, it is morally wrong to use a human being in this way, even if he would consent to it. The same goes for slavery: law does not allow someone to sell himself as a slave, even if he would do so well-informed and consciously.

A third example is put forward by Kant himself and makes it undoubtedly clear that in his view the practical imperative is not waived if the involved person consents to the action. Kant states that the practical imperative is not only relevant with respect to others, but also to oneself. In connection with this he raises the question whether suicide could be morally right. In his opinion this is certainly not the case (Kant, 1991), because this would mean that one is using one's own person as a means to an end, viz. a life which is comfortable till the end. This end of a comfortable life is reached by terminating one's life when it is no longer comfortable. In other words, one uses his own person to gain another purpose. This is according to Kant a violation of the practical imperative. From this we can learn that the consent or even explicit wish of a person does not waive the practical imperative.

Although the examples may be a little extreme, they surely make clear that informed consent as such does not make up for people being used solely as means to an end.

A second objection is that it is not wrong to use people as sole means to an end, as long as their interests are not harmed in the process. This objection which is put forward by Inez De Beaufort (1989), states – in short – that the *use* of people is not *per se abuse.* Only if their interests are at stake, could one speak of abuse.

Against this idea one could argue that, first of all, the (deontological) nature of the imperative of Kant stands in the way of it being reduced to simple balancing of interests. Kant takes the absolute position that human beings may never be used solely as means. It would not be right to state that it is yet allowable to do so as long as the interests of the people involved are not harmed too badly. Kant states:

> '.. *denn alsdenn is das praktische Prinzip . . . unbedingt, weil er gar kein Interesse zum Grunde haben kann'* ('. . . the practical imperative is absolute, because it can absolutely not be founded in interests.') (Kant, 1991).

This leaves little room for speculation.

Moreover, in medical experiments the interests of the participants are by definition at stake. This is inherent in the fact that we are dealing with an experiment. Even if by estimation risks are very low, you can never fully exclude all risks. In short, people are used as a means, and this fact does not change even if only a small risk or a limited burden is involved. On these grounds I consider this second objection not decisive.

A third objection, which I do find decisive, is the following. One cannot deny that many drugs contribute to the health of human beings. Some drugs are life-saving, others have an important role in reducing pain. The development of new drugs would be close to impossible without performing clinical experiments.

Striving for the well-being of people has always been an important point of moral attention. In as far as the development of drugs contributes to the well-being of people, there is a strong moral reason to support this development and implicitly to perform medical experiments (Waltern, 1982).

Thus it follows that there is a moral argument against performing medical experiments, as well as one in favour of them. In other words, we are stuck with a moral dilemma in the real sense of the word. In these situations it is tempting just to cut short and decide one way or the other. And indeed, some people have objected against medical experiments – at least experiments involving healthy volunteers and placebo-controlled trials – such as Hans Jonas (Schafer, 1983), whilst others are so convinced of the value of clinical research that they put aside the norm that people are not to be used solely as means. Along this vein Vere writes: 'If medicine is to advance, sacrifices by some individuals are inevitable. But it must always be remembered that if progress is not so attained, the sacrifices required by nature of us all will be far greater' (Vere, 1983). In my opinion, neither of both options is right. Both principles create obligations prima facie. This means that there are obligations which are both valid, whilst it is not immediately clear which obligation should prevail. In every individual case, we should decide which obligation ought to prevail. In making such a choice there will always be some moral pain, whichever side the balance is struck. Choosing to perform an experiment includes the use of a human being as a sole means to an end. This moral pain, Kant's pain as one might put it, can never be reduced fully. It does however create an obligation to be extremely careful in designing and performing experiments. And conversely deciding not to perform an experiment entails the possibility that valuable information may not be obtained.

In short, I conclude that the moral principle that human beings should not be used solely as means is not under any circumstance an overruling objection against clinical drug-research, even in the area of research on healthy volunteers or placebo-controlled trials. This does not mean however that this principle is not important. First of all, it creates an obligation to be very careful in designing and performing trials (Burkhardt & Kienle, 1983). Another consequence of the principle is that research that has no use is morally prohibited. I will explain these fundamental claims in the following especially with respect to a number of issues related to general practice. Furthermore, I will go into the matter of the GP as a researcher and physician, the relevance-criteria and 'seeding trials'.

The GP as a researcher

The GP has a special place in the field of health care. As a consequence of his almost unique position as a 'first-line' physician he has a special and mostly long-lasting relationship with his patients. For almost every complaint which is viewed as a medical problem by the patient, the GP will be the first – and often the only – health care worker who is consulted by the patient. Knottnerus (1988) states that in the Netherlands 85 to 90 per cent of all problems that are treated in the traditional health care system are fully dealt with by GPs. Moreover, the GP plays an important role apart from dealing with medical complaints in the strict sense. Via the GP one can obtain contraceptives, the GP is involved in pregnancies and births, as well as in dying. Besides, it is an important fact that many of the complaints that comprise the reason to consult the GP, have no medical nature, but are social or psychological. The GP is to a large extent a counsellor rather than a physician.

All of this comes down to the fact that the relationship with a GP has a special character of loyalty and trust, at least if things are well. This relationship is barely comparable to the relationship between a specialist and a patient. The specialist meets his patients mostly for a short period of time, for one special kind of complaint and often second in line. Consequently the distance between specialist and patient – allowing for exceptions will be larger than between GP and patient. Of course this special relationship between GP and patient has many advantages. Diagnostics and therapy will be more likely to be successful in a trusting atmosphere.

With respect to medical experiments however, this special relationship could be a problem. This problem is an extraordinary and additionally complicated example of the general issue concerning experiments with patients, viz. the mingling of the role of physician and researcher. This issue is doubly complicated in the case of the GP, precisely because of his special relationship with his patients.

How, for example, would a patient react when his GP, a person whom he trusts, asks him to participate in an experiment? There would be very few patients declining from such a proposal. Given their GP asks them to participate, they would suppose everything is alright. Otherwise he would not ask them! Besides, they might fear a refusal could endanger their relation with their GP. Even if the patient supposes that this will not be the case, he will be happy to stay on the safe side. Moreover, it is nice to make a friendly gesture to your own GP. In short, a patient whom is invited by his GP to participate in an experiment will be very likely to cooperate. This supposition is confirmed by research (Berden *et al.*, 1993). There is, however, a problem.

Let us return to the research protocol in the beginning of this essay. As a consequence of the fact that we are dealing with a placebo-controlled trial, quite a number of patients will leave their GP without any effective medication. They came to the physician because they had a severe lower back pain, and all they have received is a phoney pill and a phoney injection. It is not unlikely that the patient, coming home, will feel somewhat misled. Even if he gave his informed consent, as soon as he notices his pain is not lessening, there is a chance that his confidence in his GP will get a little shaken. His GP always wanted the best for him. But now, apparently, this is not quite the case. Will this also apply to other situations?

One could argue against this that patients have some kind of moral obligation to cooperate in medical experiments. It seems rather opportunistic, according to supporters of this view, to profit from experiments which have been performed in the past, and not to be prepared to participate in an experiment yourself. Whatever may be made of this argument, the fact remains that a patient who trusts his physician, may start doubting the real intentions of his GP. He may wonder whether or not his physician unconditionally gives his patients' well being the highest priority, or is he in fact for a large part also a researcher with other goals and interests?

In connection to this, I find it rather discomforting that investigation among GPs showed that for them the first criterion for not participating in research projects was the unacceptable burden they would lay on themselves; an unacceptable burden for the patient was only the second criterion. At the same time, if they were willing to participate in a research project the main criterion was that they found the research personally interesting and the burden for themselves acceptable (Kocken *et al.*, 1992).

What are the consequences of all of this? First of all, a GP should be very selective and careful when considering whether to take part in a trial (van Benthem, 1988). He will have to explore and scrutinize the protocol with respect to the question whether the research serves an important medical interest. He should have a good insight into the burden and risks for his patients, and should take special interest in the way he will inform the patients whom he asks to participate in the experiment (Lamberts, 1987). His supposition should be that a patient is liable to participate in the trial. As a matter of fact, the GP should play the role of the *advocatus diaboli*, in the sense that he has to make it very clear what the possible negative aspects of participating are or can be.

As I said, the first question is whether the research serves an important medical interest. This draws our attention to two relevant matters, i.e. the relevance of the research and so-called 'seeding trials'.

Relevance of the research

The norm that medical experiments may only be performed on condition that they serve a useful purpose has, as one consequence among others, that research should always be *relevant* research (Bergkamp, 1990). In other words, in case of a pre-registration trial, the drug to be tested should potentially offer a substantial added value to the already existing armamentarium. This may seem to be self evident, but it certainly is not. Many products that are in development are in fact 'me too's'. Now there is a lot of ambiguity in the term 'me too'. In reality there is a continuing line from products that may be considered a sensational new drug (the first aspirin, the first penicillin) through to, at the other end of the spectrum, those products which will offer nothing new with certainty. This is a continuum with a very large grey area. One can, of course, never exclude the tiniest possibility that a product is an improvement with respect to side-effects, even albeit for a very small number of patients. And on the other hand, sensational new drugs, real innovations, occur just once every five years or so.

This fact creates a problem when trying to develop the criteria for relevance. In view of the moral duty to perform only relevant research – because people are involved – it should be considered very important to take action to develop these criteria for relevance. In this essay, I shall try to contribute to this. It should be noted that this is indeed only a very modest beginning. For this purpose, I will use the perspective of the GP who is consider-ing whether or not he is willing to 'expose' his patients to a certain trial.

Key criteria seem to be that the drug at hand could constitute an interesting contribution to the number of drugs already available to the GP. It is a very well-known fact that GPs use only a small part of the drugs available in their practice. In their opinion, most of the time they can manage quite reasonably with a small amount of different drugs.

An interesting question to test the possible relevance of the product on trial could be: How big is the chance that I will actually prescribe this product if the experiments go well? I would state that if this chance is below, e.g. 10 per cent, the GP should decide not to participate in the research.

Another, more objective, approach to the relevance criteria would be the following. The GP can consider the question how many products there are already available in the relevant indication area. As a general rule I propose that if there are up to three drugs, research may be relevant; above this number the relevance is doubtful.

The next question can be whether the GP feels that there are gaps in the relevant indication area, and whether he is often dissatisfied about the available drugs, both with respect to effectiveness and side-effects. If such a gap exists, he could explore whether or not the new product might fill this gap. If this is not the case, he should not participate in the experiment.

'Seeding trials'

Seeding trials are experiments on drugs which serve to enhance the sales of a product. In these trials, drugs are used that have already been registered, and with which so-called phase IV studies are performed. GPs are very often confronted with these seeding trials. An informal estimate amounted to 1200 trials per annum in general practice. The impression was that no less than 1100 of these trials would have to be seeding trials!

However, phase IV research as such can be very useful. Often it has become apparent that the initial estimates of effectiveness and side-effects have to be corrected. Catastrophes like the thalidomide affair are a painful example of this fact, but there are also many examples on a much smaller scale. I think it would be a good idea to create an official system of post-marketing surveillance. In The Netherlands the first steps in this direction are being made.

A seeding trial however is something quite different. It does not serve to acquire insights into the effectiveness and side-effects of a drug, but mainly to improve the sales of the product. A seeding trial is a marketing instrument.

Sometimes it is stated that, although little is to be said in favour of seeding trials, neither can you really object to them. I do not agree with this view. In the case of placebo-controlled trials, or research in which patients receive therapy other than the usual one, human beings are mere means to an end. Consequently, one should have a very good reason for performing such an experiment. I do not consider a purely marketing purpose such a good reason. In this respect, I find seeding trials unethical.

One side-remark however should be made. It will not always be clear that a research project has purely marketing purposes. There may be a mingling of goals. This should be judged case by case. Of course, it is clear that a method of research which could not lead to scientifically valid results constitutes an experiment that is utterly senseless. Many seeding trials comprise such an unscientific approach.

It would be very sensible if the pharmaceutical companies would make agreements on the point of seeding trials. In many cases, the reason for performing seeding trials is that the competition does so as well.

Reviewing research in general practice

All relevant parties have an interest in careful and adequate reviewing of protocols for experiments in general practice. In The Netherlands, this view formed the basis of a cooperation of associations of GPs, of pharmaceutical professionals and the National Hospital Institute (Berden *et al.*, 1993). This cooperation resulted in the creation of a new organization called METOH (Medical Ethical Review Board of Research in General Practice). This organization coordinates a national review of protocols for experiments in general practice.

Strictly speaking, review of this research is not a legal obligation in The Netherlands. This will change when the Guidelines for Good Clinical Practice are enforced, or when the Law on Medical Experiments has passed Parliament. Although there is no legal obligation to review, most involved parties do feel the need for an adequate platform for ethical review. The fact that such a platform is lacking often results in protocols not being reviewed. Besides, there is the possibility of 'shopping' at different review boards of hospitals, e.g. in order to get the most easy approval of a protocol.

The purpose of METOH is to avoid these problems. This is achieved by the following procedure.

First of all, all relevant documents have to be available. An incomplete protocol, for example without a patient information brochure in Dutch, is not admitted for review. After all documents have been received, METOH makes a first evaluation of the relevance of the research for the general practice. This evaluation results in the codes of 'clear', 'doubtful' or 'no' relevance.

In the latter case, a protocol will be sent back to the sponsor with the question whether the sponsor is still wishing to put forward his protocol for review. If this is the case – which most of the time is not the case – the reviewing process will proceed. The same goes for protocols that get the code of 'clear' or 'doubtful' relevance. Review takes place within the Dutch Hospital Institute and is performed by an expert committee. This board is a selection from a pool of experts who are prepared to participate in a review board on a regular basis and who are specially trained for this task. If the board has no objections against a protocol – perhaps after adjustments are made – it's judgement is published in a number of important journals. In this way GPs are informed about the protocools against which the review board has no objections.

As mentioned earlier, this review facility is not obligatory. If a pharmaceutical company decides to ask participation in research which has not been reviewed, there is no legal sanction. On the other hand, one might expect physicians to object against participation in such research. If so, pharmaceutical companies will only benefit from the review of their protocols by a board of high scientific quality. This will help to avoid the turning down of protocols for the wrong reasons. And in the end one may expect an overall improvement in the quality of protocols.

Perhaps this may slightly lessen Kant's pain, although we must not expect it to disappear completely. In most experiments, people are used as means to an end. Everyone who is involved in medical experiments should always realize this and feel a little of Kant's pain.

References

Berden, H.J.J.M., Bos, M.A.J.M. & De Smet, P.A.G.M. (1993): Medisch-ethische toetsing van huisartsgeneeskundig onderzoek. *Ned. Tijdschr. Geneeskd.* **137**, 1414.

De Beaufort, I. (1985): *Ethiek en medische experimenten met mensen.* Assen: van Gorcum.

De Beaufort, I. (1989): Niet-therapeutisch wetenschappelijk onderzoek met wilsonbekwame personen. *Ned. Tijdschr. Geneeskd.* **133**, 737–740.

Bergkamp, L. (1990): Ethische en juridische aspecten van medische experimenten met mensen. In: *Handboek voor Gezondheidsethiek*, eds. I. De Beaufort en H. Dupuis, pp. 549–562. Maastricht: Van Gorcum.

Burkhardt, R. & Kienle, G. (1983): Basic problems in controlled trials. *J. Med. Ethics* **9**, 80–84.

Kant, I. (1991): *Kritik der praktischen Vernunft; Grundlegung zur Moral der Sitten*, 11th edn. pp. 51 & 61. Frankfurt: Suhrkamp.

Knottnerus, J.A. (1988): Dialectiek van het onderzoek in de huisartsgeneeskunde. *Huisarts en Wetenschap* **31**, 318–325.

Kocken, R.J., Prenger-Duchateau, A., Smeets-Rinkens, P.E.L.M. & Knottnerus, J.A. (1992): Het oordeel van huisartsen over deelname aan wetenschappelijk onderzoek. *Huisarts en Wetenschap* **35**, 32–34.

Lamberts, H. (1987): Interventie-onderzoek en informed consent: een dilemma voor huisarts en patiënt? *Huisarts en Wetenschap* **30**, 183–187.

Schafer, A. (1983): Experimentation with human subjects: a critique of the views of Hans Jonas. *J. Med. Ethics* **9**, 76–79.

van Benthem, L.H.B.M. (1988): Onderzoek naar geneesmiddelen in de huisartspraktijk. *Medisch Contact* **43**, 533–534.

Vere, D.W. (1983): Problems in controlled trials – a critical response. *J. Med. Ethics* **9**, 88.

Walters, L. (1982): Research involving human subjects. In: *Contemporary issues in bioethics*, Eds T.L. Beauchamp & L. Walters, pp. 503–509. Belmont: Wadsworth.

The ethics of animal and human experimentation, edited by P.P. De Deyn.
©1994 John Libbey & Company Ltd., pp. 269–276.

23

The moral anatomy and ethical pathology of the randomized clinical trial

Arthur Schafer

Department of Philosophy, University of Manitoba, Director, Centre for Professional and Applied Ethics, University of Manitoba, 500 Dysart Road, Winnipeg, Manitoba, R3T 2M8, Canada

Summary

The author analyses a case of research fraud which brought discredit upon the largest and, arguably, most important multicentred randomized clinical trial to have been carried out to date. Both the fraud and the rationalizations produced to justify or excuse it are critically examined in order to throw light both upon the importance of randomized clinical trials and the ethical difficulties which can arise for physicians who enrol their patients as research subjects. The role conflicts potentially involved in being both a physician and a medical investigator are discussed, as are the difficulties of obtaining genuinely informed consent from patients who volunteer to participate in clinical trials. It is argued that the risks of exploiting vulnerable patients must be balanced against (a) the good of future generations of patients and of society and (b) respect for the wishes of the patients themselves to behave altruistically.

Not infrequently, one can gain new and significant insights into an institution or a practice at the point when it breaks down, that is, when something goes seriously wrong. There occurred, recently, in Canada, a serious research fraud from which we may be able to learn some important lessons about the ethical implications of conducting randomized clinical trials.

Dr Roger Poisson, chief of oncology at St.-Luc Hospital in Montreal, was discovered deliberately to have violated the protocol of the largest, most expensive, and arguably the most important, randomized clinical trial ever undertaken. This multi-centred clinical trial (known as 'B-06') was organized by the National Surgical Adjuvant Breast and Bowel Project (known by the initials NSABP), and had as its object the assessment of the respective merits, as treatment for breast cancer, of mastectomy, lumpectomy, and lumpectomy with adjuvant radiation therapy.

Prior to the completion of the NSABP trial, in 1985, the comparative merits of mastectomy versus lumpectomy (with or without adjuvant radiation therapy) were highly controversial. Some surgeons were strongly committed to total mastectomy. Others, with equal conviction, advocated lumpectomy (sometimes called 'segmental mastectomy'). Through the altruism of thousands of women with breast cancer who volunteered to be research subjects, we now know that lumpectomy, with adjuvant radiation therapy, is best for most women (Fisher *et al.*, 1985). The result: vast numbers of women are now spared from undergoing surgery which is unnecessarily maiming.

It can be confidently asserted that only a scientifically rigorous study could have persuaded most women and their surgeons of the worth of lumpectomy. 'Common sense' seemed strongly to point in the direction of favouring total mastectomy. After all, surely one's chances of avoiding a recurrence or spread of breast cancer would be enhanced if more rather than less breast tissue were removed from the area surrounding the initial tumour. 'Common sense' was wrong in this case, as in so many others, but the challenge was to demonstrate conclusively the truth of this scientific proposition. Thus, the need to recruit thousands of women as volunteers for a clinical trial in order to generate a sufficiently impressive statistical sample, and the need to carry out the trial in the most scientifically rigorous manner possible. Patients were randomized to one or other of the three treatment arms in order to rule out the possibility of selection or other bias.

There were, in addition, carefully devised criteria of admissibility for research subjects. Participants in the trial were all women undergoing treatment for primary operable breast cancer who fulfilled a number of very specific eligibility criteria: for example, the tumour had to be confined to the breast or to the breast and ipsilateral axillary nodes on clinical examination, and the primary tumour had to be 4 cm or less in its largest dimension and movable in relation to the skin, underlying muscle, and chest wall, with no clinical evidence of skin involvement. The axilla had to be free of palpable nodes unless the nodes were movable in relation to the chest wall and neurovascular bundle (Fisher *et al.*, 1985).

Dr Poisson recruited more patients to this NSABP trial than any other single physician, a fact of which he was reported to be inordinately proud. He was awarded over a million dollars in research grants by the US National Institutes of Health, gained high status in the eyes of the cancer research community, and was listed as fourth author when the main results were published in *The New England Journal of Medicine* (Fisher *et al.*, 1985). Alas, we now know, through the investigative reporting of a diligent Chicago reporter, that Dr Poisson was able to recruit such a large number of patients only by falsifying patient data which would, if not falsified, have resulted in many of his patients being excluded from becoming research subjects in the trial. A double set of records was kept: a true record for the use of himself and his colleagues and a false record which was sent to the trial headquarters in Pittsburgh, USA.

From 1977 to 1990, a period of more than a decade, Dr Poisson falsified or fabricated some of the medical reports used in this trial. In his eagerness to enrol the maximum number of patients, Dr Poisson falsified dates of treatment and enrolled patients without always obtaining valid consent from them. More than 100 patients, who were ineligible, by the rules of the NSABP protocol, were fraudulently enrolled. For example, a woman whose cancer had spread from one breast to the other was falsely described as having cancer in only one breast, and was given postoperative radiation therapy in only one breast.

Dr Poisson's patients represented up to 16 per cent of the total number of women enrolled in the NSABP clinical trials designed not only to test the efficacy and safety of lumpectomy, but also, subsequently, of the drug tamoxifen and post-surgical chemotherapy; but his research fraud had its most significant effect on the famous (or must we now write 'infamous'?) lumpectomy trial.

Tens of thousands of women who relied upon the NSABP trial results in choosing to have lumpectomy rather than mastectomy must now feel betrayed. Did they make the wrong decision? Thousands of women currently confronting the decision of which breast cancer surgery to choose, are reported now to be experiencing dramatically enhanced anxiety levels. (Most of the women interviewed by the press have expressed their emotional upset and anger.) NSABP officials, after initially withholding information from the public about the research fraud, have now re-assessed the data, excluding that which is known to be fraudulent, and have been able to issue reassurance that the conclusions of the study are still scientifically valid. They add the further reassurance that other, independent clinical trials, conducted in other countries, have reached conclusions consistent with the preference for lumpectomy (with adjuvant radiation therapy) over total mastectomy. Nevertheless, there appears to be continuing widespread public unease, bordering on distrust of the entire scientific research community. When further cases of breast cancer research fraud come to light, as is now happening both in Canada and in the United States, public confidence withers further and the terrible anxieties associated with having breast cancer are compounded by anxieties about the integrity of scientific data.

In North America and, increasingly, in Europe, Institutional Review Boards (IRBs) are charged with the responsibility of assessing and approving the ethical propriety of all clinical trials involving human subjects. But cases such as that of Dr Poisson raise the question: once the protocol of a randomized clinical trial has been given ethical approval, how closely is the actual conduct of the trial monitored? The involvement of the Ethics Committees and IRBs seems to end once the research protocol is judged ethically sound. Evidence is now coming to light that – such are the competitive career pressures of modern medical research – much more frequent and careful audit of research practices must be carried out if both the scientific community and the general public are to be properly assured of the integrity of scientific data. More frequent audit, of course, means increased allocation of already scarce resources and increased financial expense. Some will, doubtless, object that the cost of carrying out multi-centred randomized clinical trials is already a burdensomely costly enterprise. Nevertheless, the goal of ensuring the integrity of scientific data is sufficiently important to the medical research community that, whatever the additional expense, it may simply be unavoidable.

Before turning our attention away from the sad case of Dr Poisson and his research fraud, it will be instructive to consider some of the claims made by Dr Poisson in his own defence (as reported in *The Globe and Mail*, Canada's national newspaper). Essentially, Dr Poisson portrays himself as the champion of his breast cancer patients.

'I firmly believed', wrote Dr Poisson in an open letter to the Montreal newspaper *La*

Presse, (30 March 1994) 'that a patient admitted to the protocol would be better treated, get the best possible care'. Dr. Poisson then adds that in 30 years of treating breast-cancer patients his 'goal has always been providing the best treatment available with the least amount of mutilation'. In other words, Dr Poisson justifies his research fraud, including the falsification of health records, by appealing to the principle of patient benefit. His prime concern, as a physician, was to do whatever was in the best interest of his patients. Or so he claims. And, he claims, his breast cancer patients could receive the best possible treatment and care only if they were enrolled as research subjects in the NSABP. Unfortunately, this claim does not withstand careful scrutiny.

It simply does not make sense for any doctor with a strong preference for one form of treatment (in this case, a preference for lumpectomy, the least maiming surgical treatment for breast cancer), to enrol patients in a randomized clinical trial in which many of them will be randomly assigned to receive the treatment believed by that doctor to be inferior. Thus, so far from heroically defending his patients' best interests, Dr. Poisson guaranteed that one-third of them received more mutilation than he believed medically necessary. (Recall that the three treatment arms in the NSABP trial were mastectomy, lumpectomy, and lumpectomy with adjuvant radiation therapy (Fisher *et al.*, 1985).

Ironically, the NSABP trial dragged on for years longer than had originally been anticipated because of difficulties in recruiting the large number of patients required for statistical validity. Large numbers of surgeons worried (Taylor, 1984) that patients enrolled in this trial would receive sub-optimal treatment and, therefore, refused to enrol their patients. Both camps of surgeons (the partisans of mastectomy and the partisans of lumpectomy) worried that some of their patients would be randomized to the wrong treatment arm, though of course the very reason it was vitally necessary to have the trial was to establish which form of surgery was the better and which the worse.

It is also worth noting that many surgeons reported a strong reluctance to admit to their patients, as they would have to admit if they were to enrol them as subjects in the NSABP trial, that they (the surgeons) were uncertain as to which treatment was optimal. Some surgeons rationalized their reluctance to inform potential research subjects, that is, their breast cancer patients, of their ignorance by appealing to the therapeutic benefits to patients when they are confident in the knowledgeability of their surgeon. As one surgeon commented: '. . . were I to enter my patients into the trial, I might undermine the patients' trust and faith, which are an important part of the cure'. Another reflects, with evident discomfort: '. . . how could I possibly tell the patient I don't know which operation is best? I am not uncomfortable telling her there are two options, but then she says: "Well, what do you think?" – and then what do I say? (Taylor, 1984).

More than three-quarters of those surgeons who did not enter all eligible patients into B-06 made some reference to the conflict they felt between, on the one hand, their traditional role as healer, committed exclusively to the well-being of their patients and, on the other hand, their modern role as scientific investigator committed to promoting the acquisition of scientific knowledge. (Schafer, 1982; Taylor, 1984). This reluctance to enrol patients as research subjects is scarcely surprising when one recalls that the traditional basis of a physician's authority over patients has derived from the claim to expert knowledge, combined with a moral commitment to individualized decision-making. 'The life and health of my patient will be my first consideration', or words to this effect, is the foundational principle of traditional medical ethics.

It has been noted above that Dr Poisson's unqualified enthusiasm to recruit his breast cancer patients as subjects for the NSABP trial seems inconsistent with his strongly expressed preference, from the outset of the trial, in 1976, for one treatment modality (lumpectomy) over the other (mastectomy). It is generally agreed that ethical justification for recruiting patients to a randomized trial comparing two treatments, A and B, requires that the physician-researcher must be able to say honestly to the patient/subject that there is no scientifically validated reason to predict that treatment arm A is superior or inferior to treatment arm B. (Moreover, it must also be the case that there is no alternative treatment, C, such that C is known to be superior to either A or B for this population of research subjects (Levine, 1985)). In the language of statistics, the ethical justification for beginning a randomized clinical trial requires that the investigator be able to state 'an honest null hypothesis'. Consequently, for a physician-investigator to recruit patients as subjects for a randomized clinical trial is not inconsistent with the physician's duty to provide the best possible treatment for his or her patients.

Investigators involved in the NSABP breast cancer trial of lumpectomy *vs* mastectomy could state an honest null hypothesis. That is, prior to the completion of the trial no one knew which therapy was superior. Nevertheless, there is a serious ethical problem here. Because randomized clinical trials are generally expensive to conduct (both with respect to financial costs and human resources), they are not usually initiated unless there is a substantial body of 'preliminary evidence' that the experimental treatment (in NSABP trial B-06, lumpectomy) is better than the standard treatment (in B-06, total mastectomy). This preliminary evidence may consist of clinical experience and/or data from earlier uncontrolled trials or previous but less-than-satisfactory randomized clinical trials. Thus, Dr Poisson was not unusual in having a treatment preference prior to the commencement of the randomized clinical trial which would, ultimately, provide confirmation or refutation of his preference. Animal models, clinical experience and uncontrolled trials do not add up to scientific 'knowledge', but nor can they be dismissed as a mere 'guess' or 'hunch'.

Very few patients are aware that by the phrase 'scientifically validated knowledge' the physician means 'confirmed by a controlled trial meeting the standard of significance of $P < 0.05$'. It seems more than a little arbitrary to claim that one achieves knowledge of the comparative value of competing treatments only when the results of one's experiments are 95 per cent certain. This statistical convention conceals a value judgement which might not be shared by all patients.

Indeed, it seems plausible to suppose that many patients facing the prospect of surgery for breast cancer, would expect that their doctor would share with them his/her treatment preferences even when these fall below a confidence level 95 per cent. Even when the physician's treatment preference is based on nothing more solid than uncontrolled clinical experience, most patients would consider this information relevant to their choice of treatment. It would, therefore, be inconsisent with a patient's right to give informed consent if doctors were to withhold such information from them.

The fear is that if physicians do disclose their treatment preferences, even when accompanied by a warning that the medical profession is divided on the issue and that other doctors have conflicting preferences, then few patients may be willing to have their treatment chosen by 'a flip of the coin', so to speak. (Schafer, 1985). Doctors, like Dr Poisson, who seek to recruit large numbers of their patients to randomized clinical trials, may find themselves tempted either to conceal from their patients that their treatment will be chosen by a randomizing formula (which seems to have happened in the case of some of Dr. Poisson's patients) or else to conceal from their patients information about doctors' pre-scientific treatment preferences. Since physicians would normally share such information with the patients, many of them experience this as a serious ethical problem. A clash of obligations.

When medical researchers, who are also physicians treating sick patients, tell their patients that it is not yet known which treatment is best, very few patients will be aware that the prevailing scientific convention is to withhold the title 'knowledge' from any evidence which is less than 95 per cent certain. In common (non-medical) discourse, a doctor who possessed evidence favouring treatment A over treatment B to a probability of, let us say, 70 per cent, would not be said to lack knowledge of the superiority of A over B.

Not all of Dr Poisson's patients understood that the treatment arm to which they would be assigned would, if they became research subjects in the NSABP trial, be chosen by a randomizing formula. When interviewed, several of them expressed gratitude to Dr Poisson for having chosen to give them lumpectomies rather than more radical surgery. But, of course, this was not a choice made by Dr Poisson, or any other doctor. It was the result of randomization. It would not be surprising if large numbers of patients in this randomized clinical trial or, indeed, in most randomized clinical trials, were found to be ignorant of the fact that their treatment was not selected, on an individualized basis, by their physicians. Sometimes this ignorance will result from a culpable failure on the part of investigators to inform subjects of the relevant information. (Some of Dr Poisson's patients claim that they were not so informed.) Sometimes this ignorance will result not from a failure to inform them, but from a failure properly to inform them. Patients, in other words, if they are to give validly informed consent must not only be given technical data; they must also be given information in a form which is comprehensible by them.

Patients who are very sick and/or hospitalized are vulnerable to exploitation in a variety of ways. They will often respond to medical personnel with an attitude of submissive deference, and this may prejudice their ability to assimilate the necessary information or to assert properly their own wishes. (Applebaum *et al.*, 1983). As Lurie & Shapiro (1987) report, despite the fact that they made their status as scientific investigators clear to research subjects from the outset of their study, 'they [the subjects] continued to view us as physicians first and researchers second'. Thus, when the research subjects gave what appeared to be informed consent, the validity of their consent was dubious.

Emotionally, patients are strongly conditioned to view physicians as acting primarily in their (the patient's) interest. Moreover, many patients misinterpret the nature and purpose of the entire consent procedure. As Meisel & Roth (1983) have shown, patients frequently view the process of informed consent as a requirement before receiving treatment. The knowledge that such a misinterpretation is likely, places a special obligation on researchers to follow better consent procedures which, in practice, would more adequately respect the autonomy of patients. Clearly, more empirical research is needed in this field in order for the scientific community to establish optimal methods for properly informing patients of the materially relevant information patients need in order to give genuinely informed consent.

Having said this, however, one must at the same time be aware of the need to achieve balance between hopes and fears. If one focuses exclusively on the many psychological factors which limit or vitiate patients' capacity to give informed consent to research, one then runs the opposite and equally serious risk of denying to patients the opportunity to make a generous-spirited contribution to medical knowledge by participating as research subjects (Katz, 1984). Every present patient has benefited from the medical knowledge obtained as a result of past patients' willingness to participate as subjects in earlier (randomized clinical trials. (Gilbert *et al.*, 1977). Thus, the desire to contribute, in one's turn, reflects the altogether admirable virtue of social altruism as well as fulfilling what some will regard as an obligation of justice. If we insist on imposing an excessively scrupulous standard of proof that consent is truly voluntary and informed, we risk undermining the autonomous wish of many patients to make something morally significant out of the misfortune of their disease. Moral and medical wisdom consists in striking a balance between the risk of exploiting patients, using them as a mere means to another's end (dubbed 'Kant's pain' by Huibers, in Ch. 22 (*Kant's pain*), and the risk of denying patients the right to join as co-participants with the medical research community in the valuable task of advancing medical knowledge for the benefit of future generations. There may be no easy way to escape the value conflicts inherent in the conduct of medical research on human subjects. Different societies may opt to strike the balance in one place or in another. Even within the same society, views may change over time with respect to the question of just which value should predominate when it is not possible to maximize simultaneously all the important values involved. This much seems clear. A society which seriously undervalues the importance of patient/subject autonomy will forfeit that most important of medical assets: patients' trust. Contrariwise, a society which seriously undervalues the need for scientifically rigorous research will waste its scarce medical resources and, at the same time, permit or even inflict much unnecessary suffering and death on future generations of patients.

References

Applebaum, P., Roth, L. & Lidz, C. Jr. (1983): Letter to the editor. *New Engl. J. Med.* **303**, 344.

Fisher, B., Bauer, M., Margolese, R., Poisson, R. *et al.* (1985): Five-year results of a randomized clinical trial comparing total mastectomy and segmental mastectomy with or without radiation in the treatment of breast cancer. *New Engl. J. Med.* **312**, 665–673.

Gilbert, J., McPeak, B. & Mosteller, F. (1977): Statistics and ethics in surgery and anesthesia. *Science* **198**, 684–689.

Katz, J. (1984): *The silent world of doctor and patient*. New York: The Free Press.

Levine, R. (1985): The use of placebos in randomized clinical trials. *IRB: Rev. Hum. Subjects Res.* **7**, 1–4.

Lurie, N. & Shapiro, M. (1987): Is the pursuit of scientific truth always the greatest good? Ethical issues in health care research. *Clin. Res.* **35**, 517–520.

Meisel, A. & Roth, L. (1983): Toward an informed discussion of informed consent: a review and critique of the empirical studies. *Arizona Law Rev.* **25**, 265–346.

Schafer, A. (1982): The ethics of the randomized clinical trial. *New Engl. J. Med.* **307**, 719–724.

Schafer, A. (1985): The randomized clinical trial: for whose benefit? *IRB: Rev. Hum. Subjects Res.* **7**, 4–6.

Taylor, K. (1984): Obstacles to participation in randomized clinical trials: the physician's perspective. In: *Moral priorities in medical research: the second Hannah conference*, ed. J. Nicholas, pp. 123–130. London, Ontario: The Hannah Institute for the History of Medicine.

Section V: Medical research on humans: cases of special interest

The ethics of animal and human experimentation, edited by P.P. De Deyn.

24

Clinical evaluation of antiepileptic drugs: Guidelines of the International League Against Epilepsy

Harry Meinardi

Catholic University, Nijmegen, The Netherlands

Summary

The paper examines the issue whether guidelines formulated by the International League against Epilepsy (ILAE) for Clinical Evaluation of Antiepileptic Drugs implicitly or explicitly pay attention to ethical questions. It is noted that in parallel to the guidance offered by the professional organization ILAE the WHO Regional office for Europe also embarked on drafting guidelines for the same purpose and so did the office of the European Economic Community. Only the draft of the WHO Regional Office for Europe included a separate chapter with ethical aspects. Yet all three documents dealt implicitly with ethical issues. Finally the paper concludes that one ethical issue appears not to have been touched upon, i. e. the relationship between the clinical investigators and the industrial producer of the new drug. Yet some guidelines for the control of the concurring and the diverging interest of industry and of investigators seem to be appropriate.

Introduction

Waren Reich, the editor of the first *Encyclopedia on Bioethics* which appeared in 1978, gave three reasons for a general increase of interest in bioethics:

(1) The issues of bioethics have captured the contemporary mind because they represent major conflicts in the area of technology and basic human values, those dealing with life, death and health. Although many bioethical issues have been discussed since ancient times, the introduction of modern biomedical technologies, especially since the 1950s, has intensified some age-old questions and has given rise to perplexing new problems –

the prolongation of life, euthanasia, prenatal diagnosis and abortion, human experimentation, genetic interventions and reproductive technologies, behaviour control and psychosurgery, the definition of death, the right to privacy, allocation of scarce health resources, and dilemmas in the maintenance of environmental health.

(2) There is an intense and widespread interest in bioethics because it offers a stimulating intellectual and moral challenge. In contrast to earlier eras, when ethical world views were held in common and offered a certain security for dealing with moral dilemmas, today the very tools for coping with these problems are themselves the subject of considerable controversy. There is uncertainty about moral values, ethical principles, and their priorities; the contemporary world is experiencing a philosophical upheaval; and many systems of theological thought are questioning traditional assumptions in religious ethics. Bioethics has already had a significant intellectual impact, for it has precipitated a reexamination of basic moral values and methods of applying them to practical ethical questions.

(3) The rapid growth of the field of bioethics has been facilitated by the openness to multidisciplinary work that characterizes many scholars and academic institutions today, especially in matters dealing with personal and social aspects of human behaviour.

Perhaps, apart from the reasons presented by Reich, another factor is the high level of education of the general public. The public probably is well aware that an expert can no longer be expected to encompass all there is to know. Therefore guidelines and protocols can assist those who deliver a service but can also help clients to gauge whether they are getting the treatment on which consensus has been reached.

Principles for clinical testing of antiepileptic drugs

The reasons given by the ILAE when it published its first guidelines in 1973 for use in clinical evaluation of antiepileptic drugs were as follows:

> 'With no new primary drugs for the treatment of epilepsy having been introduced in nearly a decade and several compounds languishing for years in clinical investigational status without proof of efficacy, it became apparent that a critical need existed for principles for the clinical testing of antiepileptic drugs. These principles are intended to improve the quality of the clinical evaluation of new antiepileptic drugs and to facilitate the international exchange of data supporting the investigation of new antiepileptic agents, resulting in the more rapid development and precise use of new drugs for the treatment of epilepsy.'

Sixteen years later a new set of guidelines entitled 'Guidelines for Clinical Evaluation of Antiepileptic Drugs' were published by the ILAE (1989). In its justification the following goals were presented:

(1) To offer guidance to those involved in clinical evaluation of antiepileptic drugs on the optimal and innovative use of experimental compounds.

(2) *To protect subjects and patients from undue harm without compromising the evaluation of the full potential of experimental drugs with regard to efficacy and toxicity.*

(3) To stimulate further development of better antiepileptic drugs.

For this treatise on bioethics it would be important to know which considerations led the Commission to include the protection of subjects and patients amongst the goals of these guidelines. However, to obtain this information retrospectively is a well-nigh impossible task. It is easier to look for differences in the guidelines of 1973 and 1989 as a consequence of this goal. Indeed in 1973 the emphasis for Phase I research was on determining the pharmacokinetics of the investigational substance in man. With respect to side-effects only the need to employ a double-blind paradigm is stressed, 'because subjects will be warned side-effects may occur and some subjects are bound to be suggestible'.

In 1989 it was pointed out that in Phase I the investigational drug will have to be assessed at different dosages. However, it is emphasized that doses should only be increased if it is certain that the last dose given did not cause any adverse effects. Furthermore, it is underscored that the relationship of the side-effects and the serum level of the investigational drug should be laid down. With respect to side-effects it is pointed out that not only blood pressure, blood chemistry, kidney and liver functions should be registered but also neuropsychological parameters.

In 1989, the close observation of subjects in order to detect adverse effects of the drugs is particularly emphasized.

Yet, also in the 1973 point of departure is the assumption that no new antiepileptic drug should be introduced unless it could be proved that some patients with epilepsy resistant to the available therapy could become seizure-free or at least would experience an appreciable reduction in seizure frequency. Industry proposed that there should be room for new antiepileptic drugs with similar efficacy as drugs already on the market but devoid of side-effects. In theory this is a valid request. However, the experts objected that the evaluation of such a drug would have great practical difficulties. The evaluation protocol would require the inclusion of patients free of seizures on a marketed drug, but suffering from side-effects. These patients should be willing to take the chance that the new drug might be less efficacious or at least not suited for their particular type of epilepsy. If this were the case, they would have a relapse of seizures with all its social repercussions.

Comparison of two active drugs also involves a larger number of matched pairs than the comparison of a potentially active drug against placebo. The problem of exchanging an active drug with a test-drug is that the patient, seizure-free on the active drug, might have remitted and therefore would have remained seizure free if the active drug had been exchanged with placebo. Usually drug withdrawal in seizure-free patients is only attempted after 3 to 5 years but that does not alter the fact that in some individuals withdrawal of the antiepileptic drug could have taken place earlier with impunity. Though little is known about the percentage of seizure-free patients who suffer from side-effects, the experts were afraid that it would be unethical to ask a person to run the risk of losing seizure control only in the hope that an apparently bearable adverse effect would disappear. Part of the misgivings of the experts were probably based on the background knowledge that it is sometimes very difficult to regain control of seizures when a seizure-free patient withdraws medication and suffers a relapse.

In fact, the text of the 1973 guidelines does permit the inclusion of patients whose seizures would have been controlled by available drugs, but at the cost of excessive adverse effects. Though it is not clear from the text, the commission members argued that in case of excessive adverse effects an efficacious drug would not be applied to its full potentiality and in practice the patient would therefore still have seizures. Besides, new drugs are doomed to lose a comparison between equal seizure control but less adverse effects, if one realizes that one of the very severe side-effects of a drug is the financial burden it bestows on the patient, and unfortunately all new drugs are bound to be more expensive than the older drugs.

In 1989, throughout the document, the subjects involved in the different phases of investigation are supposed to be 'with incomplete control of seizures. Incomplete control is defined as seizures despite maximum tolerable serum concentrations of standard drug therapy'.

The ILAE guidelines do not quite solve the problem of the evaluation of investigational antiepileptic drugs in women of childbearing potential. In 1973 the possibility of including these women in Phase II investigations is considered acceptable if animal studies and Phase I studies (healthy volunteers) did not reveal contra-indications. How such contra-indications could emerge from Phase I studies is not explained. Probably reference is to enzyme-induction or other mechanisms of interference with contraception. In 1989, women of childbearing potential are excluded from Phase I studies but accepted for early Phase II studies if dependable contraception is practised. In late Phase II studies, participation is only accepted if animal studies did not reveal teratogenicity. Even if this is the case, adequate contraception is an absolute requirement.

Pregnant women or women intending to become pregnant are in an unfortunate position with respect to the introduction of a new drug. In general, package inserts stipulate that the drug should not be used during pregnancy. And in fact, data upon which a different statement would be possible will remain missing until sufficient healthy children have been born from pregnancies during which the drug was accidentally used or during which the drug was used consciously disregarding the warning. In the spring of 1992, Andermann and Meinardi discussed this problem during the Second Jerusalem Conference on Pharmaceutical Sciences and Clinical Pharmacology and in the Progress Report on New Antiepileptic Drugs during the Post-conference Satellite Symposium at Eilat.

A proposition to invite women considering to become pregnant for a Phase IV (post-marketing) controlled study to verify whether the theoretical greater safety of a new drug for the child (i.e. not teratogenic in animal studies) would be confirmed in practice was rejected. The argument was that women with epilepsy usually postpone family planning until the seizures are controlled. Even though they would run a 6–9 per cent risk that the child would suffer from minor or major malformations on the medication in use, switching to a new drug with theoretically greater safety with respect to teratogenesis would introduce a difficult-to-estimate risk that their seizures would relapse if the efficacy of the new drug for these individuals did not equal that of the drug they were using.

Another proposition was to exchange, in all women of childbearing potential, the currently used drugs with a record of teratogenicity for new drugs proven safe in animal studies. For those drugs the relevant section of the package insert should then be changed into: 'When the drug is used during pregnancy it should be realized that insufficient information about the influence on the human foetus is available. Animal studies however have not shown any untoward effect on the offspring.' Representatives of the pharmaceutical industry however were of the opinion that such a change of the caution in the package insert would gain the approval of neither the drug regulatory authorities nor their company lawyers.

Another special category are children with epilepsy. Right from the beginning it was taken into account that drugs designed to control seizure types that occur only or predominantly in children can only be evaluated by admitting children to the drug trial. Nevertheless ILAE judged the target group sufficiently different to require an independent set of guidelines that had to address the specific problems stemming from the inclusion of children in a drug trial. This resulted in a document 'Guidelines for Antiepileptic Drug Trials in Children' which is to be published in 1993. In this document it is emphasized that pharmacokinetics are undergoing important changes in children and therefore the data for different age groups should be studied to obtain adequate Phase I information. However, it is considered impermissible to involve healthy children in drug trials, therefore Phase I information has to be obtained from children with epilepsy expected to benefit from the new drug. The document also recommends only the use of parallel and not cross-over studies even though larger numbers of children have to participate. Parallel studies are shorter, which is also important because of the physical changes of the child over time.

The 'Guidelines for Antiepileptic Drug Trials in Children' also address the issue that some of the important epilepsy syndromes of childhood have a low prevalence and therefore a drug trial will necessarily be conducted in several centres and quite likely in several countries. This necessitates consensus about the protocol and the evaluation procedures, not only between the research groups, but also with respect to the regulatory authorities.

With regard to a universal acceptance, guidelines produced by an international scientific organization like ILAE should be well placed. Yet the Regional Office for Europe of the WHO also embarked on *Guidelines for the clinical investigation of antiepileptic drugs* (1985). It was stressed 'that this document is not intended to have any regulatory or legal character. It is intended for the use of clinical investigators and seeks to state what may currently be regarded as sound investigational practice for this particular group of drugs. It is realized that, in various of the fields with which it deals, alternative approaches are possible and that others will be developed. The text thus has no mandatory character; it does not, for example, seek to indicate which studies should be undertaken before a drug is admitted to the market, nor does it define in which order particular investigations should be performed, except where there are purely scientific or ethical reasons to follow a particular sequence. Regulatory standards are likely to be closely similar in some respects to scientific investigational standards, but they will necessarily depend in large measure on a country's drug legislation and will therefore differ in various parts of the world.' Its last appearance was as a 'Revised Draft' in 1985.

It is interesting to note that this document did have a separate chapter dealing with ethical aspects. In fact, in that chapter the document transgresses its field by making a stand against the prophylactic use of antiepileptic drugs in persons who have sustained serious head injury. More within line is a remark about the use of placebo. The verdict was that a placebo is out of bounds if it is known that the seizures could be controlled by an available drug. This is particularly relevant with respect to a protocol introduced by the manufacturer of Felbamate in the USA. Patients whose (insufficiently efficacious) medication is withdrawn, in order to register electroencephalographically the exact place of onset of their seizures in preparation for neurosurgical removal of the focus, receive either placebo or the investigational drug after the seizure registration has taken place. After a predetermined number of seizures, the patient is returned to the preregistration regimen. The reason for this protocol is the strong interaction Felbamate has with other antiepileptic drugs. The reason for using placebo instead of randomizing between the preregistration regimen and investigational drug is the lack of power of a design comparing two (partially) active drugs.

It is possible that the WHO Regional Office for Europe never finalized the draft guidelines as the office of the European Economic Community in the meantime produced guidelines ('Note for guidance, intended to assist applicants for marketing authorization in the interpretation of directive 75/318/EEC as amended with respect to clinical evaluation of medicinal products used in epileptic disorders, and to provide guidance on clinical testing of such products). This note 'Medicinal Products for the Treatment of Epileptic Disorders' (1989 revision) also states: 'It is highly advisable to potential investigators also to consult 'Guidelines for Clinical Evaluation of Antiepileptic Drugs' from the ILAE.' With respect to the ethical considerations this note opens with an introduction saying 'The rules and norms laid down in the Declaration of Helsinki (Venice, Italy 1983) and the norms and standards of Good Clinical Practice should be strictly adhered to. Except for the very earliest phase of tolerability studies, it is generally desirable that clinical assessment of antiepileptic medicinal products be performed by experienced epileptologists with adequate support facilities. Special attention should be given to multicentre studies so that facilities, conditions and patient materials as well as the experience of the various investigators are similar in the different centres'.

Guidelines obviously are not the same as regulations. With respect to the desideratum of equivalence between the different centres participating in multicentre drug trials, obviously there will be a difference between countries that include special centres for epilepsy in their health system and countries where epilepsy is only taken care of by general neurologists or paediatricians.

On reviewing these guidelines on evaluation of antiepileptic drugs, one ethical issue appears not to have been touched upon, i.e. the relationship between the clinical investigators and the industrial manufacturer of the new drug. It is striking that also none of the speakers of a 1993 Antwerp Conference on Experimental Animals and Human Subjects was assigned this topic as far as can be gauged from the titles of their presentations. Yet this is a problem with ethical implications that should be faced.

The assertion that it is not in the interest of a physician to introduce the magical cure that eliminates all diseases, as it will reduce him to beggary while the industrialist will bathe in riches, is obviously balderdash. There is plenty of emotional reward for the physician who has been instrumental in curing a previously intractable case. However, for drug evaluation, pharmaceutical companies approach authoritative physicians, considered to be opinion leaders in their specialty. As this collaboration will become increasingly fruitful as both parties gain experience, industry will return again and again to the same physician. It is clear that currently such collaborations involve financial ties between industry and the investigator. Both parties are aware that financial incentives should not bias results. Indeed the actual investigation uses blinded techniques, but once the code is broken, the interpretation and presentation of results is not bias protected. In fact, human nature being distrustful, even unimpeachable scientists who often collaborate with industry notice that their papers are regarded with suspicion as their colleagues surmise that they have become puppets of industry. One option to solve this problem would be the creation of a research fund for drug evaluation and a surtax on all drugs sold to finance this fund. However, such a solution has the drawback that poor companies thus would have the opportunity to develop new drugs at the expense of richer companies. The problem of a surtax is also that politicians sometimes tend to forget the purpose for which the tax money is collected and divert it to other, politically more savoury objectives, as reputedly happened to gasoline taxes originally intended for maintenance and improvement of the road system.

Some guidelines for control of the concurring and the diverging interests of industry and investigators seem to be appropriate. Apparently some are being developed (see the book edited by Porter & Malone (1992)). However these are not guidelines of the ILAE with which this chapter has been concerned.

References

Commission on Antiepileptic Drugs of the International League Against Epilepsy (1973): Principles for clinical testing of antiepileptic drugs. *Epilepsia* **14**, 451–458.

Commission on Antiepileptic Drugs of the International League Against Epilepsy (1989): Guidelines for clinical evaluation of antiepileptic drugs. *Epilepsia* **30**, 400–408.

Commission on Antiepileptic Drugs of the International League Against Epilepsy (1994): Guidelines for antiepileptic drug trials in children. *Epilepsia* **35**, 94–100.

Medicinal Products for the Treatment of Epileptic Disorders (1989 Revision). Feiden, *Arzneimittelprüfrichtlinien* (1.Erg.lfg.1991).

Porter, R.J. & Malone, T.E. eds. (1992): *Biomedical research: collaboration and conflict of interest.* Baltimore: Johns Hopkins University Press.

Reich, W.T. ed. (1978): *Encyclopedia of bioethics.* New York: The Free Press.

World Health Organization, Regional Office For Europe (1985): *Guidelines for the clinical investigation of antiepileptic drugs* (Draft).Copenhagen: WHO.

The ethics of animal and human experimentation, edited by P.P. De Deyn.

25

Endoscopic techniques in surgery: ethical aspects

Robrecht Van Hee

Department of Surgery, University of Antwerp, Universiteitsplein 1, B-2610 Wilrijk, Belgium

Summary

Endoscopic surgical techniques have gained wide acceptance in surgical practice in the last 5 years. Great advantages in using these techniques soon became apparent for the patient as well as for the surgeon. The ethical consequences of the rapid acceptance of these new techniques may however have been overlooked. Only very limited prospective studies were performed to compare statistical results of open and endoscopic surgical interventions. Scarce randomized trials even had to be abandoned. On the other hand too liberal extension of the indications for some types of surgery became possible and have already been noted. Competition between surgeons, as well as between institutions, induced immediate use of the techniques without adequate training. The instrument industries play an important role in sponsoring and technical education programmes of endoscopic surgery. Surgeons should be aware of the ethical dangers these kinds of sponsorships may represent in the future.

I shall withhold myself from stonecutting and leave this to the expert: a statement by Hippocrates (*c.* 460–*c.* 377 BC) from the 4th century BC and written down in the so-called Hippocratic Oath, probably one of the most universal medical–ethical texts that has come down to us (Lindeboom, 1948). This sentence describes very clearly the specialistic nature of certain manual surgical practices which have been applied to the sick and injured since time immemorial. It is clear that the specific nature of these interventions entails ethical connotations regarding patients, as well as the physicians who perform them not only from the inclusion of this quotation in the Hippocratic oath; it has been obvious in every new development of surgical techniques throughout the centuries. This also applies, undoubtedly to the most recent surgical development of endoscopic techniques in the surgical treatment of disorders. In order to be able to deal with some of these ethical reflections regarding scopic surgery, a short assessment of these techniques is necessary.

Until the middle of the last century, surgeons were limited to the treatment of external conditions such as fatty bumps, haemorrhoids, abcesses, gangrene, fractured or dislocated limbs, etc. After the introduction of anaesthesia in 1846, internal organs became accessible for surgery. Also by the introduction of aseptic and antiseptic techniques a breakthrough in medicine occurred in the last quarter of the 19th century, which flourished especially in the big surgical schools of Vienna, Paris, Berlin, Boston, etc. In Berlin, in 1882, Carl Langenbuch performed the first successful gall-bladder removal (Langenbuch, 1882); in Vienna, Theodor Billroth developed the first stomach resection, different types of intestine anastomoses etc. (Billroth, 1881). A few decades later at the *lé Charité* hospital in Berlin, Ferdinand Sauerbruch performed the first lung operation (Sauerbruch, 1904), while in the United States, Harvey Cushing brought brain surgery to previously unknown flourishing (Van Hee, 1993). Each time, depending on the pathology under treatment, minor or major incisions had to be made in the abdomen or the chest. Since the turn of the century the successes of cystoscopy in enabling a view into the internal of the bladder led to the first hesitant attempts to look directly for disorders in the abdomen: it was the Swede Jacobeus who in 1911 announced the first results of this so-called laparoscopy in humans. In the 1930s, visibility in the peritoneal cavity was much improved by inflating with carbon dioxide. A special needle with a spring, developed by Veress for the treatment of pneumothorax, was used to insert the gas (Veress, 1938). From the 1960s on, gynaecologists started using the technique of laparoscopy for the diagnosis of abdominal disorders. They performed the first abdominal surgery, i.e. diathermic section, the elipsing of the ovaries. Semm, in the 1970s, definitely started laparoscopic surgery techniques (Semm & Mettlere, 1980). Not only for gynaecological surgery but also for appendectomy, it was Semm who developed the bases (Semm, 1983). The first tidings about complications of laparoscopy (Loffer & Pent, 1975), and also the first results of numerous gynaecological surgical procedures (Mintz, 1976) appeared in the 1970s, and gave the impetus for further animal research on laparoscopic possibilities of surgical intervention in the abdomen. Thus, Ko & Avians from Chicago, and Cuschieri & Nathanson from Dundee developed (the former on dogs, the latter on pigs) more or less simultaneously the technique of laparoscopic gall-bladder removal (Macintyre & Wilson, 1993). It is assumed that Mouret in France was the first to perform, in 1987, a successful cholecystectomy in humans (Mouret, 1991a). Not more than a year later, all over the world, but especially in France, many teams applied this technique so that information about the first series of patients emerged in 1989 (Reddick & Olsen, 1989; Dubois *et al.*, 1990; Périssat *et al.*, 1990; Nathanson *et al.*, 1991). The development in the medical world since the 1989 publications, defies all imagination: many spoke justly about a second surgical revolution (Lerut, 1992), comparing it to the explosion of surgical techniques at the end of the previous century, after the introduction of asepsis and anaesthesia.

What are the reasons why in only 4 years endoscopic surgical techniques developed at full speed and met with such wide acclaim? Essentially, it is the very limited impact that the endoscopic approach has on the human body as compared to open techniques. To paraphrase Sir Winston Churchill's statement on the battle of Britain, one can say that never before have such impressive results with a new surgical technique been achieved with so little means (Mouret, 1991b).

Some basics of this so-called mini invasive technique should be briefly explained. After inserting carbon dioxide in the body cavity concerned, a various number of perforating pins or trocars will be inserted, through which either the optical equipment or surgical instruments can be inserted. A laparoscope is screwed to a camera, which is connected to video equipment. This will enable the surgeon to follow movements and surgery performed in the inside of the abdominal or thoracic cavity directly on a screen. The array of surgical instruments, increasingly developed by the industry in the last few years, enables the surgeon to perform all kinds of operations in the body cavity: as mentioned before, removing the appendix or gall-bladder, but also repair of an inguinal or diaphragmal hernia, removing a lung segment or an affected piece of bowel, etc. Because the entire operation is performed through a number of small openings in the abdominal or thoracic cavity, only a little bit of muscle fibre in the wall of the trunk is sectioned, which allows much faster recovery of body movements in the patient. At the same time, the general condition of the patient is normalized much faster, which enables quick discharge from the hospital. The quicker recovery of the patient, entailing less time lost from work, has immediate and important economical implications. Where the occupational disability of the so-called open removal of the gall-bladder used to be 6 weeks, the laparoscopic technique is accompanied by interruption of work of an average of 11 to 12 days (Cuschieri *et al.*, 1991; Peterson *et al.*, 1983).

It is not amazing that not only the medical world as well as the instrument industry, but even more the patient himself, want to urge this transition to endoscopic surgery techniques. And exactly there hide the ethical dangers, associated with such a quick innovation. The problems comprise different fields, i.e. the demonstration of the statistical significance of the medical advantages of the new method; the acceptance of these new surgical techniques by skilled surgeons; their performance by the present academic and non-academic community; the commercial pressure of the instrument producing industry as well as the training of candidate specialists in these new techniques.

Let us elaborate on these different points. First of all, *the scientific demonstration of the soundness of endoscopic techniques.* Where laparoscopic techniques in gynaecological surgery proved to entail no higher mortality risk (Peterson *et al.*, 1983), this was by no means clear for gall-bladder removal or stomach surgery. On the contrary, open gall-bladder removal or cholecystectomy was a standard procedure with a negligible mortality risk, in large series varying between 0 and 0.4 per cent (Ganey *et al.*, 1986; McSherry, 1993), and an extremely small risk for complications (Meyer *et al.*, 1967; Gilliland & Traverso, 1990). The small risks of the traditional technique made the attempts to reduce the incision to a so-called mini-laparotomy rather useless because the superiority of the new technique could not be demonstrated (Olsen, 1993). On the other hand, in the development of new endoscopic techniques, emphasis is put on the surgical feasibility of the procedure rather than on long-term results in operated patients. From the start, as already mentioned, there were positive results reported on short term as well in pilot series (Reddick & Olsen, 1989; Dubois *et al.*, 1990; Périssat *et al.*, 1990; Nathanson *et al.*, 1991), and recently, in larger European and American patient groups (Barkum *et al.*, 1993; Gadacz, 1993; Périssat, 1993). Compared to the open technique the mortality rate seemed to be even lower, fluctuating between 0.04 and 0.12 per cent (Deziel *et al.*, 1993; Dunn, 1991). Results on long term effects are scarce, and only the data for gall-bladder removal are published. However, the first-year results would not differ too much from those of open techniques (Wilson & Macintyre, 1993b). Still, most series undoubtedly keep underestimating the mortality and morbidity risks and all suffer from so-called positive reporting, more so because the present reports came exclusively from large specialized centres, and these results will certainly not be achieved by other hospitals. On first sight, it seems easy to resolve this problem by means of prospective randomized clinical trials in which open and closed techniques could be compared. However, the decision to set up such trials does not take into consideration the actual wish of patients whom are aware of the cited advantages of endoscopic techniques, nor the surgeon's ascertainment that laparoscopically operated patients painlessly walk around in their room the next day. Not surprisingly, large-scale multicentre trials, as set up in the UK and in Germany, were doomed to fail, and had to be terminated prematurely (Neugebauer *et al.*, 1991). Fortunately, smaller randomized studies seem to point to the advantage of laparoscopic techniques (Kunz *et al.*, 1992). By 1993, it was generally regrettable that no larger trials support these new surgical techniques, perpetuating that 'operations introduced on the basis of a prospective randomized trial are rather the exception than the rule' as Macintyre and Wilson justly quote (Macintyre & Wilson, 1993).

As a second point in this discourse, *it is striking how extremely fast these endoscopic surgery techniques have been adopted by the surgical community*. Where at first surgeons were cautious regarding these new techniques, possibly for fear of degradation of their own trusty surgical clientele (Terblanche, 1991), it is at present assumed that at least for gall-bladder removal, about 80 per cent of these interventions are performed in a laparoscopic way (Kalser *et al.*, 1993). Not only were surgeons supported in their choice by positive reports from almost all international centres (Meyers *et al.*, 1991; Schirmer *et al.*, 1991; Cholelithiasis European Consensus Conference, 1992), not in the least from Belgium (Dallemagne *et al.*, 1991), also socio-economic and technical aspects contributed to the decision of many surgeons to acquire these techniques. The plethora of surgeons, that characterizes the Western countries during past few years, undoubtedly led many surgeons to quick acceptance of these new endoscopic techniques. It is indeed striking how laparoscopic surgery of gall-bladder, appendix or stomach struck home faster with general surgeons than such interventions on female genitalia ever did with gynaecologists. Could it be the continuously diminishing role played by the general surgeon because of the expansion of surgical specialties; or, especially in Belgium, the almost logarithmically increasing number of surgeons; or is it the urge for innovation, technicity, and use of video-controlled equipment, which made so many surgeons simultaneously abandon familiar open surgical techniques, to pursue closed endoscopic surgery? Or, has it been the fear of many surgeons also of losing the surgical aspects of endoscopy to gastro-enterologists and endoscopists, physicians who, at least in most European countries, have almost totally mastered the endoscopic diagnosis of the digestive tract?

My own inquiry about the reasons for selecting one or other technique demonstrated that surgeon-related motivations were more important than pressure from patients or general practitioners. Both seemed, certainly in the beginning, inadequately informed with regard to endoscopic techniques, and their advantages. With regard to the acceptance of a new technique in the world of medicine it is very striking that in several countries, especially in France and Belgium, surgeons at non-university hospitals used endoscopic surgery techniques earlier than their colleagues at university or academic hospitals. Here also certain economic or personal motives may have enhanced the surgeon's choice for the new endoscopic technique. Moreover, it is striking that in both types of hospitals, the local ethical review boards were not consulted before introducing this new technique, which at that moment had not yet won its spurs. Lately, the academics especially warned against lax indication in surgery of diaphragmal hernia, a pathology for which the number of interventions in Belgium quadrupled in 2 years time according to the Belgian third party payers' data (Dallemagne, 1993).

Aside from medical and patient-related aspects of endoscopic surgery, *commercial and industry-related elements play a significant role.* As in the pharmaceutical sector, there are at present enormous efforts and investments made by the instrument industry in order to conquer a more or less competitive part of this new market. It is however worth considering that sound judgement and daring, which some American industries displayed in the initial development of equipment, led to the evolution which we now witness. When Mouret from Lyon compared endoscopic equipment with stapling devices for intestinal anastomosis, developed by a USA-based company, he stated: 'Lorsque Léon Hirsch [of the mentioned industry] a développé et diffusé le Stapling, qui croyait que ces machines venues d'Europe de l'Est, avaient un quelconque avenir? Et en 1985; lorsqui'il a décidé d'étudier la technologie des trocarts, qui croyait à le coelioscopie digestive? Je vous assure que nous étions dans le monde, moins que les doigts de la main. J'en étais un, Léon Hirsch en était un autre' (Mouret, 1993).

Undoubtedly, it was due to fast industrial development and distribution of equipment that these endoscopic techniques could be used worldwide in such a short time. Evidently, this technological development brought grist to the industry. In a few years time, almost every hospital in Belgium was supplied with so-called 'endoscopic towers', equipment essential to perform endoscopic surgery with a cost price of 1.5 to 2 million Belgian francs each. On top of that are the disposable trocars or perforating pins, which are principally a patient-related and chronic financial burden on the hospital and its surgeons. To paraphrase Gérard Champault from Paris: 'le salaire d'un chirurgien en hôpital général équivaut en ce moment à 50 trocarts,' which might indicate the poor wages of the Parisian surgeon as well as the expense of the trocars (Champault, 1993).

It goes without saying, that several instrument companies are involved in keen competition. Sometimes less correct interactions occur between surgeons and industry. Industry sponsors surgeons, who at present are confronted with a dramatic shortage of research resources; industry also assists in the education of assistants, etc. Often such cooperation leads to a productive relationship. However, Keeman from Amsterdam justly warns of illicit forms of sponsoring and adds this: 'it is important that physicians show great care so that they do not put themselves in a compromising or even ethically indefensible position' (Keeman, 1993). It is important that national and international scientific authorities and medical faculties do not lose sight of their directional tasks.

The training of surgeons was already mentioned as being an important part in successfully and safely perform-ing these new techniques. In the Anglo-Saxon countries, the Royal Colleges of Great Britain and Australia, as well as the American Society of Gastrointestinal Endoscopic Surgeons gave clear guidelines with regard to performing this surgery. The surgeon who applies these endoscopic techniques should be a trained general surgeon who has acquired knowledge of diagnostic laparoscopy, and has attended a course or workshop in surgical-endoscopic techniques.

Up to now, such guidelines do not exist in Belgium. The danger exists that surgeons will make their first attempts of laparoscopic gall-bladder or stomach surgery directly on patients. A survey among British surgeons showed that, although 99 per cent of those interrogated found that specific training is a must, 20 per cent of the responders mastered the technique from experience on patients (Wilson & Macintyre, 1993a). This percentage is without any doubt even higher in Belgium. Fortunately, *the first training centres are now arising throughout Belgium*, some organized by universities and hospitals, others by the instrument industry. They use artificial models which imitate closed body cavities which allow training in all kinds of interventions and stitching. In a second term, attendants exercise *in vivo* techniques on anaesthesized research animals. Thus, as far as funds are made available within the plan of 'Advanced Academic Training', these demonstrations will be expanded in a joint venture with the industry.

Evidently, some surgeons may be too old or too specialized in a certain branch of surgery for this in-service training. The British survey mentioned above pointed out that this was only the case for 15 out of 103 questioned (Wilson & Macintyre, 1993a), which immediately shows the benefit of these organized courses for board-certified surgeons as well as for residents in training.

Summarizing, we can say that in a short time endoscopic-surgical techniques, also called mini-invasive surgery, have earned their definite place in medicine. This places surgeons and society in front of a number of medical ethical questions with regard to indication of intervention, with regard to training of the surgeon and the assistant surgeon in these new techniques, and with regard to the relation between the instrument industry and the surgeon. We may only hope that the surgical community will find an adequate answer to these novel ethical problems.

References

Barkum, J.S., Barkum, A.N., Meakins, J.L. & the Mill Gill Gallstone Treatment Group (1993): Laparoscopic versus open cholecystectomy: the Canadian experience. *Am. J. Surg.* **165,** 455–458.

Billroth, C.A.T. (1881): Offenes Schreiben an Herrn Dr. L. Wittelshöfer. *Wien. Med. Wochenschr.* **31,** 161–165, 1427.

Champault, G. (1993): 'Money-money': réponse à la réponse. *Assoc. Franç. Chir.* (Bulletin) 618.

Cholelithiasis European Consensus Conference, Strasbourg, December 1991 (1992): Summary. *Presse Méd* **21,** 453–456.

Cuschieri, A., Dubois, F., Mouiel, J. *et al.* (1991): The European experience with laparoscopic cholecystectomy. *Am. J. Surg.* **161,** 385–387.

Dallemagne, B. (1993): Personal communication. The Congress of the Royal Belgian Society for Surgery, Brussels 12–14 April, 1993.

Dallemagne, B., Weerts, J.M., Jehaes, C., Markiewicz, S. & Lombard, R. (1991): Laparoscopic Nissen fundoplication: preliminary report. *Surg. Laparosc. Endosc.* **1 (3),** 138–143.

Deziel, D.J., Millikan, K.W., Economon, S.G. *et al.* (1993): Complications of laparoscopic cholecystectomy – results of a national survey of 4292 hospitals and analysis of 77,604 cases. *Am. J. Surg.* **165,** 9–14.

Dubois, F., Icard, B., Berthelot, G. & Levard, H. (1990): Coelioscopic cholecystectomy. Preliminary report of 36 cases. *Am. Surg.* **211,** 60–62.

Dunn, D.C. (1991): Voluntary confidential audit of outcome of surgery. *Br. Med. J.* **303,** 1272.

Gadacz, Th.R. (1993): US experience with laparoscopic cholecystectomy. *Am. J. Surg.* **165,** 450–454.

Ganey, J.B., Johnson, P.A., Prillaman, P.E. & McSwain, G.R. (1986): Cholecysectomy: clinical experience with a large series. *Am. J. Surg.* **151,** 352–357.

Gigot, J.F. and the Belgian Group for Endoscopic Surgery (1992): Laparoscopic cholecystectomy: which results in the current practice of general surgeons? Presented at the Third World Congress of Endoscopic Surgery, Bordeaux, June 18–20.

Gilliland, T.M. & Traverso, L.W. (1990): Modern standards for Comparison of cholecystectomy with alternative treatments for symptomatic cholelithiasis with emphasis on long-term symptom relief. *Surg. Gynecol. Obstet.* **170,** 39–44.

Jacobeus, H.C. (1911): Kürze Übersicht über meine Erfahrungen mit der Laparoskopie. *Münch. Med. Wochenschr.* **58,** 2017–2019.

Kalser, S.C. & the Planning Committee of the NIH Consensus Conference (1993): National Institutes of Health consensus development conference statement on gallstones and laparoscopic cholecystectomy. *Am. J. Surg.* **165,** 390–398.

Keeman, J.N. (1993): De industrie en de heelkunde, hoe ver gaat de samenwerking? *Ned. Tijdschr. Heelk.* **2,** 69–70.

Kunz, R., Orth, K., Vogel, J. *et al.* (1992): Laparoscopic cholecystectomy versus mini-laparotomy cholecystectomy. Results of a prospective randomized trial. *Chirurg.* **63,** 291–295.

Langenbuch, C. (1882): Ein Fall von Extirpation der Gallenblase wegen chronischer Cholelithiasis. Heilung. *Berl. Klin. Wochenschr.* **48,** 725–727.

Lerut, T. (1992): Editorial. *Acta Chir. Belg.***92**, 63–65.

Lindeboom, G.A. (1948): *Hippocrates.* Antwerpen: Het Kompas & Amsterdam: L.J. Veen.

Loffer, F.D. & Pent, D. (1975): Indications, contra-indications and complications of laparoscopy. *Obstet. Gynecol. Surv.* **30,** 407–426.

Macintyre, I.M.C. & Wilson, R.G. (1993): Laparoscopic cholecystectomy. *Br. J. Surg.* **80,** 552–559.

McSherry, Ch. (1993): Open cholecystectomy. *Am. J. Surg.* **165,** 435–439.

Meyer, K.A., Capos, N.J. & Mittlepunkt, A.I. (1967): Personal experiences with 1,261 cases of acute and chronic cholecystitis and cholelithiasis. *Surgery* **61,** 661–668.

Meyers, W.C., Branum, G.D., Farouk, M. & the Southern Surgeons Club (1991): A prospective analysis of 1518 laparoscopic cholecystectomies. *N. Engl. J. Med.* **324,** 1073–1078.

Mintz, M. (1976): Le risque et la prophylaxie des accidents en coelioscopie gynécologique. Enquête portant sur 100.000 cas. *J. Gynecol. Obstet. Biol. Reprod.* **5,** 681–695.

Mouret, G. (1991a): From the first laparoscopic cholecystectomy to the frontiers of laparoscopic surgery: the future perspectives. *Dig. Surg.* **8,** 124–125.

Mouret, P. (1991b): Philosophie de la chirurgie coelioscopique. In: *Chirurgie digestive par voie coelioscopique*, eds. P. Testas & B. Delaitre, pp. 7–8. Paris: Maloine.

Mouret, Ph. (1993): Lettre ouverte à Gérard Champault. *Assoc. Franç. Chir*, (Bulletin) p. 618.

Nathanson, L.K., Shimi, S. & Cuschieri, A. (1991): Laparoscopic cholecystectomy: the Dundee technique. *Br. J. Surg.*. **78**, 155–159.

Neugebauer, E., Troidl, H., Spangenberger, W., Dietrich, A. & Lefering, R. (1991): The cholecystectomy study group. Conventional versus laparoscopic cholecystectomy and the randomized controlled trial. *Br. J. Surg.* **78**, 150–154.

Olsen, D.O. (1993): Mini-lap cholecystectomy. *Am. J. Surg.* **165**, 440–443.

Périssat, J. (1993): Laparoscopic cholecystectomy: the European experience. *Am. J. Surg.* **165**, 444–449.

Périssat, J., Belliard, R., Collet, D., Dost, C. & Bikandou, G. (1990): Cholécystectomie par laparoscopie. La technique opératoire. Les résultats des 100 premières observations. *J. Chir (Paris)* **127**, 347–355.

Peterson, J.B., Destefano, F., Rubin, G.L., Greenspan, J.R., Lee, N.C. & Ory, H.W. (1983): Deaths attributable to tubal sterilisation in the United States, 1977 to 1981. *Am. J. Obstet. Gynecol.* **146**, 131–136.

Reddick, E.J. & Olsen, D.O. (1989): Laparoscopic laser cholecystectomy. *Surg. Endosc.* **3**, 131–133.

Sauerbruch, E.F. (1904): Über die physiologischen und physikalischen Grundlagen bei intrathorakalen Eingriffen in Meiner pneumatische Operationskammer. *Verh. dtsch. Ges. Chir.* **32 (2)**, 105–115.

Schirmer, B.D., Edge, S.B., Dix, J. *et al.* (1991): Laparoscopic cholecystectomy. *Ann. Surg.* **213**, 665–677.

Semm, K. & Mettlere, L. (1980): Technical progress in pelvic surgery via operative laparoscopy. *Am. J. Obstet. Gynecol.* **131**, 121–127.

Semm, K. (1983): Die endoskopische Appendektomie. *Gynäkol. Praxis* **7**, 131–140.

Terblanche, J. (1991): Laparoscopic cholecystectomy: a new milestone or a dangerous innovation? *Hepatobiliary Surg.* **3**, 177–180.

Van Hee, R. (1993): De evolutie van de heelkunde tijdens de laatste 100 jaar. In: *Société Royale Belge de Chirurgie, 1893–1993. Koninklijk Belgisch Genootschap voor Heelkunde*, eds R. Van Hee & P. Mendes da Costa, pp. 11–42. Wetteren: Universa Press.

Veress, J. (1938): Neues Instrument zur Ausführung von Brust-oder Bauchpunktionen. *Dtsch. Med. Wochenschr.* **41**, 1480–1481.

Wilson, R.G. & Macintyre, I.M.C. (1993a): Impact of laparoscopic cholecystectomy in the UK: a survey of consultants. *Br. J. Surg.* **80**, 346.

Wilson, R.G. & Macintyre, I.M.C. (1993b): Symptomatic outcome after laparoscopic cholecystectomy. *Br. J. Surg.* **80**, 439–441.

The ethics of animal and human experimentation, edited by P.P. De Deyn.
©1994 John Libbey & Company Ltd., pp. 295–301.

26

Psychiatric patients as research subjects

Paul Cosyns

Department of Medicine, University of Antwerp Universiteitsplein 1, B-2610 Wilrijk, Belgium

Introduction

In principle there is no fundamental difference between psychiatric patients and other medical patients. Also, the ethics of clinical scientific research and biomedical experimental methods is principally the same for all patients. Medicine has been divided into several disciplines and subdisciplines, for reasons that are inherent to the nature of the discipline, but which do not bear upon patients.

There hides a subtle danger in categorizing separately patients with mental disorders under the denomination 'psychiatric patients'. Thus they are defined as being 'different' from other patients in their being more vulnerable and less capable of handling situations and taking decisions concerning their own health and/or welfare. They are regarded as a group that can take no valid decision concerning their own health because of their disturbed thinking and they should be able to enjoy special protection from the medical team. Their psychiatric disorder makes them vulnerable for exploitation by others and they should be protected against this. A paradoxical consequence of this well-meant protection ideology is the increasing loss of autonomy in this group of patients. During the second half of the 20th century, psychiatry as a discipline has reintegrated this repulsed group of patients into medicine in a fully fledged way. Patients suffering from psychiatric disorders should be treated like other patients. We cannot turn back the clock for the purpose of the ethical discussion, and go on stigmatizing this group as being different from the others.

Besides, talking about psychiatric patients as if they were a homogeneous group is an arbitrary and totally wrong concept. We come across persons with depressive disorders, schizophrenic disorders, sexually deviant behaviour, anxiety disorders, toxicomanic tendencies, mental handicaps, . . . Each of these disorders are further divided into several clinical entities with their own aetiology, different severity and course. Therefore, it is irresponsible to make global statements about psychiatric patients as a group. Basically they are not 'different', but they have their own characteristics and accents so that the ethical discussion is put in a special light.

In this contribution, attention is focused on the special characteristics of these patients, and psychiatry as a medical discipline.

The following problems are discussed:

- the lack of *in vitro* and animal models for psychiatric disorders;
- empirical and experimental methods;
- scientific and heuristic theories;
- the principle of autonomy;
- the utalitarian principle;
- informed consent.

The lack of *in vitro* and animal models for psychiatric disorders

The possibilities of *in vitro* or animal research in psychiatry are very limited. There are few useful animal models for psychiatric disorders. The study of psychopathological phenomena cannot proceed along this way, a way that has been so yielding for medicine in general. Psychiatry has to experiment earlier with humans because the studied phenomena cannot be reproduced in animals. Psychosurgery can serve as an example. In 1935 the famous neurophysiologist Fulton gave a lecture about frontal lobectomy in monkeys, and only a year later the book of the neurosurgeon Egas Moniz was published, who in the meanwhile had leucotomized 20 psychiatric patients (Moniz, 1936). During this period more patients than monkeys were treated with this experimental procedure. More animal experimental research probably could have detected the side-effects subsequently observed, but the curative effects of this innovating procedure for depression, psychoses or obsessive–compulsive neuroses could only be examined in humans.

Psychopharmacology can serve as an example also. In psychopharmacology, the biological aspects of psychopathological phenomena are studied, and it forms the basis of a spectacular development in treating possibilities in psychiatry (Gallant & Eickelman, 1987). Schizophrenia can indirectly be studied *in vitro* or *in vivo* through the central dopaminergic system; affective disorders (depressions) through the serotoninergic and noradrenergic system. But this approach has limitations for depressive disorders, e.g. we have not been able to identify a specific clinical entity in humans which corresponds to decreased serotonin or noradrenalin turnover, and the anti-depressive strength of the new very specific serotonin re-uptake inhibitors is no better than that of the aspecific tricyclic anti-depressives, which have been known for a long time already. Recent research further showed that serotonin also plays a role in other disorders such as obsessive-compulsive disorder, panic disorder and possibly eating disorders.

From these examples, it is clear that psychic phenomena are too complex to be reduced to simple biological variables which can be experimentally examined. This biological psychiatry research is definitely valuable, and therapeutically yields to psychopharmacology, but as an explanation for psychic and psychopathological phenomena it remains very limited.

Empirical *vs* experimental methods

Psychiatry, compared to other branches of medicine, remained 'empirical' longer and only evolved to the experimental model later. The term 'experimental' is used in the context of the clinical attitude by which the physician repeats well-known routine treatments as long as they 'work', without trying to provoke new observations. Only if they fail, novel treatment strategies are tested in a haphazard and intuitive way, without a clear research method (Fagot-Largeault, 1993).

The experimental method was conceptualized in medicine in 1886 by Claude Bernard (1959) in his masterly *Introduction à l'étude la Medicine Expérimentale*. In this experimental point of view only knowledge which can be sufficiently stated by facts is retained as valuable; and new knowledge is only accepted after careful experimental testing of the underlying hypothesis.

Two factors restrain the use of this experimental method in psychiatry. First of all there is a restricted usefulness of *in vitro* animal research in the study of mental disorders. Secondly the experimental method is focused on explaining phenomenon, searching for aetiological relationships according to the logic of science. But psychic phenomenon normally cannot be objective such as is demanded for experimental scientific research. Many studied psychic phenomenon are intersubjective in origin and only become clear in the relationship between two persons. The investigator forms a complete part of the situation and can not remain objective as if he were not involved in it. This approach, inherent in social science, is focused on understanding and making meaningful relationships rather than explaining causal relationships.

Scientific and heuristic theories

Medical activity is as well defined as a whole of scientific knowledge (medical science), and as an art (medicine). Physicians are supposed to treat patients by means of scientifically based methods. Here arises a problem in psychiatry because the scientific base of most psychotherapeutical methods is weak or nonexistent. Psychotherapy is definitely more an art than a science. There exist over 100 psychotherapy schools, and each of them has its own theories of health and disorder, objectives, and therapeutical techniques and interventions (Karasu, 1991). The theoretical framework of these psychotherapy schools is usual little scientific but primarily heuristic, i.e. discoveries and new opinions are derived from statement, explanation and interpretation. Psychotherapies pose a lot of ethical issues of which insufficient scientific foundation is only a special aspect (Lakin, 1988).

The principle of autonomy

A fundamental ethical obligation of the physician is respecting a patient's personality, his autonomy and capacity of self-determination. Nevertheless the word 'autonomy' or independence as counterpart to dependence means something else to a lawyer than to a psychiatrist. Autonomy is not inborn, it is obtained during the development of a person. After birth we are in a situation of dependence, and developing independence in the form of expression of free will is an attainment, a goal to reach for rather than an absolute moral value. Patients who suffer and need help should feel that they are comprehended by their physician, and as Dyer (1988) puts it 'autonomy is the goal of therapeutic relationship. It is not the base of our ethical concern for our fellow human beings'.

The utilitarian principle

The ethical basis of biomedical experimental research lies in extending medical scientific boundaries and improving treatments and preventing diseases. Besides the possible individual benefit for a person involved in research, the use for the whole community remains centrally; namely maximal benefit for most people. We must honestly admit that the eventual benefit of most experimental investigations is namely reserved for prospective patients rather than for the actual persons involved in the investigation. Nevertheless, the latter cannot be withdrawn from appropriate treatment for their disease because of participation in an experimental investigation and hereby they must not take unreasonable risks. The ethical reflection should be so much sharper when the collective benefit is bigger than the individual. The principles of autonomy of the patient and of collective (and occasionally individual) benefit from an underlying ethical dilemma of the so-called informed consent of the person involved in experimental research.

Informed consent

The informed consent has three parts (Parizeau, 1993; Wing, 1991):

- expression of free will by the human research subject;
- information from the physician;
- capability (to act and to decide) of human research subjects.

In biomedical experiments human persons involved are regarded as research subjects and not as research objects. According to the theory of Kant, human research subjects should not be treated as a means to gain knowledge but always as an end in itself. The rule of consent enables us to respect the principle or Kantian categorical imperative of 'respecting a person'. This presumes for human research subjects the ability of expressing their free will. Besides prisoners, who are on principle excluded from biomedical examinations, there are also compulsorily admitted patients. They are juridically not fully free but this should not be a reason for depriving this group of patients of the advantage of biomedical research. Psychopharmacology can again be quoted as an example. We have knowledge of antidepressives, anxiolytics, antipsychotics (neuroleptics), hypnotics but not yet of antiaggressives. Nevertheless these are in progress and will at the appropriate time be tested on an adjusted population of severely behaviourally disturbed aggressive patients or psychiatric disturbed delinquents.

With the investigator's obligation of giving information to human research subjects arises a difficult question of 'how complete should this information be'? Complete enough to enable the human research subject to make an informed decision whether he is going to participate to the research or not. On the other hand this information should not induce fear so that it endangers confidence in the physician. By this question of consent the physician will make sure that the patient has well understood the information. The problem posed by consent for experimental investigation is in essence not very different from that of current treatment proposals for which every patient should also give his consent. Opinions differ on who should give the information in research, and who should receive the 'informed consent': the physician in charge of the patient or the independent physician involved in the investigation. In our opinion the physician in charge is suited for this because he ultimately has the responsibility for the treatment and the confidence of the patient (see the penultimate paragraph of this chapter).

The problem of competence is difficult to solve for a number of psychiatric patients, who because of their pathology are not capable of expressing their will totally freely. Their consent to or rejection of participation is more a consequence of their pathology than an expression of their ability of self-determination. But can we assume that no examination on schizophrenic disorders should take place because these patients cannot give full consent? This would be unjust and the answer is definitely 'no' (Gallant & Eickelman, 1987; Fagot-Largeault, 1993). Physicians have an ethical and deontological obligation to experiment within consensually defined limits.

Psychiatrists attach a different meaning than lawyers to the concept of 'competence'. It is not an absolute characteristic that could be present in one person and absent in another. It can be situation- and/or problem-related, and a patient can be capable of taking one particular decision but not another. This ability can change or fluctuate with time in response to the psychiatric condition (Dyer, 1988).

Who decides instead of the *de facto* incompetent patient if he has an advantage in participating in a proposed research? Normally, we consult the close relatives and/or legal representative of the patient. In an institutionalized patient the physicians will also be involved in taking the decision. Even with an incompetent patient who cannot give full consent, the investigator will always if possible ask his assent. An incompetent patient who explicitly refuses to participate in a study is not considered.

The key position of the Commission for Medical Ethics which has to be consulted and that gives approval for the examined protocol concerning possibly incapable patients, should be underlined. The Commission ensure that:

(1) human research subjects are sufficiently protected against possible damage;

(2) the research is relevant for the group of patients;

(3) the methodology is scientifically sound.

In general is assumed that incompetent patients can be considered for therapeutic research but opinion is divided when it is non-therapeutic. Several professional organizations have accepted the following guidelines for psychiatrically incapable patients:

- the risk to patients is not higher than minimal;
- the research concerns the medical problems of involved patients and cannot be performed on competent patients;
- human research subjects do not explicitly resist doing the test;
- relatives give informed consent;
- the Commission for Medical Ethics gives its approval for the protocol.

Conclusions

1. The necessity of a valid informed consent is in practice the central problem for experimental investigation in psychiatric patients. Nevertheless, this problem is not different from daily clinical psychiatric practice when the patient's consent is required for the proposed psychiatric treatment. The physician should ask and receive approval from a Commission for Medical Ethics if in the case of innovating clinical research or experimental protocols. It does not seem necessary or desirable to make a separate arrangement for the psychiatric patient as an experimental subject. Such an attitude only adds to stigmatizing and discriminating against this group of patients.

2. Physicians are obliged to enlarge their medical knowledge and to perform experimental research on problems inherent to incompetent patients, who because of their pathology are not capable of expressing their free will. Experimental research should be possible within consensually-restrained limits.

3. Throughout the last years several scientific and/or professional organizations have increasingly developed guidelines concerning various problems such as treatment of affect-ive disorders, eating disorders, toxicomanias (providing methadone), the indication for psychosurgery, and implanting brain cells. Such guidelines refer to ethical principles as well as to scientific data and must help physicians to treat their patients correctly. On the other hand, they should not have an obligatory or enforcing character or be in the way of further development of innovative treatments. Whether this tendency to self-regulation should be complemented by legislation remains an open question.

4. As important as the concept 'autonomy' is to the lawyer, so the concept 'trust' is to the psychiatrist. Both psychiatric treatment and experimental research are unconceivable without a relationship of trust between a physician and his patient. If this is absent, the patient becomes 'non-compliant' and cannot give his consent. This interactional relationship of trust should be protected throughout the whole research procedure. Only with such a relationship of trust will the patient be able to perform his right of self-determination and eventually agree to participate in the study.

5. Experimental biomedical research problems concern the whole society and is not only restricted to medical clinical practice. They presume the existence and accomplishment of a climate of trust between the public and the physician: a trustful relationship between physicians and patients, and between physicians and society. Good functioning and competent Commissions for Medical Ethics play an important role in this. Trust is no automatic datum of a medical situation but should be obtained by the physician. For him this is an important ethical obligation because he must obtain this confidence by practising his profession, and he must be worth it.

References

Bernard, C. (1959): *Introduction à l'étude de la médecine expérimentale.* Paris: Librairie Delagrave.

Dyer, A.R. (1988): *Ethics and psychiatry, toward professional definition.* p. 176. Washington: American Psychiatric Press.

Fagot-Largeault, A. (1993): Expérimentations humaine. In: *Les mots de la bio-ethique..* eds. G. Hottois & M.H. Parizzau, pp. 219–228. Bruxelles: De Boeck Université.

Gallant, D.M. & Eickelman, B. (1987): Ethical dilemmas in neuropsychopharmacologic research. In: *Psychopharmacology: the third generation of progress.* Ed. H.Y. Meltzer, pp. 1–15. New York: Raven Press.

Karasu, T.J. (1991): Ethical aspects of psychotherapy. In: *Psychiatric ethics.* 2nd edn, eds. S. Block & P. Chodoff, pp. 136–166. Oxford: Oxford University Press.

Lakin, M. (1988): *Ethical issues in the psychotherapies.* Oxford: Oxford University Press.

Moniz, E. (1936): *Tentatives opératoires dans le traitement de certaines psychoses.* Paris: Masson.

Parizeau, M.H. (1993): Consentement. In: *Les mots de la bio-ethique* . eds. G. Hottois & M.H. Parizeau, pp. 88–95. Bruxelles: De Boeck Université.

Wing, J. (1991): Ethics and psychiatric research. In: *Psychiatric ethics.* 2nd edn, eds. S. Block & P. Chodoff, pp. 415–434. Oxford: Oxford University Press.

The ethics of animal and human experimentation, edited by P.P. De Deyn.
©1994 John Libbey & Company Ltd., pp. 303–320.

27

Research involving children – scientific and ethical aspects

Robert Clara

Professor Emeritus of Paediatrics, University of Antwerp, Verdussenstraat 8, 2018 Antwerpen, Belgium

Summary

Human experimentation is the central pillar of modern medicine. The harm being risked must be the minimum necessary for the benefit of the patient, and the study should have both scientific value and scientific validity. Therefore, strict guidelines for the conduct of human experimentation should be provided. Research involving children is necessary, because children are biologically different from adults; many diseases occur exclusively in children and certain processes can only be studied in childhood.

The hazards of experimentation may be greater in younger age groups who are not mentally and emotionally capable of understanding the nature and purpose of the experimental procedure and protocol. Research on children places a special responsibility on those who do and monitor research because of the children's vulnerability and their inability to give full informed consent.

Experimentation in children can be allowed when the following premisses are accepted: that research involving children is important for the benefit of all children; that the degree of benefit resulting from the research is important in relation to the risk of disturbance, discomfort or pain; that there is approval from an ethics advisory committee; that special safety requirements are applied; that the informed consent of the children (assent) if possible, and their parents or guardians, has been obtained.

Introduction

The child's agreement should be required at a very early age (7 years?). Procedures with more than minimal risk are only allowed when the intervention holds out the prospect of direct benefit for the individual subject.

Research in children is a scientific and moral obligation. For the investigator there is a dual responsibility – to children and their parents – and he must assume a greater responsibility to ensure that the means and ends of the project are necessary, worthy, and possible at minimal risk. The only real protection for the individual lies in the scrupulousness, conscience and personal integrity of the investigator.

The ethics of experimentation with human subjects

Basic issues

Human experimentation is the central pillar of modern biomedicine. Knowledge gained from research on animals would be irrelevant to medicine if it were not tested in human beings, and the sophisticated and often expensive forms of diagnosis and therapy that for many people have come to characterize contemporary medicine are merely the fruits of human research. Standing, then, in the pivotal position between basic research and animal laboratories, on the one hand, and routine clinical application in the health-care system, on the other, is the complex social practice known as human experimentation (Capron, 1978).

It is easy to forget how new medical science really is. The revolutionary advances based on knowledge of physiology and biochemistry have only emerged in the past 60 years, and they came from research. The basic work could be done with test-tube preparations and laboratory animals, but eventually human subjects had to be involved. Man is 'the final test site,' as Beecher (1966) once put it as a pioneer amongst physicians concerned with the ethics of research (Barber, 1976).

Historical background

If research employing human subjects is undeniably as old as medicine itself, systematic experimentation became an integral part of medical practice only in modern times, with the development of medical science.

There are two major reasons for the general recognition that experimentation with humans is a subject for concern. First there is the increased power, scope and funding of biomedical research. The other reason involves the change in values: an increased emphasis on equality, participation, and objection to arbitrary authority.

The extreme example of neglecting accepted ethical principles in the pursuit of scientific knowledge is the atrocities committed by Nazi physicians in the concentration camps during World War II. From this, a panel of judges outlined ten principles that must be observed in the conduct of human clinical experimentation in order to satisfy moral, ethical, and legal concepts. They became known as the Nuremberg Code of 1947 (Friedman, 1992).

A year after the Nuremberg Code, in 1948, the World Medical Association introduced the declaration of Geneva. Sixteen years later, in 1964, and still under the influence of the horrific accounts of brutal human experiments on concentration camps inmates, the World Medical Association codified under the Declaration of Helsinki efforts to protect research subjects. The medical community endorsed the principles expressed in the Declaration of Helsinki (1964), which was revised in Tokyo (1975) and in Venice (1983). Increased attention and concern has been widely and continually displayed in the mass media. This concern has perhaps been especially focused on three *causes célèbres* during the last 10 years: the thalidomide disaster in Germany and elsewhere; the Southam and Mandel case in New York State in which live cancer cells were injected into geriatric patients without their informed consent, and the Willowbrook experiment conducted in the Willowbrook State Hospital of New York (Krugman, 1971), on 800 institutionalized retarded children who were either injected with or given oral doses of live hepatitis virus material to induce the disease and test the effectiveness of a vaccine for hepatitis. Consent was requested and given by parents, although this vulnerable group of children was put at considerable intentional risk by physicians.

Finally, there have been expressions of concern from within the biomedical community itself. In the United States, very distinguished moral influence was given by Beecher (1966), and Pappworth (1967) in the UK has made somewhat similar statements about shortcomings in this area.

Conceptual clarifications

When dealing with a patient, therapy refers to a set of activities that are designed solely to relieve suffering and to restore or maintain a patient's health and that have a reasonable chance of succes. Human experimentation, or research using human beings, is a scientific activity whose primary purpose is to develop or contribute to the knowledge of physiological or psychological processes involved in human function.

A prime source of confusion on this point arises from the fact that physicians, in the course of regular care and management, sometimes try new and unproved procedures on their patients, especially in desperate situations when existing modalities have been ineffective. It seems proper to term this 'experimentation', even though it may occur as an isolated innovation rather than as part of a well-regulated clinical trial; yet the intent of the physician is plainly different from that prevailing in other types of research. Consequently, a distinction may be drawn between such beneficial experimentation, and experimentation in which the sole purpose is non-beneficial – to acquire knowledge rather than to improve the subject's condition.

Beneficial experimentation

Beneficial experimentation is sometimes called 'therapeutic experimentation'. The term 'beneficial' refers merely to the intent with which an experiment is performed, not to its outcome; also 'non-beneficial' should not be equated with 'useless', because the intention is information of use to science and not any direct benefits to the subject.

Non-beneficial experimentation

In non-beneficial (non-therapeutic) research, the sole purpose of a study is to provide information required by the researchers, and the study does not provide any therapy to the research subjects. It may, however, provide indirect benefits to the subjects, since improved medical care may result from the study. Non-therapeutic research is often done to help understand normal and abnormal human function. In the actual conduct of medicine, beneficial and non-beneficial experimentation are often intermingled with each other and with non-experimental procedures. Non-beneficial research may in fact have unintended helpful consequences for its subjects, or some of them may at some future date be ill with the same condition again and be aided by the knowledge gained from the experiments; yet this does not place the research, if it was undertaken for scientific purposes, into the category of intended beneficial experimentation.

Basic ethical issues

The basic ethical problem in human experimentation – as well as the central social issue – is that experimentation is the use of one person by another to gain knowledge or other benefits that may be only partly good, if at all, for the former person; that is to say, the experimental subject is not simply a means but is in danger of being treated as a mere token to be manipulated for research purposes. While many would agree that human clinical experimentation is indispensable to the progress of medical science, and to the subsequent improvement in the art of medical practice, the rights and welfare of every human subject are equally a first priority. As long as these two basic principles are not in conflict with each other, there should be no ethical problems in dealing with human clinical experimentation.

One of the guiding principles in the practice of medicine is *primum non nocere* – first, do no harm. This commandment cannot be read literally, of course, since every medical intervention contains the potential for some harm. Yet a strict reading would suggest that the phrase means that the harm being risked must be the minimum necessary for the benefit of the patient.

For a study to be ethical, it must have scientific worth. If a study involving human subjects is poorly or improperly designed, such that it will not result in reproducible scientific facts relevant to the question under study, then by definition it is unethical and all other ethical considerations become irrelevant.

In such a situation, any risks to the subjects, no matter how trivial, cannot be justified. To protect subjects, a study of scientific worth and merit must have two components – *validity* and *value*. A study is scientifically valid when it is designed to yield reliable information concerning the hypothesis being examined according to accepted principles of research practice. While a study may be scientifically valid, it may be of no scientific value because the hypothesis itself is trivial or meaningless. Therefore, in an ethical review, a research protocol should have both scientific value and scientific validity.

Guidelines for the conduct of experiments with human subjects

Human experimentation is no longer a matter of occasional interest to a few physicians, but is a major social activity in which large numbers of people are involved under the aegis of profit-making as well as academic institutions, and on which future progress in pharmacology, genetics, and all areas of the life sciences depends. Therefore, strict guidelines for the conduct of human experimentation should be provided.

First, an experiment should be based on laboratory and animal experimentation and other scientifically established facts, so that the point under inquiry is well-focused and has been advanced as far as possible by non-human means. It is a rare instance when animal experiments are not possible before human experimentation. Historically, however, there has often been more concern for animal welfare than for the welfare of sick patients.

Second, an experiment should follow proper scientific and medical procedures. The means employed to perform tests and observe phenomena should be capable of yielding the data that the research intends to provide. In most instances, this will mean that the experiment should be built around a testable hypothesis, and conducted according to the criteria for validity already described. Some human research, however, does not proceed on the basis of a testable hypothesis. Epidemiological studies or tests designed to yield profiles of the 'normal' range for various characteristics in a population are acceptable forms of human research although not directed at proof of a particular point.

Third, an experiment must be carried out by persons who are scientifically qualified, and the devices used must be those contemplated in the research design. It is surprising how often this requisite of experimentation is not fulfilled in actual practice.

Fourth, all foreseeable risks and reasonably probable benefits to the subject of the investigation and to science, or more broadly to society, *must be carefully assessed*, and the comparison of these projected risks and benefits must indicate that the latter clearly outweigh the former. Moreover, the probable benefits must not be obtainable through other less risky means.

Fifth, participation by a subject in an experiment, *should be halted immediately if the subject finds continued participation undesirable* or a prudent investigator has cause to believe that the experiment is likely to result in *injury, disability, or death to the subject.*

Sixth, compensation for research-related injuries must be available, and the investigator must be prepared to treat the subject for any adverse outcome related to the study.

Seventh, experimentation may go forward only with the informed and voluntary consent of the subject. The concept of informed consent is a troublesome one. The investigator wants to have enough subjects and is afraid of scaring them off. Patients are likely to be concerned about their own condition, may feel powerless with respect to the physician or hospital and often have difficulty understanding medical language or concepts. Difficulties arise because of the inevitable and gross inequality between the two parties interested in consent to a medical procedure. One is fit and medically knowledgeable, the other sick and medically ignorant (Rennie, 1980). If efforts to educate patients in order to obtain their informed consent are, indeed, not harmful and are morally and legally necessary, how effective are these efforts? Cassileth *et al.* (1980) found that by the time patients had completed their consent forms, their memory of the information given to them was inadequate and often faulty, although they themselves claimed to have understood the forms. Gray *et al.* (1978), who examined 1,526 consent forms used for research procedures, likewise found that only 7 per cent were written in language as simple as *Time* magazine, and 77 per cent were 'difficult' (at the level of a research journal) or worse. Is there really such a thing as informed consent? Should it protect the patient or the doctor? If the motives of those conducting clinical trials were altruistic – to improve the quality of care and add to our knowledge – the patient's rights would never be seriously endangered. But there is always the nagging anxiety that one of the less laudable motives of clinical researchers is to benefit their careers by increasing the number of their publications. For this reason alone, all trial protocols should be scrutinized by funding bodies and local ethical committees. That aside, what arguments are there for and against full informed consent? In favour is the need to respect another's right to self-determination. Also, information about the trial will improve the patient's knowledge and understanding of the illness and treatment. Against informed consent is the difficulty for patients to comprehend the nature of their disease, the uncertainty about its treatment, and the need for randomization. There is also the risk of undermining the confidence of patients faced with a diagnosis of potentially fatal disorders but who are then told that the doctors do not know the best treatment (Baum, 1986).

Social control: the effects of peer-group review

Peer-review committees have the power to approve, modify, or reject on ethical grounds, and before they are carried out, all research proposals involving the use of human subjects. Practically speaking, the review boards assess risks, document informed consent, monitor studies and protect the privacy and confidentiality of subjects.

Lewis (1982) mentions three negative aspects of the establishment of these committees. The first problem is that the approval of a research project by a research ethics committee is a process which has acquired an intrinsic value. Such approval is a valuable commodity because it is required by outside bodies who are not directly concerned with the investigator–subject relationship: grant-giving bodies and the editors of medical journals. The problem with this is that whatever the committee considers to be a reasonable investigation then gains currency as being ethical in absolute terms. A second problem relates to the 'institutionalization of ethics' in medical research: in approving an investigation, the committee agrees to shoulder a portion of the investigator's responsibility. The investigators or their assistants have a measure of responsibility lifted from them and begin to act as if their actions were directed by a higher authority. A third problem relates to procedure. Committees are by nature bureaucratic, and process applications using guidelines which tend to become stereotyped. Most, although not all, research ethics committees insist that every subject taking part in research projects gives informed consent to the research in writing. In most situations there can be no objection to this. However, in some circumstances written consent can be distressing to the subjects, and hence become the antithesis of 'ethical'. In patients with a fatal disease where trials compare two accepted therapies could not the committees dispense with written consent?

How effective are the review committees in handling the protocols that do come before them? Two hundred and ninety-three questionnaire respondents told Barber *et al.* (1976) that, in 34 per cent of the institutions, the committees had never required any revisions, rejected any proposals or had any proposals withdrawn in anticipation of rejection for ethical reasons; 31 per cent reported revisions, 32 per cent outright rejections and 19 per cent withdrawals. Either some of these committees have very few ethical problems coming before them or they are ineffective. The peer-review groups seemed weak in other ways. In some institutions there was no face-to-face discussion among the reviewers. Only 22 per cent of the committees had members from outside the institution. In practically none of the institutions was there continuous monitoring of studies that were approved. In general ethical peer-review is hampered by the fact that each committee operates in isolation and must consider every new issue on its own and without the benefit of precedents. The major weakness in the system is the lack of keen interest in, and support of, the review committees on the part of most working biomedical investigators. Research is their business; research is their mission and predominant interest, not applied ethics or active advocacy of patients' rights.

Dilemma of therapy and science: policy recommendations

Barber *et al.* (1972) suggests two broad areas for policy changes. First is the area of socialization. In the light of its high moral aspirations and claims, the biomedical research community is not taking its obligation to train its prospective members in the medical school in research ethics *as seriously as it ought to* ; as seriously, for example, as it takes its obligation to train them in scientific knowledge and research techniques. Of the more than 300 investigators who responded to questions in this area, only 13 per cent reported they had been exposed in medical school to part of a course, a seminar or even a single lecture devoted to the ethical issues involved in experimentation with human subjects; only one respondent said he had taken an entire course dealing with the issue. Second, in the area of peer-review, it is clear that better policy requires that absolutely *all* research be screened and that such procedures as continuing review and formal appeal be used *everywhere.* Biomedical research is in a considerable measure so esoteric an activity that a great deal of the social control that guides it should be in the hands of the biomedical research community itself. Yet, like all other specialized and esoteric social activities, biomedical research is too important to the larger society to be left entirely to its experts. *In part it needs to be effectively and continuously scrutinized and controlled by outsiders.* An effective system of control, including both insiders and outsiders, will protect all the parties at interest, all the values, and both science and human therapy.

The design of experiments

Clinical trials can be grouped into two major classifications: randomized and non-randomized studies. A *randomized* trial is defined as an experiment on patients in which the therapies under investigation are allocated by a chance mechanism. An important feature of this chance or random assignment of treatment is that neither the patient nor the physician knows the treatment to be used before the patient is formally entered in the experiment. Randomized clinical trials are comparative experiments that investigate two or more therapies.

Non-randomized clinical trials usually involve only one therapy on which information is collected prospectively. An evaluation is generally based on a comparison of the new data with historical control data that were not collected specifically for the comparison. Many difficulties are involved in comparing prospective data with historical control data because of possible biases from many different sources. These potential biases are usually of such magnitude that the results of non-randomized studies are often ambiguous and not universally accepted unless the therapeutic effect is very large. These same biases are not present to the same degree, if at all, in randomized trials (Zelen, 1979). Nevertheless, many investigators and patients are reluctant to participate in randomized clinical trials. This reluctance arises in part from the regulations for informed consent, which require that patients give informed consent, before being entered into a study by a clinical investigator. The informed-consent procedure requires the treating physician to inform the patient that the treatment is chosen by randomization. Sometimes the randomization process is described to the patient as 'choosing the treatment by computer' or 'tossing a coin'. How can a physician, committed to doing what he thinks is best for each patient, tell the patient that he is choosing the treatment by something like a 'coin toss'. How can he give up the option to make changes in treatment according to patient responses? And how can he justify asking the next patient to participate in a randomized clinical trial, when one treatment is beginning to look better than another, but with less certainty than is traditionally required for statistical significance? Only after completion of the study will the actual treatment be known to both the physician and the patient. Ethically, a physician should only participate in such studies if he or she believes that all treatments under study have potentially equal therapeutic benefits.

Zelen (1979) proposed a new design for randomized trials with the novel feature that before consent is obtained, both patient and doctor know whether an experimental treatment has been assigned. Eligible patients are randomized into two groups: group G1 is called 'do not seek consent' which means that they are not asked for their consent to enter the clinical trial and they receive the best standard treatment (A); patients randomized to group G2 are asked for their full informed consent to participate in the trial and receive the experimental treatment (B). If they do not agree to receive treatment (B) then they receive treatment (A). The obvious advantage in this design is that the doctor has only to discuss a single treatment with his patient, and so will not appear compromised because he is uncertain and apparently subjecting his patient to 'a flick of the computer switch'. The patient is spared the need to agree in advance to a randomized allocation of treatment (Cancer Research Campaign Working Party in Breast Conservation, 1983).

The ethics of research involving children

Need and value of involving children in clinical research

First, children are *not* simply small adults, but are biologically different in many ways, so that knowledge acquired from adult subjects often cannot be applied to children without testing them (Fost, 1978). Immature and term infants have responses to pharmaceutical agents that are different from the responses in older children and adults. The use of certain sulphonamides and large doses of vitamin K lead to kernicterus. Chloramphenicol in doses tolerated by older persons leads to an increase in infant mortality. Therefore, research on the treatment process as well as on normal function is essential (Cooke, 1977).

Second, there are many diseases that occur *exclusively* in children, so that advances in understanding may be absolutely dependent on the use of children.

Third, the study of normal infants, including usual feeding methods, is necessary to prevent harm as well as to do good. If some interventions are inappropriate, harm may result, including disability or death or both. Oxygen administered to the immature infant may be necessary for survival, but, if in excess, may produce blindness. Water in excess causes harm, and serious harm results if not administered in adequate amounts.

Fourth, new immunization procedures in general should first be tested on animals, then on adult volunteers, then on older children able to take part voluntarily in the research, and only then on younger children. However, there are instances where this sequence might be inappropriate: for instance, in the development of a vaccine against respiratory syncytial virus where few uninfected subjects may be available above infancy.

Fifth, certain processes and circumstances can only be studied in children. These are metabolic problems unique to the developing infant: growth, the effects of sweets that cause caries, reactions to TV programmes, the development of children with mentally ill mothers, etc.

Sixth, bloodsampling in normal infants, where the investigation seems to be of no direct benefit to them, is the only way *to obtain standards* to which to relate the data of sick babies.

Risk of research in children

Risk means the risk of causing physical disturbance, discomfort or pain, or psychological disturbance to the child or his parents, rather than the risk of serious harm, which no ethical committee would countenance in any case (British Paediatric Association, 1980).

(1) *The hazards of experimentation may be greater* in younger age groups. Physical injuries that might be trivial in a mature person (such as radiation of the growing portion of a long bone) can become magnified when occurring early in the developmental process.

(2) Events that may have little *psychological significance* for an adult such as a short hospitalization or repeated venepunctures, may have profound detrimental effects on a child. There are major psychological constraints to work with children, whether they are healthy children or otherwise. Motivation and co-operation can be difficult to inspire. Young children, particularly, may be shy, diffident, or fearful. This is not to say that optimum motivation cannot be achieved, but that tests have to be more personalized, and large groups may be inappropriate (Pearn, 1984).

(3) The problem of *kindness deserves special attention.* Just because a research subject is young, there is no reason why the normal practice of good manners and courtesy should not prevail. To be courteous to a child, especially from the powerful and privileged position of a researcher, takes more time, requires greater sensitivity, and more awareness of the special place of children, than it does to be courteous to an adult.

(4) Mental and emotional *incapacity of children to understand the nature and purpose of the experimental procedure and protocol* and to weigh the risks it may entail for them should be considered. Uncoerced informed consent, the keystone of protection of human subjects, is often unattainable from the minor.

Defining 'benefit'

Non-beneficial research

(a) The procedure is of no benefit to the subject but may benefit the health and welfare of other children. A special case, but an important one, is if the subject suffers from a disorder and the research aims to benefit others suffering from a similar disorder.

(b) The procedure is of no benefit to the subject but may add to basic biological knowledge, e.g. normal values, growing.

Beneficial research

The procedure is of potential benefit to the subject.

Historical background

Under which conditions is participation of children in research ethically acceptable and under which conditions may such research be authorized by the subjects or their parents? The prevailing codes of ethics governing the use of human subjects for experimentation are curiously ambivalent about children. The progenitor of these codes, The Code of Nuremberg, if taken literally, would exclude children as subjects, for it requires the voluntary consent of the subject 'as absolutely essential', without any provision for proxy consent. The World Medical Association's Declaration of Helsinki, on the other hand, states that for non-therapeutic research involving legally incompetent subjects, 'the consent of the legal guardian should be procured'. This position has been adopted by the American Medical Association: minors or mentally incompetent persons may be used as subjects only if: (a) the nature of the investigation is such that mentally competent adults would not be suitable subjects; (b) consent, in writing, is given by a legally authorized representative of the subject under circumstances in which an informed and prudent adult would reasonably be expected to volunteer himself or his child as a subject. This position, permitting non-therapeutic research on the basis of proxy consent of the legally authorized representative, was accepted by the US Department of Health, Education and Welfare (now the Department of Health and Human Services) in 1981 (Curran, 1981). The US National Commission for the Protection of Human Subjects of Biomedical Research established guidelines published in 1978 which examined the ethical problems of research in children. The commission paid particular attention to informed consent and risk–benefit assessment (Curran, 1978). In Britain, the British Paediatric Association in 1980 published 'Guidelines to aid ethical committees considering research involving children'. Moreover, the Council for International Organizations of Medical Sciences (CIOMS, 1982), in co-operation with WHO, has after many years' work, submitted the Proposed International Guidelines for Biomedical Research. This contains a section concerning research on children.

Ethics committees and research in children

There are three main guardians of the ethics of research: the integrity of the investigator, the research ethics committee, and the editorial scrutiny of the journal to which the results are submitted. Research on children places a special responsibility on those who do and monitor research because of children's vulnerability and their inability to give full informed consent (Robinson, 1987). The ethical obligation of the individual researcher to take the case to a higher objective authority is never more important than in research involving children. Judgment by a peer-group that is collectively disinterested from the point of view of the proposed research but not from the point of view of the child is extremely valuable. It is essential that at least one member on such a committee acts specifically as if he or she were in the place of the child and is mindful of the intrinsic rights of each future potential child subject. Although the accepted ethical codes of clinical research are generally followed, grey areas may exist when a clinician is both the personal 'service' doctor and the 'research' doctor, i.e. when his clinical treatment of his patients is at the same time clinical research. Research ethics committees pronouncing on the rights of child patients may be controlled by national or federal government. The British Paediatric Association has set up a Standing Ethics Advisory Committee (1980). The function of this Committee is to offer advice on the ethics of research projects involving children. The Committee responds to requests for advice from individuals planning research projects, from local ethical committees, or from editors of journals, but its opinions are not binding. Approval of research projects remains the responsibility of statutory local ethical committees. The Committee will establish some uniformity of policy for research in children throughout the country. In the USA, the National Commission for the Protection of Human Subjects of Biomedical and Behavioral Research was given a strictly advisory role. In Sweden, an ethical board was attached to the State Medical Research Council which although not required to make individual ethical decisions – which are the responsibility of the faculty boards – should rather coordinate such decisions to work out consistent criteria for evaluating experiments on human beings. This group currently consists of the chairmen of the local committees and representatives of other institutions. The group has worked out directives for the ethical committees (Giertz, 1983).

Guidelines of research involving children

Experimentation in children can be allowed when the following premisses are accepted:

- that research involving children is important for the benefit of all children and should be supported and encouraged, and conducted in an ethical manner;
- that research should never be done on children if the same investigation can be done on adults;
- that research which involves a child and is of no benefit to that child (non-therapeutic research) is not necessarily either unethical or illegal;
- that the degree of benefit resulting from a research should be assessed in relation to the risk of disturbance, discomfort or pain – the 'risk–benefit ratio';
- that there is the approval of an ethics advisory committee;
- that special safety requirements are applied. As well as the obvious humanitarian reasons, this is because no assumptions can be made that children will act predictably. The unexpected is more likely to happen with children than with adults as subjects. Children may be especially susceptible to agents used in research. Although most potential difficulties can be averted by adult research first, unexpected reactions or biological sensitivities can arise;
- that provision is made to protect the privacy and confidentiality of children and their parents, and that the subjects are selected in an equitable manner;
- that informed consent of the children (assent), if possible, and their parents or guardians has been obtained;
- that payment to subjects must never be made under any circumstances if children are involved. This is not to say, of course, that the normal expenses of a research subject should not be met.

At the heart of the legal and ethical controversy are two central issues: proxy consent and the relevance of risk–benefit assessment.

Informed consent

Special status of 'captive subjects'

In a sense, children fall into the class of 'captive subjects', as do prisoners, students, and the members of minority groups within larger totalitarian societies, and an over-compensatory approach must be adopted to make sure that their special position of dependence is not abused.

Informed consent by proxy (parental permission)

The matter of informed consent has received more attention since 1980 than any other ethical issue in research (Papadatos, 1989). The assumption that parents can provide uncoerced informed consent for their children rests at least on the presumption that they can provide it for themselves. There is evidence that educated, competent adults are frequently not adequately informed to give meaningful consent, so their ability to speak for others may be questioned. The barriers may not be so much a lack of intelligence or motivation on the part of the patient or physician, as more complex forces may interfere, such as the anxiety of illness, the intimidating milieu of the hospital, and a sense of awe, trust and dependence on the physician – all of which may conspire to make solicitation of consent a ritual wherein few are meaningfully informed. In addition to these general barriers to informed consent, there are aspects peculiar to the parent–child relationship that complicate the matter further. The perceived vulnerability of the child may evoke excessive anxiety, which further clouds judgment. Even if these were overcome, the practice of proxy consent rests on other notions under challenge: the claim that one person may ever consent to a non-therapeutic intervention being performed on another; the assumption that adults can reliably assess what is in a child's best interest; and the faith that they are capable of acting in a person's best interest, even if it can be accurately identified. An adult might gladly consent to a venepuncture, a procedure of minimal risk and annoyance, but for a child the same event could be a major psychological trauma (Jonsen, 1978). The US Department of Health, Education and Welfare defined the basic elements of information for consent as the following:

(a) fair explanation of the procedures to be followed and their purposes;

(b) description of any attendant discomforts and risks that can reasonably be expected;

(c) description of any benefits to be expected;

(d) disclosure of alternative procedures that might be advantageous for the subject;

(e) written information in simple language which the parents keep;

(f) assertion that the person is free to withdraw his consent and discontinue participation in the project;

(g) the possibility to answer any questions related to the procedures;

(h) an interval of at least 1 day between giving information and obtaining consent;

(i) the request for consent should be made by the investigator himself;

(j) the responsibility of the investigator for the ethics of his research cannot be emphasized too strongly. A parent's consent (or a child's assent) can never be used to produce ethical justification for a project otherwise unacceptable.

There is no doubt that risks of harm in everyday activities are by far greater than risks involved in properly conducted clinical research. Many routine clinical procedures done without sufficient thought, for little purpose other than keeping the records tidy, are far worse than many research investigations.

Assent

The word 'assent' is chosen to distinguish the child's agreement from a legally valid consent, and to recognize that it is more limited than the consent of adults. Children mature in their ability to understand and to engage in various activities. The USA Commission believes that the ethical principle of respect urges acknowledgment of that development of ability. It suggests, somewhat arbitrarily but still on the basis of common experience, that the age of 7 may be an appropriate time to begin requiring parents and investigators to seek the child's assent. If the child is between 7 and 14 his unwillingness to take part in non-therapeutic research should be binding, but his parents could override his unwillingness to take part in therapeutic research. Over 14 the young person's view should be paramount, though parental consent is still legally required until 16 for therapeutic and until 18 for non-therapeutic research. In Sweden there has been no wish to stipulate any particular age when the child should be consulted: this should be decided from case to case, according to its age and state of development and the kind of situation involved. However, the child should, at a very early age, be allowed to influence its situation in matters of personal concern. The proposed legislation states that the guardian, of course, should not try to relieve himself of responsibility for the child by allowing the latter to decide to a degree that is beyond its maturity. If a child assents, the parent's consent should also be obtained. An exception to this rule may be made in research projects with insignificant risks and minimal inconvenience.

Risk–benefit assessment

As risk assessment is the fundamental step in an Institutional Review Board's (IRB's) approval of a project, the judgment of IRB members about the degree of risk is critical to their role in judging the ethics of research. However, data on the risk inherent in many paediatric procedures are limited to listings of complications and case reports, neither of which provide the frequency of morbidity and mortality associated with the procedures. Reliable information on the frequency of both the physical and psychological risks intrinsic to such research procedures as tympanocentesis, arterial puncture, skin biopsy, gastric or intestinal intubation, use of a metabolic bed, and bone scan are absent from the paediatric literature. We base our classification on the study done by Janofsky & Starfield (1981) and the British and American definitions of risk estimation (Nicholson, 1986).

Procedures with negligible or minimal risk

The definition of minimal risk corresponds to the probability and magnitude of physical or psychological harm that is normally encountered in daily life, or in routine medical, dental or psychological examination of healthy children. Research (therapeutic and non-therapeutic) that does not involve greater than minimal risk to children may be conducted, provided that all guidelines of research involving children are met, and the requirements for permission and assent have been fulfilled.

Examples of procedures with negligible or minimal risk are:

(a) part of the ordinary care of the infant or child (weighing, measuring, feeding): for example test weighing a breast-fed baby, as part of a study aimed to promote breast feeding;

(b) non-invasive collection of samples, e.g. urine, faeces, saliva, hair, or nail clippings, or, at birth, cord blood or placental tissue;

(c) invasive collection of samples, e.g. blood, cerebrospinal fluid, biopsy tissue, taken from a child who is undergoing treatment, if the sample used for research is an additional amount to that required on clinical grounds;

(d) antecubital venipuncture, skin biopsy (punch), confinement to a metabolic bed for 24 hours, bone scan, intramuscular placebo injection, and 24 hour hospitalization for infants and children regardless of age;

(e) a bare majority of the investigators questioned by Janofsky & Starfield felt that the risk of gastric or intestinal intubation, questioning a child about sexual practices, and questioning a child about illicit drug use are less than minimal for children aged 7 to 18.

Examples. In cystic fibrosis, research might be considered reasonable which involved an affected child having a sweat test that needed twice as much sweat as required for purely diagnostic purposes. During the course of an operation for hernia, a fragment of skin from the incision might be required for research involving tissue culture. The risk could be judged negligible.

Procedures with more than minimal risk

(a) Such research is allowed when the intervention holds out the prospect of direct benefit for the individual subject. Greater risks can be tolerated when, for example, all available treatments for a disorder have been exhausted and a procedure under investigation for safety and efficacy is available, or when a new procedure appears to be more efficacious or less dangerous than a standard one. The procedure under investigation must have a ratio of anticipated benefit to risk at least as favourable as other treatment alternatives, as well as the alternative of providing no treatment at all. Risks of venipuncture of femoral, internal jugular and external jugular veins for ages newborn to 1 year, and arterial puncture for ages newborn to 18 years, are rated as greater than minimal, and the risk of gastrointestinal intubation is rated as greater than minimal for ages newborn to 6 years (minor increase over minimal risk).

Two procedures, femoral venipuncture and internal jugular venipuncture done between birth and 1 year, are judged as greater than minor increase over minimal risk. It is obvious that 'weighing' of risks and benefits is not a strictly quantitative activity, although statistical data about risks and benefits might be helpful. Rather, the acceptability of benefits and risks is a matter of discretion; parents, researchers, therapists, reviewers, and, in some circumstances, the child must judge.

(b) The most difficult problem raised by research involving children is: is it ethical to expose a child to risks that are *more than minimal* when the interventions dictated solely for research purposes are not intended to benefit the individual subject? Many children suffer from debilitating disorders and fatal diseases whose aetiology is poorly understood and for which there are no or, at best, inadequate therapies. Studies performed on these children could advance the understanding of the disease and might lead to the development and improvement of therapies. The affected children themselves may be the only sources of that information. On the other hand, the prospects of an effective therapy might be so remote that, barring a breakthrough, they may never be beneficiaries of improved understanding of their condition. Indeed, it may be wholly unlikely that they could be helped, as in the case of most mental disability or many neurological disorders; still, the condition from which they suffer incurably might be prevented in the future. Given such situations, an absolute prohibition of studies that might entail more than minimal risk to these children seems unreasonable (Curran & Beecher, 1969).

The USA Commission allows that children might be entered in research entailing more than minimal risk and promising no individual benefit when (a) the risk entailed represents 'a minor increase over minimal risk', (b) the experience presented by the intervention is 'reasonably commensurate with those inherent in the actual or expected medical, psychological or social situation' of the subject, and (c) the research is likely to yield generalizable knowledge about the subject's condition that is 'of vital importance for the understanding and amelioration of the condition' from which that class of subjects suffers. In this recommendation, the Commission offers two important and equally necessary considerations about risks in this sort of research. First, it states that any additional risks must represent but a minor increase over minimal risk. 'Minor increase' over minimal risk refers to risks of harm or discomforts that pose no significant threat to the child's well-being. Thus, a biopsy, a spinal tap, or the dose of an acceptable level of a radioisotope, while surpassing the risks of daily life, are unlikely to cause any serious harm. Second, these risks must be 'reasonably commensurate with the subject's own experiences.' The children envisioned in these recommendations will be children whom, because of their illness, will be subject to frequent diagnostic, palliative, and therapeutic interventions. In the course of their care, they will undergo certain painful, uncomfortable, or risky interventions. The Commission suggests that any research procedures resemble, in ways that the children can identify, the experiences with which they are familiar. Within such a research design, the research must constitute an experience that, while possibly unpleasant, is not foreign to the child. Commensurability is intended to enhance the child's understanding and tolerance of the research procedure – not to add to its riskiness.

Research on embryos and foetuses

Consideration of the right of newborn infants merges imperceptibly into consideration of the rights of the foetus and the embryo. For the last 15 years the human embryo and foetus have been central figures in bioethical discussions. New techniques for prenatal diagnosis – for example, ultrasonography, amniocentesis, and foetoscopy – provide early information about the clinical status of the foetus to both prospective parents and physicians. New diagnostic and therapeutic techniques made the human foetus seem more like a distinguishable patient, especially during the second and third trimesters of pregnancy. Fifteen years after the delivery of the first test-tube infant, the questions of in vitro fertilization, embryo transfer, experiments with live embryos etc. are still vigorously debated. The importance and size of the ethical issues concerning experimentation with embryos and foetuses are so great, that a special article is needed to analyse all these problems which would fall outside the scope of this book.

Closing remarks

Research in children is a scientific and moral obligation. It would be unethical not to do it. In the biomedical area there are two very clear sets of values. One is the physician's value of humane therapy and the second is the fact that the researcher is a scientist and wishes to be an original and distinguished discoverer. There is the value of science. This is the dilemma of therapy and science. A major consequence of all successful research on human subjects has been the enormous benefits to the health and welfare of those who enjoy modern medical care. However, there have also been some unintended and undesired side effects, in both the medical and moral realms. Chief among the undesired moral side effects has been the failure to achieve the highest, and in a few cases even adequate, standards of professional moral concern for the human subjects being used in this necessary biomedical experimentation. In the area of research with human subjects the medical investigators are not alone; there is a tendency in other fields too for humane concerns to be left at the laboratory door. Psychologists and sociologists have often been accused of circumventing the requirement for consent and of applying unethical ma-nipulative techniques in their investigations of human behavior, and neither profession has welcomed scrutiny from outsiders or restrictive regulation. The issue goes beyond research ethics, however. Many professions now command knowledge that has great potential usefulness for human welfare but bestows power that can be abused. Because professional power is of such major public consequence, it must be subject to significant public control (Barber, 1976).

Infants and children require special consideration. For them, informed consent is usually impossible, as it is for the mentally retarded and other legally non-competent groups. They are particularly helpless, vulnerable, and liable to exploitation. They rely on their parents for love and protection, and to ask parents to agree to their child's participation in an experiment places a heavy burden on them. For the investigator, there is a dual responsibility – to children and to their parents – and he must assume a greater responsibility to ensure that the means and ends of the project are necessary, worthy, and possible at minimal risk. In this, his sense of conscience and compassion should inevitably make experimentation with children much more difficult than with adults who have consented of their own free will. The only real protection for the individual lies in the scrupulousness, conscience and personal integrity of the investigator. In practice, this is best served by the investigator also being responsible for the care and welfare of the child – that is, the paediatrician.

References

Barber, B., Lally, J., Makarushka, J. & Sullivan, D. (1972): Experimenting with humans: problems and processes of social control in the biomedical research community. In: *The challenge of life*. Eds. R.M. Kunz & H. Fehr, pp. 357–373. Basel and Stuttgart: Birkhäuser Verlag.

Barber, B. (1976): The ethics of experimentation with human subjects. *Sci. Am.* **234**, 25–31.

Baum, M. (1986): Do we need informed consent? *Lancet* ii, 911–912.

Beecher, H.K. (1966): Ethics and clinical research. *N. Engl. J. Med.* **274**, 1354–1360.

British Paediatric Association (1980): Guidelines to aid ethical committees considering research involving children. *Arch. Dis. Child.* **55**, 75–77.

Cancer Research Campaign Working Party in Breast Conservation (1983): Informed consent: ethical, legal and medical implications for doctors and patients who participate in randomized clinical trials. *B.M.J.* **286**, 1117–1121.

Capron, A.M. (1978): Human experimentation: basic issues. In: *Encyclopedia of bioethics*, ed. W.T. Reich, pp. 692–699. New York: Free Press.

Cassileth, B.R., Zupkis, R.V., Sutton-Smith, K. & March, V. (1980): Informed consent – why are its goals imperfectly realized? *N. Engl. J. Med.* **302**, 896–900.

CIOMS, c/o WHO (1982): Proposed international guidelines for biomedical research involving human subjects (with section concerning children). Geneva: WHO.

Cooke, R.E. (1977): An ethical and procedural basis for research on children. *J. Pediatr.* **90**, 681–682.

Curran, W.J. & Beecher, H.K. (1969): Experimentation in children. A reexamination of legal ethical principles. *JAMA* **210**, 77–83.

Curran, W.J. (1978): Research on children. *N. Engl. J. Med.* **299**, 1001–1002.

Curran W.J. (1981): New ethical-review policy for clinical medical research. *N. Engl. J. Med.* **304**, 952–954.

Fost, N.C. (1978): Children and biomedicine. In: *Encyclopedia of bioethics*, ed. W.T. Reich, pp. 150–156. New York: Free Press.

Friedman, R.J. (1992): Scientific and ethical considerations in human clinical experimentation. *South. Med. J.* **85**, 919–922.

Giertz, G. (1983): Ethical aspects of paediatric research. *Acta Paediatr. Scand.* **72**, 641–650.

Gray, B.H., Cooke, R.A. & Tannenbaum, A.S. (1978): Research involving human subjects. *Science* **210**, 1094–1101.

Janofsky, J. & Starfield, B. (1981): Assessment of risk in research on children. *J. Pediatr.* **98**, 842–846.

Jonsen, A.R. (1978): Research involving children: recommendations of the national commission for the protection of human subjects of biomedical and behavioral research. *Pediatrics* **62**, 131–136.

Krugman, S. (1971): Experiments at the Willowbrook State School. *Lancet*, **ii**, 966–967.

Lewis, P.J. (1982): The drawbacks of research ethics committees. *J. Med. Ethics* **8**, 61–64.

Nicholson, R.H. (1986): *Medical research with children. Ethics, law and practice.* Oxford: Oxford University Press.

Papadatos, C.J. (1989): Guidelines for medical research in children. *Infection* **17**, 411–417.

Pappworth, M.H. (1967): *Human guinea pigs: experimentation on man.* London: Routledge & Kegan Paul.

Pearn, J.H. (1984): The child and clinical research. *Lancet*, **ii**, 510–512.

Rennie, D. (1980): Informed consent by 'well-nigh abject' adults. *N. Engl. J. Med.* **302**, 917–918.

Robinson, R.J. (1987): Ethics committees and research in children. *B.M.J.* **294**, 1243–1244.

United States Department of Health and Human Services (1982): Final regulations amending basic HHS policy for the protection of human research subjects. *Federal register* 46 (16), Book 2, 8333–8392.

US National Commission for the Protection of Human Subjects of Biomedical and Behavioral Research (1978): Protection of human subjects: research involving children: report and recommendations. *Federal Register* 43, 2084–2114.

Zelen, M. (1979): A new design for randomized clinical trials. *N. Engl. J. Med.* **300**, 1242–1245.

The ethics of animal and human experimentation, edited by P.P. De Deyn.
©1994 John Libbey & Company Ltd., pp. 321–337.

28

Research on the terminally ill: AIDS and cancer

George J. Annas*

Health Law Department and Law, Medicine of Ethics Program, Boston University Schools of Medicine and Public Health, Boston, Massachusetts, USA

Since World War II there have been persistent efforts at both the national and international level to develop rules to protect the rights and welfare of subjects of human experimentation†. These efforts have focused primarily on codifying the rights of subjects, and protecting their welfare by prior peer review of research protocols. In recent years research regulations have been under attack by politicians, drug companies, researchers, and advocacy groups. In less than half a century, human experimentation has been transformed from a suspect activity into a presumptively beneficial activity. With this transformation, traditional distinctions between experimentation and therapy, subject and patient, and researcher and physician have become discouragingly blurred. Issues of power, money, control and fear of death have often been more central than protection of the rights and welfare of research subjects.

Special problems regarding rights and welfare of subjects have been recognized in research involving vulnerable populations, including pregnant women and foetuses, child-

* This article is based on a lecture Professor Annas gave the Schroeder Scholar-in-Residence at Case Western Reserve University School of Law and is reprinted from *Health Matrix: The Journal of Law-Medicine* (1992) 2, 119–140. The Schroeder Scholar-in-Residence programme honors the founder of the Case Western Reserve University Law-Medicine Center, Professor Emeritus Oliver C. Schroeder, Jr., by bringing to the law school each year a distinguished scholar who conducts faculty workshops, meets with students, and delivers a formal public address, known as the Schroeder Lecture.

† See generally *The Nazi doctors and the Nuremberg Code: human rights in human experimentation* (George J. Annas & Michael A. Grodin, eds., 1992) [hereinafter *Nazi doctors*]; Bernard M. Dickens, *et al.*, Editor's introduction to research on human populations: national and international ethical guidelines, *Law Med. & Health Care* 157 (1991).

ren, prisoners, and mentally impaired people. But as premature death becomes a rarity in developed countries, and death itself becomes more alien and feared, the most vulnerable research subject, the one most consistently transformed into an object (a mere means to an end), has become the terminally ill patient. How did terminally ill patients come to be so sought-after as research subjects? Can current international research guidelines protect their rights and welfare in research trials? And if not, what additional steps are required to protect the rights and welfare of this uniquely vulnerable population?

A careful examination of the international research guidelines set forth during the past 50 years leads to the conclusion that a project that began as one to protect both the rights and welfare of human research subjects is now concentrated on rights protection in the developed nations, and on welfare protection in the developing nations. In both settings the basic rationale for these two diverging models is the same: desperation fuelled by fear of death!*.

The Nuremberg Code

The Nuremberg Code was formulated by United States judges sitting in judgement of Nazi physician-experimenters following World War II. The Nazi experiments involved systematic and barbarous interventions in which death was the planned endpoint. The subjects of these experiments were concentration camp prisoners, mostly Jews, Gypsies and Slavs!†. The judges at Nuremberg viewed human experimentation as suspect, and the Nuremberg Code itself resulted from horrendous non-therapeutic, non-consensual prison research.

The Nuremberg Code, despite its inherent limitations, remains the most authoritative legal and ethical document governing international research standards, and one of the premier human rights documents in world history. The judges based the Nuremberg Code on a natural law theory, deriving it from universal moral, ethical and legal concepts. The Code protects individual subjects first by protecting their rights. Voluntary, informed, competent, and understanding consent is required by the first principle of the Code, and principle 9 gives the subject the right to withdraw from the experiment. The consent of the subject is necessary under the Nuremberg Code, although consent alone is not sufficient. The other eight provisions of the Code are related to the welfare of

* The most quoted words in experimental medicine are not from any legal or ethical canon, but from *Hamlet*, 'Diseases desperate grown by desperate appliance are relieved, or not at all.' William Shakespeare, *Hamlet*, act 4, sc. 2 (Edward Hubler, ed., Signet Classic, 1963). As with terminal illnesses such as cancer and AIDS, the best strategy regarding the protection of research subjects is prevention. The King's 'desperate diseases' speech begins with his musings on Hamlet, as he says

> How dangerous is it that this man goes loose!
> Yet must not we put the strong law on him:
> He's loved of the distracted multitude,
> Who like not in their judgement, but their eyes

Id.

The same thing may be said about human experimentation. It is loved by the public, but primarily because it is little understood, and its promise of 'miracle' cures seems real. Nonetheless, the dangers to human rights and welfare of research subjects are such that we must 'put the strong law on him' and develop and enforce reasonable research regulations.

† *Nazi Doctors*

subjects, and must be satisfied *before* consent is even sought from the subject. The subject cannot waive these provisions. The requirements of the provisions include a valid research design to procure information important for the good of society that cannot be obtained in other ways; the avoidance of unnecessary physical and mental suffering and injury; the absence of any *a priori* reason to believe that death or disabling injury will occur; risks that never exceed benefits; and the presence of a qualified researcher who is prepared to terminate the experiment if it 'is likely to result in the injury, disability, or death of the experimental subject'!*.

The Declaration(s) of Helsinki

Physician-researchers viewed the Nuremberg Code as confining and inapplicable to their practices, because it was promulgated as a human rights document by judges at a criminal trial, and because the judges made no attempt to deal with clinical research on

* The Nuremberg Code:

1. The voluntary consent of the human subject is absolutely essential.

This means that the person involved should have legal capacity to give consent; should be so situated as to be able to exercise free power of choice, without the intervention of any element of force, fraud, deceit, duress, overreaching, or other ulterior form of constraint or coercion; and should have sufficient knowledge and comprehension of the elements of the subject matter involved as to enable him to make an understanding and enlightened decision. This latter element requires that before the acceptance of an affirmative decision by the experimental subject there should be made known to him the nature, duration, and purpose of the experiment; the method and means by which it is to be conducted; all inconveniences and hazards reasonably to be expected; and the effects upon his health or person which may possibly come from his participation in the experiment.

The duty and responsibility for ascertaining the quality of the consent rests upon each individual who initiates, directs or engages in the experiment. It is a personal duty and responsibility which may not be delegated to another with impunity.

2. The experiment should be such as to yield fruitful results for the good of society, unprocurable by other methods or means of study, and not random and unnecessary in nature.

3. The experiment should be so designed and based on the results of animal experimentation and a knowledge of natural history of the disease or other problem under study that the anticipated results will justify the performance of the experiment.

4. The experiment should be so conducted as to avoid all unnecessary physical and mental suffering and injury.

5. No experiment should be conducted where there is an *a priori* reason to believe that death or disabling injury will occur; except, perhaps, in those experiments where the experimental physicians also serve as subjects.

6. The degree of risk to be taken should never exceed that determined by the humanitarian importance of the problem to be solved by the experiment.

7. Proper preparations should be made and adequate facilities provided to protect the experimental subject against even remote possibilities of injury, disability, or death.

8. The experiment should be conducted only by scientifically qualified persons. The highest degree of skill and care should be required through all stages of the experiment of those who conduct or engage in the experiment.

9. During the course of the experiment, the human subject should be at liberty to bring the experiment to an end if he has reached the physical or mental state where continuation of the experiment seems to him to be impossible.

10. During the course of the experiment, the scientist in charge must be prepared to terminate the experiment at any stage, if he has probable cause to believe, in the exercise of the good faith, superior skill, and careful judgement required of him, that a continuation of the experiment is likely to result in injury, disability, or death to the experimental subject. *Nazi Doctors*, p. 2.

children, patients, or mentally-impaired people. The World Medical Association has consistently tried to marginalize the Code by devising The Declaration of Helsinki, a more permissive alternative document, first promulgated in 1964, and amended three times since. This document is subtitled 'recommendations guiding doctors in clinical research' and is just that, recommendations by physicians to physicians. The Declaration's goal is to replace the human rights-based agenda of the Nuremberg Code with a more lenient medical ethics model that permits paternalism. US researcher Henry Beecher probably best expressed medicine's delight with the Declaration of Helsinki's ascendancy when he said in 1970: 'The Nuremberg Code presents a rigid act of legalistic demands ... The Declaration of Helsinki, on the other hand, presents a set of guides. It is an ethical as opposed to a legalistic document and is thus more broadly useful than the one formulated at Nuremberg . . .!*

The core of the Declaration of Helsinki divides research into therapeutic ('Medical Research Combined with Professional Care') and non-therapeutic, eliminating the necessity for subject consent in some cases!†. The major addition to the 1975 version (mirroring developments in the United States and elsewhere) was the encouragement of formal peer review of research protocols. For example, a new 'basic principle' provided that: 'The design and performance of each experimental procedure involving human subjects should be clearly formulated in an experimental protocol which should be transmitted to a specially appointed independent committee for consideration, comment and guidance'.!‡

The movement to displace the consent requirement of the Nuremberg Code with prior peer review by a medical committee found its greatest success in the 1975 Declaration. For example, the physician need not obtain the subject's informed consent to medical research combined with professional care if he submits his reasons for not obtaining consent to the independent review committee!§.

Council for International Organizations of Medical Sciences and the World Health Organization

Scientific organizations were even more hostile to the Nuremberg Code than were the world's physicians. In 1967 the president of the Council for International Organizations of Medical Sciences (CIOMS), for example, said that 'On the whole [the 1964 Declaration of Helsinki] corrects what in the Nuremberg Rules was circumstantial, related to Nazi crimes, and places these Rules more correctly in the context of generally accepted med-

* Quoted in W. Refshauge, The place for international standards in conducting research for humans 55 *Bull. World Heath Org.* 133–135 (Suppl. 1977). See also the comparison made by the world's leading liver transplant experimenter, Thomas Starzl: 'The Helsinki Declaration was shorter [sic] and easier to read.' Thomas Starzl, *The puzzle people: memoirs of a transplant surgeon*, p. 146, 1992.

† *Nazi doctors*, pp. 335–336.

‡ *Nazi doctors*, p. 334.
Principle I.2 of the 1989 revision of the Declaration (Helsinki IV) provides that the experimental protocol 'should be transmitted for consideration, comment and guidance to a specifically appointed committee independent of the investigator and the sponsor, provided that this independent committee is in conformity with the laws and regulations of the country in which the research experiment is performed'. *Id.* at 159.

§ Sharon Perley, *et al.*, *The Nuremberg Code: An International Overveiw*, In: *Nazi Doctors*, p. 159.

ical traditions"[*].

Shortly thereafter, officials in the World Health Organization (WHO) were informed by officials at the National Institutes of Health that WHO grant proposals would not be considered unless they were approved by a WHO ethical review committee. WHO had no such peer review committee, and set about to form one. This was followed by a 1978 agreement between WHO and CIOMS to 'develop guidelines to assist developing countries in evolving mechanisms that would ensure the observance of principles of medical ethics of biomedical research'[†]. The result was a 1982 document (currently under revision) designed to provide guidance to developing countries.

Remarkably the 1982 Guidelines contain the statement: 'Both the Nuremberg Code and the original Declaration of Helsinki of 1964 have been superseded by Helsinki II [1975]'[‡]. Helsinki II did supersede Helsinki I, but it could not, of course, supersede the judgement at Nuremberg. The Nuremberg Code is based on international natural law and ethics that even the prior positive law to the contrary in Nazi Germany could not supersede. Thus the Nuremberg Code is *the* basis for international law and ethics in the area of human experimentation, and lowering its standards can be accomplished neither by vote of a group of researchers, nor by legal rule in any individual country. In this regard, individual countries can only legitimately *add* protections to the Nuremberg Code.

Nonetheless, the heart of the WHO/CIOMS project seems to compromise the Nuremberg Code's requirement for consent of the research subject as an integral part of international law and ethics. Instead, the 1982 Guidelines rely heavily on 'an independent impartial prospective review of all protocols'[§]. For the first time in an international document, special attention is given to children, pregnant and nursing women, and mentally ill and mentally impaired people. However, adults in developing countries, perhaps unintentionally, are given the same uncomprehending status as children and the mentally ill[¶]. For example, the rights of subjects are subordinated to the view that researchers and community leaders have of their welfare. Thus in developing countries it is suggested:

> [W]here individual members of a community often do not have the necessary awareness of the implications of participation in an experiment so as to adequately give informed consent, the Guidelines suggest that the decision on whether or not to participate should be elicited through the intermediary of a trusted community leader ... [T]he intermediary should make it clear ... that participation is entirely voluntary and that he may abstain or withdraw from the experiment at any time[++].

* Refshauge, p. 137.

† Michael Grodin, Historical Origins of the Nuremberg Code, in *Nazi Doctors*, pp. 135–160.

‡ WHO/CIOMS (1982): *Proposed International Guidelines for Biomedical Research Involving Human Subjects*, Geneva: CIOMS, p. 23 [hereinafter *Proposed guidelines*]. This language was deleted from the August 1992 redraft of the revisions.

§ *Id.* p. 15.

¶ Carel B. Ijsselmuiden & Ruth R. Faden, Research and informed consent in Africa: another look, **326,** *N. Engl. J. Med.* 830–832 (1992).

++ *Id.* pp. 26–27. *See also* Perley *et al.*, p. 163. Substantially similar language remains in the August 1992 redraft.

On the other hand, the standards for 'externally sponsored research' done in developing countries are appropriately strict. Such research must meet not only the ethical standards of the host country, but also the ethical standards of the initiating country*. If this standard (No. 28) is taken seriously, following the rights and welfare requirements of the Nuremberg Code would be required in most instances of United States and European-sponsored research in developing countries. Nonetheless, CIOMS greatly confuses the very concept of international law and ethics, seemingly encouraging countries to find their lowest common denominator in subject protection.

A 1992 draft revision of the 1982 Guidelines opens with a recharacterization of human research in developing countries. It states that there is a 'positive duty to do good,' and that 'Research is being seen as a good in itself, and as the discharge of an ethical responsibility'†. This is, to my knowledge, the first time research has been privileged over treatment, and virtually no explanation is presented in the document for this radical assertion. If the developed countries have ethical responsibilities to the developing countries (and I believe they do), then the responsibilities of providing food, clothing, housing, education, and basic medical care must all have a much higher priority than providing research protocols. Thus, what seems at the centre of this reconceptualization of research is not the 'discharge' of an 'ethical obligation', but gaining access to a population of research subjects for research that will primarily benefit citizens in the developed world‡.

In summary, although the concept of vulnerable populations has been recognized, there are no international research guidelines that provide special rules or protections for the terminally ill, and there are no specific rules for research on terminal illnesses such as cancer and AIDS. We have witnessed a general trend away from the Nuremberg Code toward considering the protection of *either* rights (consent) or welfare (prior peer review) sufficient for human subject protection. With regard to research on terminal illnesses such as AIDS and cancer in the developed countries, this usually means that the research will be seen as therapy, and patients (subjects) who have the disease will be expected to protect themselves through the mechanism of informed consent. In developing countries, on the other hand, research on AIDS may be characterized as 'community-based', and prior ethical review seen as sufficient protection for the rights and welfare of community members. In both cases the primary justification for research on terminal illnesses is the same: desperation in the face of death.

Research on dying patients: AIDS and cancer

Perhaps the primary reason that existing national and international research guidelines have little practical relevance for individuals with terminal illnesses is that the terminal diagnosis itself determines both what researchers and physicians deem 'reasonable', and what the subjects (patients) themselves find acceptable – even desirable. Many researchers themselves fear death, and believe that terminally ill patients really can't be hurt (they are 'going to die anyway') and therefore have 'nothing to lose'. Prior peer

* *Proposed Guidelines*, pp. 31–32.

† This April 1992 draft language was dropped in the August 1992 redraft, and hopefully will not be resurrected in the final document.

‡ See, e.g., Lawrence K. Altman, Aids vaccine to be tested on human volunteers, bypassing animals trials, *New York Times*, Nov. 11, 1191, p. A7.

review of protocols under such circumstances becomes pro forma and provides no meaningful protections for subjects. Likewise, terminally ill patients who are told that medicine has 'nothing to offer' them have come to view experimental protocols as treatment. Therefore, instead of being suspicious of experimentation, patients may *demand* access to experimental interventions as their right. Under such circumstances informed consent alone provides no meaningful protection.

Psychiatrist Jay Katz has noted that when medicine seems impotent to fight the claims of nature, 'all kinds of senseless interventions are tried in an unconscious effort to cure the incurable magically through a 'wonder drug', a novel surgical procedure, or a penetrating psychological interpretation'[*]. Although physicians often justify such interventions as simply being responsive to patient needs, 'they may turn out to be a projection of their own needs onto patients'[†]. Similarly, transplant surgeon Francis Moore has observed of transplant experiments based on the 'desperate remedies' rationale: 'There must be some likelihood of success before the desperate remedy becomes more than a desperate search for an opportunity to try a new procedure awaiting trial'[‡]. AIDS activist Rebecca Pringle Smith put it similarly, 'Even if you have a supply of compliant martyrs, trials must have some ethical validity'[§].

Susan Sontag has noted that cancer and AIDS have become linked as perhaps the two most feared ways to die in the developed world. In her words, 'AIDS, like cancer, leads to a hard death . . . The most terrifying illnesses are those perceived not just as lethal but as dehumanizing, literally so'[¶]. And although philosopher Michel Foucault was not speaking of the medicalization of death by cancer or AIDS, he could have been when he chronicled how the power of government over life and death has shifted in the past two centuries. 'Now it is over life; throughout its unfolding, that power establishes its domination; death is power's limit, the moment that escapes it . . .'[**]. In human experimentation on the terminally ill we have Foucault's vision of public power played out in private: researchers take charge of the bodies of the dying in an attempt to take charge of the patients' lives and prevent their own personal deaths, and death itself[††].

The Nazi doctors' chief defence at Nuremberg was that experimentation was necessary to support the war effort. Now combating disease has itself become a 'war', as we speak of a 'war on cancer' and a 'war on AIDS'. And in that war, patients, especially terminally ill patients are conscripted as soldiers. As former editor of the *New England Journal of Medicine*, Franz Ingelfinger, put it: '[T]he thumb screws of coercion are most relentlessly applied' to 'the most used and useful of all experimental subjects, the patient with disease'[‡‡]. But as Sontag reminds us, war metaphors are dangerous in disease because they

* Jay Katz (1984): *The silent world of doctor and patient*, p. 151.

† *Id.*

‡ Francis D. Moore (1989): The desperate case: care (costs, applicability, research, ethics), *JAMA* **261**, 1483–1484.

§ Quoted in Joseph Palca (1989): AIDS drug trials enter new age. *Science* **246**, 19–20.

¶ Susan Sontag, *Illness as Metaphor; and, AIDS and its Metaphors* 126 (1989).

** Michel Foucault: *The history of sexuality*. p. 138 (Robert Hurley trans., 1990).

†† *Id.* p. 143.

‡‡ F.J. Ingelfinger (1972): Informed (but uneducated) consent. *N. Engl. J. Med.* **287**, 465–466.

encourage authoritarianism, overmobilization, and stigmatization. In her words:

> No, it is not desirable for medicine, any more than for war, to be "total". Neither is the crisis created by AIDS a "total" anything. We are not being invaded. The body is not a battlefield. The ill are neither unavoidable casualties nor the enemy. We – medicine, society – are not authorized to fight back by any means whatever . . ."*.

Cancer

In the early 1980s the President's Commission for the Study of Ethical Problems in Medicine and Behavioral Research attempted to get agreement on categorizing Phase 1 drug studies with anti-cancer agents. Are they research or therapy? Federal Food and Drug Administration (FDA) regulations state that Phase 1 studies are intended to have no therapeutic content, but are to determine 'toxicity, metabolism, absorption, elimination, and other pharmacological action, preferred route of administration, and safe dosage range'†. Nonetheless, National Cancer Institute (NCI) researchers insisted that Phase 1 cancer studies, using cancer patients as subjects, should be described as therapeutic. The Assistant Secretary of the Department of Health and Human Services (HHS) wrote to Congress in 1981:

> Notwithstanding the fact that some individuals within HHS may not concur, the official position of the Department, including NCI, NIH, and FDA, is to regard Phase 1 trials of anti-cancer drugs as *potentially* therapeutic. The often small, but real possibility of benefit must be weighed against the nearly 100 per cent probability of death if experimental therapy is not attempted for the advanced cancer patients who participate in Phase 1 studies‡.

The President's Commission never received a better answer to its inquiry, and this answer is not helpful. In a sick person, virtually any intervention, even a placebo, can be described as 'potentially therapeutic', and once this misleading label is applied, the nonbeneficial Phase 1 study is *de facto* eliminated and transformed into 'experimental therapy'. Any distinction between experimentation and therapy is lost. Under these circumstances the President's Commission could only bow weakly to informed consent: 'It is important that patients who are asked to participate in tests of new anti-cancer drugs not be misled about the likelihood (or remoteness) of any therapeutic benefit they might derive from such participation'§.

American oncologists use so many approved drugs for unapproved uses that it seems fair to conclude that for most cancers there are no standard treatments, and sound scientific studies are needed. A 1990 survey, for example, found that fully one-third of all the drugs used on cancer patients are of unproven safety and efficacy for the purpose for which

* Sontang, pp. 182–183.

† *President's Commission for the study of ethical problems in medicine and biomedical and behavioral research, protecting human subjects*, **65** (1981) [hereinafter *President's Commission*].

‡ *Id* (quoting letter from Edward N. Brandt, Jr., Assistant Sec. for Health, Dept. of Health and Human Services, to the Hon. Henry A. Waxman, Chairman, Subcomm. on Health & Environment (Nov. 20, 1981, pp. 3–4).

§ *President's Commission*, pp. 43.

they are given; and unapproved use is even more prevalent for malignancies that have metastasized than for earlier cancers*. Unapproved chemotherapy for patients being treated with palliative intent is twice the rate for curative intent, indicating an appropriately higher degree of risk-taking for quality of life enhancement. Oncologist Charles Moertel, commenting on the study, noted that the major beneficiaries of such an approach to cancer treatment are the 'appointment book of the oncologist' and 'the pharmaceutical companies and their stockholders'†. In short, business ethics seem to be supplanting medical ethics. As to the argument that oncologists are just responding to the demand of dying patients, Moertel responded: 'This argument abandons the scientific basis for medical practice and could just as well be used to justify quackery. Also, one wonders how many patients with advanced pancreatic cancer, for example, would really demand cytotoxic drugs if the sheer futility of such therapy was honestly explained'‡.

If we accept patient demand as sufficient justification to mistreat them, it is a short step to say that the patient should have the right to demand to be killed by his physician. In fact, this very argument was made in early 1992 in the *New England Journal of Medicine*, where another oncologist noted that cancer chemotherapy, while it can prolong life, often makes the patient's dying 'unbearable'§.

He went on to argue that, 'since we physicians brought the patient [subject] to the state she is in, we cannot abandon her by saying that euthanasia violates the purpose of our profession'¶. The use of killing as 'damage control' for a physician-created harm to patients is chilling. It is far better to avoid the harm than to use it to justify killing. The quest to master terminal illness may, however, make killing by physicians seem reasonable**.

The 'desperate remedies' rationale used to justify experimentation on the terminally ill is seriously flawed. There are fates worse than death, and many Americans have written living wills and health care proxies to *prevent* their lives from being prolonged under certain circumstances††. Likewise, the horrible and prolonged deaths of Barney Clark and William Schroder on the permanent artificial heart ensured the end of all further experiments with the Jarvik 7‡‡. Although the device can obviously prolong life, it cannot do so at an acceptable level of quality. The conclusion is clear: dying patients are real people, not objects, who value quality over quantity of life, and cannot be legally or ethically

* Thomas Laetz & George Silberman (1991): Reimbursement policies constrain the practice of oncology, *JAMA* **266**, 2996–2997.

† Charles G. Moertel (1991): Off-label drug use for cancer therapy and national health care priorities. *JAMA* **266**, 3031.

‡ *Id.* See also Cornelius O. Granai (1992): Ovarian cancer – unrealistic expectations. *N. Engl. J. Med.* **327**, 197.

§ Guy I. Benrubi (1992): Euthanasia: the need for procedural safeguards. *N. Engl. J. Med.* **326**, 197.

¶ *Id* pp. 198.

** See, e.g. Physician-philosopher Leon Kass, who has argued. 'We do not yet understand that the project for the mastery of nature and the conquest of death leads, only to dehumanization; that any attempt to gain the tree of life by means of the tree knowledge leads inevitably also to the hemlock . . .' Leon R. Kass, *Suicide Made Easy: The Evil of 'Rational' Humaneness*, Commentary, Dec. 1991, pp. 19, 24.

†† See Nancy M.P. King (1991): *Making sense of advance directives.*

‡‡ George J. Annas (1987): Death and the magic machine: informed consent to the artificial heart. *W. New Engl. L. Rev.* **9**, 89.

used simply as a means to an end. Individuals do have a right to refuse *any* treatment or experiment. But respecting patient autonomy does *not* require that we accept demands for mistreatment, experimentation, torture, or whatever the dying might want, anymore than we must accede to demands to illegal (but effective) drugs like heroin and LSD, unlicensed practitioners, or a physician-induced death.

Closely related to the difficulty of distinguishing research from treatment is distinguishing the role of the researcher from the role of the physician when these two conflicting roles are merged in one person. For example, in a 1992 article on cancer and AIDS research two prominent commentators seem to assume that 'cancer researchers' are properly seen as doctors providing 'treatment' to 'patients'*. Little attention has been paid to the researcher's inherent conflict of interest. It is unlikely that patients can ever draw the distinction between physician and researcher, because most simply do not believe that their physician would either knowingly do something harmful to them, or would knowingly use them simply as a means for their own ends. Cancer researchers, however, know better. James F. Holland, for example, has said simply, 'Patients have to be subsidiaries of the trial . . . I'm not interested in holding patients' hands. I'm interested in curing cancer . . . Every patient becomes a piece of scientific data'†. As candid as Holland is, it seems almost certain that his patients come to him for a cure, and look upon him as their physician – not simply as a researcher. In such a circumstance, the Helsinki Declaration's theoretical division between therapeutic and non-therapeutic research is meaningless.

Finally, we should emphasize that which has generally been marginalized: most studies on the terminally ill, including cancer and AIDS clinical trials, are funded by private drug companies that have tremendous financial stakes in their success. Clinical investigators may even 'own equity interest in the company that produces the product or may serve as paid consultants and scientific advisers', roles that at least call their objectivity into question‡. Medical ethics is being eroded by a new commercialism in medicine. This fact has led most leading medical journals in the United States to require financial disclosure prior to publication of research results. However, neither Institutional Review Boards (IRBs) nor individual subjects are routinely informed of the financial aspects of proposed clinical trials, even though the finances often create major potential conflicts of interest among the sponsor, the researcher, and the patient-subject.

One need not search far for examples. In early February 1992, the stock of US Bioscience lost $550 million in value on one day after the FDA review panel refused to recommend approval of its drug, Ethyl (a drug said to protect healthy cells from the toxic effects of cancer chemotherapy)§. One week later another United States biotechnology company lost half of its value in one day when a clinical trial of one of its cancer drugs was halted

* David J. Rothman & Harold Edgar (1992): Scientific rigor and medical realities: placebo trials in cancer and AIDS research. In: *AIDS: the making of a chronic disease*, eds. E. Fee & D. Fox, pp. 194–206.

† Dena Kleiman (1986): In search for cancer cure, patients come second. *New York Times*, Feb. 18, pp. B1, B7.

‡ Arnold Relman (1992): What market values are doing to medicine. *The Atlantic Monthly* **99**, 103.

§ Michael Waldholz (1992): U.S. bioscience holders are latest to get costly lesson, *Wall St. J.*, Feb. 4. p. B. 6.

because of adverse effects on the subjects*. Financing may be *the* major change in clinical trials over the past two decades, and this change has not been mirrored in research regulations. New research findings are often reported first on the financial pages of newspapers, and only later in the medical literature. It thus came as little surprise in March 1992 when Dow Corning openly declared that its decision to discontinue the manufacture of silicone breast implants was made strictly 'on the basis of business'†.

AIDS

AIDS has always been perceived as the disease in which there literally is *no* distinction between treatment and experimentation. This is because there is no cure for AIDS. The disease primarily strikes the young, leading to a death that is premature by virtually any calculation, and existing treatments that can prolong life are far from satisfactory. In addition, many people with the disease have no access to health care, so the only way they can obtain medical care is to enrol in an experimental drug trial. Thus, although theoretically wrong, ACT-UP's (AIDS Coalition to Unleash Power) political slogan 'A Drug Trial is Health Care Too', tragically is factually correct in many US settings. However, the slogan serves to wrongly conflate experimentation with therapy, and to encourage people with AIDS to seek out experimentation as treatment, and physician-researchers to see AIDS patients as potential subjects who have 'nothing to lose'.

As the *Wall Street Journal* editorialized in 1988, supporting a loosening of FDA testing procedures for people with cancer, Alzheimer's disease, and AIDS: 'AIDS patients have driven home to the US medical and political establishment what enormous risks human beings in death's grip will take to gain relief or respite'‡.

This editorial identified the *problem* and illustrated why regulation is necessary. The FDA is not in the business of regulating 'hope' for 'relief or respite', but of determining whether 'relief or respite' from particular drugs and devices is likely. Deregulation of human experimentation cannot produce new drugs or treatments. Money can, however, be made by pharmaceutical companies by exploiting our fear of death and desperation. It seems fair to conclude that virtually all of the drugs that have been developed for AIDS treatment have been over-priced, and financially exploitative of those with AIDS§.

* Floyd Norris (1992):Drug's test pains MGI investors *New York Times*, Feb. 11, p. C1; James P. Miller (1992): MGI Pharma suffers 52 per cent fall in stockprice, *Wall St. J.* Feb. 11, p. B3.

† Philip J. Hilts (1992): As it quits implant business, maker says product is safe, New York Times, March 20, p. A12. See also, Michael Waldholz (1992): An unapproved drug for Alzheimer's gets a big marketing push, *Wall St. J.*, Aug. 25, p. A1.

‡ New ideas for new drugs, *Wall St. J.*, Dec. 28, 1988, p. A16. See also, Andrew Pollack (1992): Gene therapy gets the go-ahead, *New York Times*, Feb. 14, p. D1; Mireya Navarro (1992): Into the unknown: AIDS patients test drugs, *New York Times*, Feb. 29, pp. 1, 29. See also Rothman & Edgar, pp. 205.

§ See, e.g. Forcing poverty on AIDS patients, *New York Times*, Aug. 30, 1988 p. A18 (editorial); Maher (1989): Pitiless scourge: separating out the hype from the hope on AIDS, *Barron's*, March 13, pp. 6, 22; Eric Savitz (1991): No magic cure: the war on AIDS produces few gains, except on Wall Street, *Barron's* Dec. 16, p. 10.

Again, business ethics seem to be supplanting medical ethics.

Although the cover story is compassion, the movement to loosen FDA's research rules should be seen for what it is: a political strategy by a free market administration bent not on helping people with AIDS, but on exploiting the AIDS epidemic to loosen drug regulations and maximize profits for the pharmaceutical industry*. For example, Jay Plager, counsellor to the former Undersecretary of the Department of Health and Human Services, asserted that one purpose of early drug release regulations is to give 'desperately ill patients the opportunity to decide for themselves whether they would rather take an experimental drug or die of the disease untreated'†.

And former FDA Commissioner Frank Young said of AIDS that 'there is such a degree of desperation, and people are going to die, that I'm not going to be the Commissioner that robs them of hope'‡. The FDA must concentrate on using science to identify beneficial treatments, not on using faith healing to promote hope that an unproven drug might be beneficial. There is some evidence that AIDS activists now recognize this. At the July 1992 International AIDS conference in Amsterdam, for example, ACT-UP member Mark Harrington said he believed that regulatory reforms often 'go for naught'. In his words, 'What is the point of streamlining access and approval when the result is merely to replace AZT [with] mediocre, toxic, expensive drugs?'§ Harrington urged others to follow his example and volunteer for experiments involving basic science¶.

Of course, it remains unethical to conduct a clinical trial in a manner in which no reliable data can be generated. As Anthony Fauci, director of the National Institute of Allergy and Infectious Disease, has properly noted, the primary goal of clinical trials is 'not to deliver therapy. It's to answer a scientific question so that the drug can be available for everybody once you've established safety and efficacy'**. On the other hand, community activists have made some important points regarding AIDS, and some rules for AIDS research in the United States are appropriately changing. Three are of note: (1) Representatives of the gay rights and AIDS communities are being asked to join governmental scientific advisory panels which set research priorities; (2) people with AIDS are being placed on local IRBs to evaluate community-based AIDS research protocols; and (3) end points involving quality of life instead of death are being explored in evaluating the results of AIDS drug trials††. Emphasis on quality of life measures seems especially rele-

* See generally George J. Annas (1989): Faith (healing), hope and charity at the FDA: the politics of AIDS drug trials. *Vill. L. Rev.* **34,** 771.

† Robert Pear (1987): U.S. to allow use of trial drugs for AIDS and terminal ills. *New York Times*, May 21, p. A1.

‡ Philip M. Boffey (1988): FDA will allow AIDS patients to import unapproved medicines. *New York Times*, July 24, pp. A1, A19.

§ Quoted in Lawrence K. Altman (1992): At AIDS talks, reality weighs down hope, *New York Times*, July 26, p. A1.

¶ *Id.*

** Joseph Palca (1989): AIDS drug trials enter new age. *Science* **246,** 19.

†† Carol Levine *et al.* (1990): Building a New Consensus: Ethical Principles and Policies for Clinical Research on HIV/AIDs, IRB, 1(22 (report which indicates an emerging consensus of the formation and conduct of

vant in diseases like AIDS and cancer where brief increases in longevity may be possible only at the cost of severe suffering.*

Strategies such as promoting unproven AIDS drugs by press conference and press release, and changing research rules for political gain, foster false hope and financial exploitation. Terminally ill AIDS and cancer patients can be harmed, misused, and exploited. It has even been persuasively argued that we as a society have developed a 'cure or kill' attitude that permits us to use the terminally ill as 'volunteers' for our experiments designed to banish death:

> Our quest for a formula that will banish death seems to make it acceptable to try questionable regimens on the aged and terminally ill . . . Those who insist on using the dying as experimental subjects . . . see death as abnormal and dying patients as subhuman. We cast the terminally ill in modern rites of sacrifice, putting patients of experiments . . . through what one might see as torture in the hope of postponing the inevitable†.

Of course, consent is no justification for the torture or inhumane treatment of human beings. We must stop treating terminally ill cancer and AIDS patients as subhuman by offering them questionable experiments in the guise of treatment. We cannot justify this behaviour on the basis of either their demand for it or our belief that the ultimate good of mankind will be served by it. Researchers who believe their subjects cannot be hurt by experimental interventions *should be disqualified* from doing research on human subjects on the basis that they cannot appropriately protect their subjects' welfare with such a view. Likewise, subjects who believe they have 'nothing to lose' and are desperate because of their terminal illness should also be disqualified as potential research subjects because they are unable to provide voluntary, competent, informed or understanding consent to the experimental intervention with such a view. It should be emphasized that these are proposed *research* rules that would not necessarily apply to treatment in a doctor–patient relationship untainted by conflicts of interest.

What should be done generally?

Action to protect research subjects in our new age of cancer and AIDS seems reasonable on both the international and national levels. On the international level we have already seen that the Nuremberg Code, the Helsinki Declaration, and WHO/CIOMS guidelines are almost universally seen as advisory and ethical only. They have no legal status in most individual countries, and they provide no mechanism for accountability or sanction of researchers who disregard their precepts. Moreover, the content and structure of medical research has changed radically in the past decade, as we have moved away from medical ethics towards commerce and business ethics. It would, therefore, seem reasonable at this time to seek more definitive action or international research rules from the United Nations. Although the United Nations never formally adopted the Nuremberg Code, its

[contd] clinical trials for AIDS research. *Evaluation Rev.* **14**, 502 (1990) (discusses the development and design of the Community Research Initiative of New York City, an IRB that reviews community-based AIDS research).

* Office of Technology Assessment, Congress of the United States (1990): *Unconventional cancer treatments* p. 228.

† Ralph Brauer (1988): The promise that failed. *New York Times*, Aug. 28, sec. 6 (magazine) pp. 34, 76.

consent principle did become an important part of the United Nations International Covenant on Civil and Political Rights, which was promulgated in 1966 and adopted by the United Nations General Assembly in 1974*. Article 7 of this covenant states: 'No one shall be subjected to torture or to cruel, inhuman or degrading treatment or punishment. In particular, no one shall be subjected without his free consent to medical or scientific experimentation'†.

Most physicians would, of course, be shocked at having anything they do to patients considered 'torture or cruel, inhuman or degrading treatment'. They would thus view the Covenant's provisions much the same way they view the Nuremberg Code: as a criminal law document not applicable to anything done in the doctor–patient relationship. It should be noted, however, that in Nazi Germany no distinction between torture and experimentation was possible, and many contemporary experiments produce 'unbearable' suffering.

Because none of the existing conventions of the United Nations deal in a detailed manner with human experimentation, M. Cheriff Bassiouni has proposed that the United Nations adopt a specific criminal Covenant on Human Experimentation:

> Section 1. Acts of Unlawful Medical Experimentation
>
> 1.0 The crime of unlawful medical experimentation consists of any physical and/or psychological alterations by means of surgical operations or injections, ingestion or inhalation of substances inflicted by or at the instigation of a public official, or for which a public official is responsible and to which the person subject to such experiment does not grant consent as described in Section 2.
>
> Section 2. Defense of Consent
>
> 2.1 For the purpose of this Article a person shall not be deemed to have consented to medical experimentation unless he or she has the capacity to consent and does so freely after being fully informed of the nature of the experiment and its possible consequences.
>
> 2.2 A person may withdraw his or her consent at any time and shall be deemed to have done so if he or she is not kept fully informed within a reasonable time of the progress of the experiment and any development concerning its possible consequences‡.

Professor Bassiouni believes this draft Code was rejected because some member countries thought it might impinge upon the practices of their pharmaceuticals industry§. If true, this is a serious condemnation of the drug companies involved. It also makes clear the need to include privately funded research in the Code as well. The Code's purpose is to articulate *human* rights that *all* members of the human community share by virtue of being human¶. Human rights are more important than either medical or business ethics,

* Perley *et al.*, p. 153.

† G.A. Res. 2200 A, UN GAOR, 21st Sess., Supp. No. 16, at 49, UN Doc. A/0316 (1966).

‡ M. Cheriff Bassiouni, *et al.* (1981): An appraisal of human experimentation in international law and practice. *J. Crim. Law & Criminology* **72,** 1597–1666.

§ Perley, p. 166.

¶ Ruth Macklin, Universality of the Nuremberg Code, in *Nazi Doctors*, pp. 240–257.

and are *not* a matter of 'internal affairs'. Because the United Nations is the only credible international body capable of articulating an international code of conduct for human experimentation, an international Covenant on Human Experimentation based on the Nuremberg Code, covering all non-therapeutic research, and all therapeutic research on competent individuals, should be adopted. Additional provisions regarding children, the mentally impaired, and the terminally ill [see *infra*] should be included.

An international tribunal for human experimentation should also be established. Such a tribunal could be established to enforce a United Nations-adopted Code, initially limited to civil sanctions, and financed with a small percentage of the human research budget of member states. Without an international tribunal with the authority to judge and punish violators of international norms of human experimentation, we are left where we began: international norms of human experimentation are relegated to the domain of ethics, and are ignored or subverted in that domain. This is because without the possibility of judgement and punishment, there is no international law worthy of the name, only international ethics.

An international tribunal will not be established overnight; therefore, we should agree to voluntarily take some steps immediately. With regard to human rights, we should insist on informed consent from all potential subjects capable of giving it. With regard to human welfare, we must be much more insistent that nonresearchers and nonphysicians make up a significant proportion (at least half) of all ethical review committees. This step will not solve the power problems inherent in expertise, but will help expose the extent to which the agenda of the researcher/scientist diverges from that of the nonexpert citizen. In addition, all research protocols should be made public, and the financial arrangements and sources must be made available to both review committees and subjects to expose (and hopefully curtail) conflicts of interest. All meetings of such review committees should be open to the public, because openness helps to dilute the power of expertise and democratically enfranchise the public.

The special problems of terminally ill research subjects

Because the voluntary and understanding nature of consent of the terminally ill subject is compromised, and because this population is especially subject to exploitation by researchers who are often unrealistically optimistic in their expectations and believe their subjects cannot be harmed, adoption of the following additional safeguards is suggested. The primary goals of these safeguards should be to protect the quality of life of conscious patients, and to protect the unconscious from being used simply as objects for the ends of others.

Proposed regulations governing research on terminally ill patients

1. For the purpose of these regulations a 'terminally ill patient' is one whose death is reasonably expected to occur within six months even if currently accepted and available medical treatment is used.

2. In addition to all other legal and ethical requirements for the approval of a research protocol by national and local scientific and ethical review boards (including IRBs), research in which terminally ill patients participate as research subjects shall be approved only if the review board specifically finds that:

(a) The research, if it carries any risk, has the intent and *reasonable probability* (based on scientific data) of improving the health or well-being of the subject, or of significantly increasing the subject's length of life without significantly decreasing its quality;

(b) There is no *a priori* reason to believe that the research intervention will significantly decrease the subject's quality of life because of suffering, pain, or indignity attributable to the research; and,

(c) Written informed consent will be required of all research participants over the age of 16 in research involving any risk, and such consent may be solicited only by a physician acting as a *patient rights advocate* who is appointed by the review committee, is independent of the researcher, and whose duty it is to fully and objectively inform the potential subject of all reasonably foreseeable risks and benefits inherent in the research protocol. The patient rights advocate will also be empowered to monitor the actual research itself.

3. The vote on and basis for each of the findings in subpart (2) shall be set forth in writing by the review board, and be available to all potential subjects and the public.

4. All research protocols (including the financial arrangements between the sponsor and the researcher) involving terminally ill subjects shall be available to the public, and the meetings of the scientific and ethical review boards on these protocols shall be open to the public.

The major features of this proposal are worth emphasizing. The first is that so-called non-therapeutic research may not be performed on terminally ill patients at all unless there is no risk to the patient. Nor may 'potentially', or 'hopefully' or 'possibly' therapeutic research be performed – the research must have 'the intent and *reasonable probability* (based on scientific data) of improving the health or well-being of the subject . . .' The fact that there is no treatment for the condition does *not* make any intervention 'therapeutic' or even 'probably' therapeutic. Phase 1 cancer drug research, for example, may not be performed on terminally ill subjects under these guidelines because there is no reasonable probability that it will benefit the subjects. Second, for subjects over the age of 16, only the subjects themselves are permitted to give consent for any research that involves any risk. Unless the condition is unique to children, no experimentation should be done on children until it has been demonstrated to meet the 'reasonable probability' standard in adults. Proxy consent is acceptable only for *no* risk research (such as observation and monitoring studies, blood sampling, and research involving comatose patients). Third, the researcher is disqualified from obtaining the subject's consent. This task must be performed by an independent physician acting as a patient rights advocate, and whose primary obligation is to protect the rights and welfare of the potential research subject. Finally, the protocols, their financing, votes on them, and meetings concerning them, shall be open to the public.

These steps should help to protect both the rights and welfare of the terminally ill. Changes in codes and procedures alone, however, will not be sufficient to clarify societal goals for research and the practice of medicine, to define the meaning of progress, or to delineate the appropriate content of the practice of medicine. Resolving these central questions requires a recognition on the part of both society and medical practitioners that immortality is not a reasonable goal for medicine or humanity*, that there are fates worse than death, and that quality of life is more important than quantity of life†.

We can harm the terminally ill by treating them as objects with nothing to lose. They are our most vulnerable population, and need much more protection than they are currently afforded. It will take reality-based care for the dying, rather than fantasy-based experiments on the dying, to reclaim medicine's commitment in The Declaration of Geneva: 'The health of my patient will be my first consideration'‡.

* See, e.g. Hans Jonas (1992): The burden and blessing of mortality, *Hastings Center Rep.* **Jan.–Feb.**, pp. 34, 39.

† See, e.g. Daniel Callahan (1990): *What kind of life: the limits of medical progress.*

‡ World Medical Association, Declaration at Geneva, 1948.

The ethics of animal and human experimentation, edited by P.P. De Deyn.
 pp. 393–358.

29

Ethical aspects of exposure to toxic chemicals and the use of human subjects in the process of risk assessment

William F. Tordoir

Shell Internationale Petroleum Maatschappij B.V., Health, Safety and Environment Division, Occupational Health and Toxicology Division, HSE/2, PO Box 162, 2501 AN The Hague, The Netherlands

Summary

Legislative requirements for risk assessment and risk management of new and existing chemicals will soon be implemented in the Member States of the European Union. It can be expected that there will be an increasing scientific interest and an economic incentive to improve the interpretation of toxic hazards identified in animal experiments in terms of human hazards and human risks, for workers, consumers and members of the public exposed to chemicals.

As has been the case for several decades, there will be scope for the well controlled and ethical use of human subjects in toxicological experiments to achieve this improved interpretation. The basic ethical criterion of beneficence (or non-maleficence) and the concept of minimal risk have been used by authoritative organizations to provide guidance on the requirements and restrictions for ethically acceptable research with human volunteers in 'non-therapeutical biomedical research'.

Such experimental work done for the benefit of workers, consumers or members of the public is discussed and examples are provided.

Another requirement resulting from the new legislation is the need for quality assurance of risk assessment and risk management. Health and exposure monitoring of workers, consumers and members of the public will contribute to quality assurance. Although many ethical and social requirements have to be met for an acceptable procedure, it is important to realize that this health and exposure monitoring is not an experiment. Conversely, it may be an experiment if these quality assurance tools are not part of risk assessment and risk management. The scope for health and exposure monitoring of workers, consumers and members of the public is discussed and examples are provided.

Introduction

In this chapter we shall review ways and means to identify and assess the risks to human health by exposure to chemical substances and preparations (the European Union term for mixtures of chemical substances) with particular attention to the ethical use of human subjects. As exposure to cosmetics and toiletries is particularly intense and a voluntary, deliberate act, this will receive special attention. Therapeutic substances and preparations will be dealt with elsewhere in this book and therefore fall outside the scope of this chapter. Pesticides, however, will be included as these can be considered as a special kind of industrially produced substances or preparations intended to be biologically active, in contrast to industrial chemicals and cosmetics. Sometimes pesticides are used for treatment of dermal or internal pests; in those cases they will be considered as therapeutic drugs.

The identification or examination of the toxic properties of chemicals mentioned above is normally carried out in the animal model. There are, however, sometimes indications and situations which 'invite' human experimentation. The ethical acceptability of this experimentation is the central theme of this chapter. If the risks of exposure to chemicals have not been adequately assessed and if proper protective measures have not been taken, one could consider such a situation as an experiment, although of a totally different nature. Those involved would not have realized this and certainly would not have had the intention of carrying out or of participating in an experiment. For a proper opinion and judgement of the acceptability of human experimentation, either deliberate or unintentional, it is necessary to be aware of and understand the full context. It is therefore essential to examine the procedures for risk assessment and risk management before we can address the three main fields in which human subjects are involved in the investigation of the toxic properties of chemical substances and preparations, i.e. occupational health, product safety and environmental health.

In doing so, health and exposure monitoring of exposed populations will be discussed. This is an essential part of the whole process of risk assessment and risk management, but it should not be confused with the experimental use of human subjects.

Risk assessment and risk management

The processes of risk assessment and risk management comprise an iterative, systematic, well-structured sequence of several steps which, when applied according to the 'rules', will guarantee an adequate protection of human health against the toxicological hazards of a chemical. A similar process is also applied to protect the environment against the ecotoxicological hazards of chemicals, but these will, of course, not be addressed here. Although the term 'risk management' is considered by some to be a better description of the whole multi-step process, this term is currently used by the European Commission to cover the control of risks and associated activities, such as information and training aimed at protection against risks. The term 'risk assessment' – which in fact deals with only one step – is used by the Commission as the umbrella term for the steps up to the control of risk.

After more than two decades, in which the investigation of the toxicity and the collection of toxicity data for new chemicals were central in regulations initiated by the European Community (EC), attention has broadened during the last few years to the preparation of a systematic inventory of the toxicity of existing chemicals and to the logical and inevitable phase of risk assessment, both for new and existing chemicals.

The Commission Directive 93/67/EEC of 20 July 1993 deals with the principles of risk assessment of *new* chemicals; it is based on the Seventh Amendment of Council Directive 67/548.

For *existing* substances the Council Regulation (EEC) No. 793/93 of 23 March 1993 requires a systematic data collection and an evaluation of the risks to man and the environment. The Commission Regulation (still in draft) on the risk assessment on existing substances provides more detailed requirements.

These legal instruments have had and will continue to have, a major impact on the chemical industry in Europe.

Hazard identification

The first step of the risk assessment process is hazard identification.Toxicity tests are carried out on experimental animals and in in-vitro systems to unravel acute, sub-acute, sub-chronic and chronic toxicity. The nature of these tests and the sequence in which they are carried out is prescribed by the EU for new chemicals; the amounts placed on the market create regulatory triggers for different levels of prescribed testing. Guidelines on the strategy for additional testing, over and above that required by these amount-related triggers, have been developed recently for new chemicals and are likewise under development for existing chemicals. The results of many years of work on the development and validation of a large number of toxicity tests have been evaluated by the Organization of Economic Cooperation and Development (OECD) which has published agreed guidelines on test methodology; these are regularly updated and when appropriate, new guidelines are issued. All testing is done according to Good Laboratory Practice guidelines.

As explained above, amount-related regulatory triggers and/or triggers resulting from the steps in the risk assessment process, in particular from the hazard identification itself and/or from the expected/established exposure patterns, cause the appropriate toxicity tests to be carried out in the appropriate sequence. In this way, all possible manifestations of the toxic properties related to the various biological 'end points' in experimental animals become gradually known and understood.

Exposure assessment/measurement

In the second step, personal exposure is predicted, assessed or measured by personal monitoring (using personal samplers to measure concentrations representative of those in inhaled air, or by measuring skin deposition/contamination) or by biological monitoring techniques which measure the chemical and/or its metabolites in human excreta, blood or tissues. Biological monitoring provides information on the total absorbed/internal dose from all routes of uptake.

Health characteristics of the population at risk

Although it is sometimes overlooked, it is useful to assess at this stage the existence of any particular susceptibilities in the exposed population. For instance, malnutrition or chronic infections may make a group of exposed people more susceptible than the 'standard' healthy individual. Such increased susceptibility should be taken into account during risk characterization.

Risk assessment or risk characterization

The third step is the risk assessment (*sensu stricto*), which in EU documents is referred to as 'risk characterization'. In this step the intrinsic toxicity, insofar as it is known from the experimental animal tests and the use of certain in-vitro systems, in particular dose-effect and dose-response curves, is compared with the expected or known exposures whilst any particular susceptibilities of the population at risk are taken into account. If available, data from experiments with human volunteers and from health monitoring will also be included.

Provided that sufficient and reliable data are available, this process will lead to a judgement on the *nature* of the toxic effects that may occur and on the *probability* of occurrence. At one end of the spectrum there is a high probability of the occurrence of life-threatening effect(s); obviously at the other end there is the low probability of occurrence of minor non-adverse health effects. If the toxicity data are insufficient for an appropriate risk characterization, additional data will have to be generated.

Risk acceptance

Subsequently a judgement has to be formed about the acceptability of the expected risk. Accepted health standards, such as threshold limit values (TLVs) or maximum allowable concentrations (MACs), may be helpful in forming that judgement in the case of occupational exposure. However, in many cases such standards are not available and the risk acceptance step must be elaborated for that particular case.

Risk management

If the risk is deemed not to be acceptable, (additional) control measures have to be taken to eliminate or reduce exposure. There is an accepted hierarchy of control measures, in order of preference:

- replacement by a less hazardous chemical;
- technical measures to reduce exposure;
- organizational measures to reduce exposure;
- adaptation of work practices resulting in a lower exposure;
- the use of personal protection equipment.

Other components of risk management are information and training.

For consumers and workers the label is the primary source of information on the hazards and safe handling. In addition, for workers, Material Safety Data Sheets and/or Workplace Information Sheets should be available. They should also receive training in the proper use and maintenance of personal protection devices.

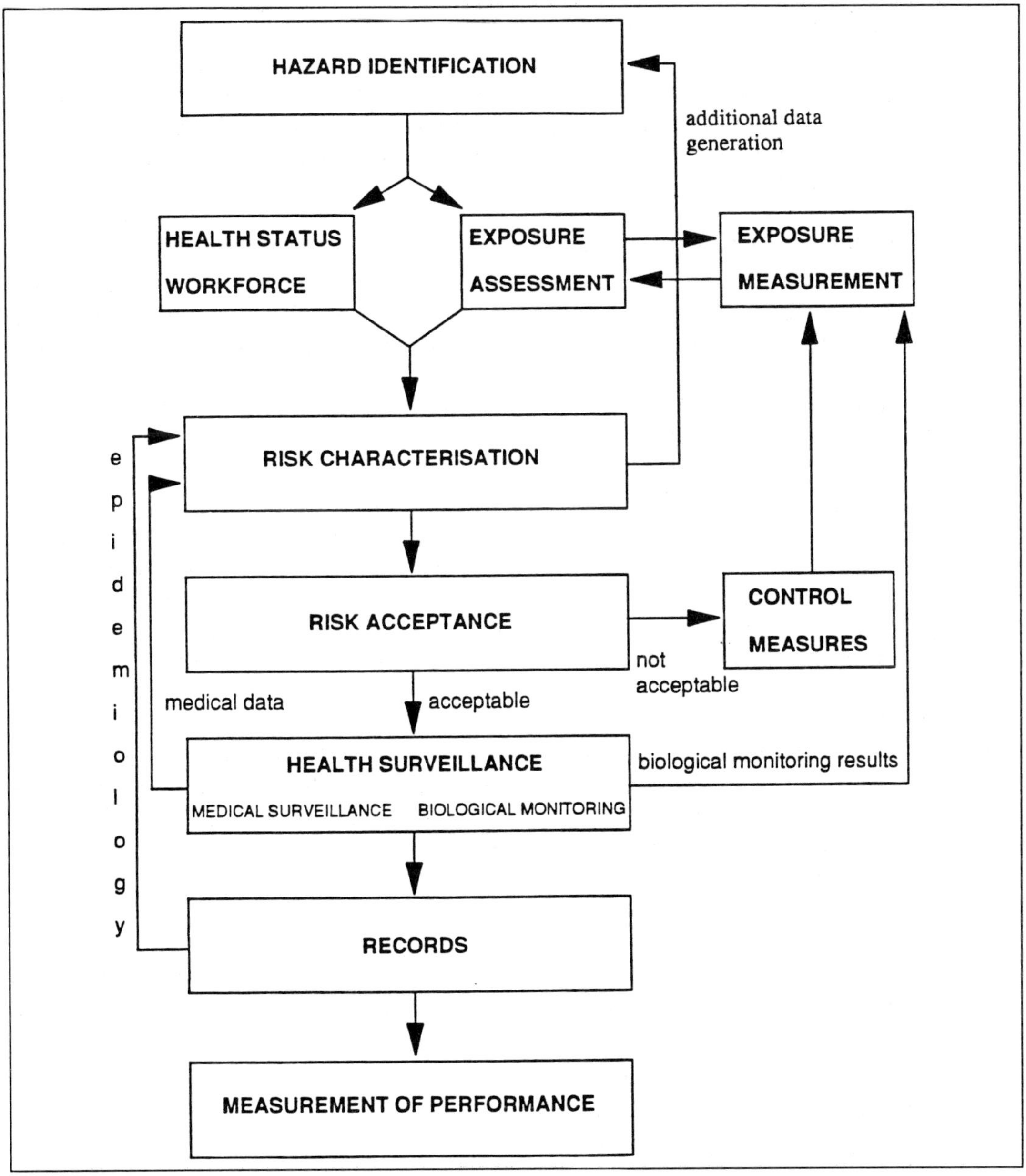

Fig. 1. Schematic presentation of the health risk assessment and health risk management process.

Feedback loops – health surveillance

To improve the reliability of the risk assessment and risk management indicated above, a number of feedback loops should be introduced (see Fig. 1). The effectiveness of the technical and organizational control measures can be checked immediately by measuring the resulting reduced concentrations in ambient air and/or personal exposures, and by using this information for going through the risk-assessment procedure once more.

Another way of checking the effectiveness of the control measures is by performing biological monitoring on the exposed individuals to measure the total absorbed dose (via all routes of exposure). This feedback loop, together with the one provided by the exposure measurements using industrial hygiene methods (see above), provides essential information for a repeat of the risk-assessment procedure. Medical surveillance of exposed individuals is usually limited to occupationally exposed workers, although it has been carried out in exceptional cases with consumers and members of the public. The objective is to identify any exposure-related health effects, preferably at an early stage when there are either only non-adverse biological effects or early minor adverse effects which can be treated successfully. Biochemical effect monitoring which addresses the occurrence of early biochemical effects, such as changes in enzyme concentrations, DNA or haemoglobin adducts, etc. plays an increasingly important role in this respect. The information obtained from medical-surveillance programmes should of course also be fed into the risk assessment process.

The ultimate check on the quality of the risk-assessment and risk-management procedures is to carry out an epidemiological study on the morbidity and/or mortality of the population at risk. This can only be done if data on exposure and health effects have been collected in such a way that subsequent epidemiological analysis is feasible.

Ethical considerations

One could take the position that by exposing workers, customers or members of the general public to chemicals, without going through the above steps of risk assessment and risk management, a form of human experimentation is carried out in which the subjects are not even volunteers.

Although there is of course no intention of conducting such an experiment, the character of experimentation remains if the risks of such exposures have not been reliably predicted and controlled.

Criteria for the acceptability of the use of human subjects

According to existing and developing legislation in the EU, new and existing chemical substances and preparations must be systematically and thoroughly evaluated for their toxic hazards and risks in order to make possible an adequate risk-management approach.

In risk assessment a distinction should be made between, on the one hand, the *experimental study* of the toxicity before or after large scale manufacturing and introduction onto the market, and on the other, the health *monitoring* of occupationally exposed workers during manufacturing and of persons exposed directly as consumers, or indirectly as members of the public, to substances or preparations present in one or more of the environmental compartments.

In the case of toxic-hazard identification there is a limited scope for experiments with human volunteers; however, the health-monitoring activities should not be seen as experiments – provided that indeed the health risk assessment and health risk management procedures have been adequately followed – but as part of a safeguarding or quality assurance activity.

The scope for using human subjects in experiments to improve hazard identification is, in essence, defined by the International Covenant on Civil and Political Rights, adopted by the General Assembly of the United Nations in 1966, of which article 7 states 'No one shall be subjected to torture or to cruel, inhuman or degrading treatment or punishment. In particular, no one shall be subjected to medical or scientific experimentation'.

The fundamental document in the field of ethics in biomedical research preceding the Covenant mentioned above was the Declaration of Helsinki, promulgated in 1964 by the World Medical Association and since revised several times, most recently in 1989 in Hong Kong. This adapted Declaration of Helsinki provides, in addition to the 'Basic Principles' (Section I) which are always applicable, in Section III some guidance for non-therapeutic biomedical research involving human subjects:

> '1. In the purely scientific application of medical research carried out on a human being, it is the duty of the doctor to remain the protector of the life and health of that person on whom biomedical research is being carried out.
>
> 2. The subjects should be volunteers – either healthy persons or patients for whom the experimental design is not related to the patient's illness.
>
> 3. The investigator or the investigating team should discontinue the research if in his/her or their judgement it may, if continued, be harmful to the individual.
>
> 4. In research on man, the interest of science and society should never take precedence over considerations related to the well-being of the subject.'

Since the late 1970s, the Council for International Organizations of Medical Sciences (CIOMS) and WHO have undertaken a further examination of the ethical requirements and constraints related to biomedical research involving human subjects and issued in 1982 their *Proposed International Guidelines for Biomedical Research Involving Human Subjects*. These proposed guidelines were widely distributed and carefully reviewed. Amended guidelines were presented at the CIOMS Conference on 'Ethics and Research on Human Subjects – International Guidelines', held in Geneva in 1992 and subsequently published in the proceedings (CIOMS,1993). The guidelines are based on three general ethical principles: respect for persons, beneficence (sometimes expressed as non-maleficence) and justice.

The Royal College of Physicians of London accepts a concept of minimal risk in healthy volunteer studies, as any activity or even inactivity is associated with some risk. However, a risk greater than minimal is not acceptable. Thus only substances of low toxicity, and so predicted to have a low hazard, are given to healthy volunteers; administration in graded doses would provide additional reassurance. Furthermore, the probability of the occurrence of an adverse effect should be considered and not only its possible seriousness (Royal College of Physicians of London, 1986).

In contrast to the above-cited sources for guidance, which provide advice of a rather general nature, advice on the acceptability of the use of radioactive substances in research with human volunteers is very detailed, and precise dose ranges and their associated risks are given (Gezondheidsraad, 1980).

Table 1. New and existing chemicals. Scope for experiments during the hazard identification phase and options for health monitoring during manufacturing and marketing

Hazard identification			Health monitoring		
Workers	Consumers	Public	Workers	Consumers	Public
Toxicokinetic studies at non-toxic dose levels for: • hazard interpretation across species • development of biological monitoring tests Toxicodynamic studies at non-toxic dose levels for: • development of biochemical effect monitoring • evaluation of adequacy of expected no-effect levels or health standards • evaluation of safe handling procedures	• Skin irritation • Skin sensitization • Eye irritation • Upper respiratory tract irritation • Biological monitoring • Biochemical effect monitoring • Evaluation of safe handling/use procedures	Little scope for additional experimentation; usually data are available from studies with animals/workers/consumers	Periodically: • medical examinations • biological monitoring • biochemical effect monitoring • morbidity pattern analysis (epidemiology) • mortality pattern analysis (epidemiology)	Occasionally: • health effect studies • biological monitoring • biochemical effect monitoring	Exceptionally: • health effects study Periodically or occasionally: • biological monitoring • biochemical effect monitoring

In Section III of the Declaration of Helsinki ('Non-therapeutical biomedical research involving human subjects'), the basic ethical principle of '*beneficence*' or '*non-maleficence*' as explained in the CIOMS proceedings and the concept of minimal risk as accepted by the Royal College of Physicians were presumably the most important criteria for determining the ethical acceptability of experiments with human subjects for identifying hazardous chemicals, in addition to all other guidelines which obviously also apply.

The basic ethical principles of beneficence (or non-maleficence) and minimal risk proscribe the deliberate infliction of harm on persons; they determine thereby the scope for the experimental use of human subjects for the improvement of hazard identification.

It may therefore be assumed that, generally speaking, ethical review committees will accept experiments with dosages that in animal experiments have been found to be safe. Adverse and irreversible health effects will not be acceptable; non-adverse and transient effects may be acceptable, depending on the circumstances. Such effects would in most cases be restricted to manifestations of topical irritation (skin, eyes, upper respiratory tract) or very mild systemic effects such as a slight headache.

The scope for using human subjects to improve the hazard identification of chemicals is thus strictly limited, but the benefits from an ethical use of human subjects in terms of safeguards and reassurance are significant.

Table 1 provides an overview of the scope for experiments with human volunteers in the hazard identification phase and the options for health-monitoring activities, each for the benefit of workers, consumers and members of the public. The only difference between new and existing chemicals in this respect is that the experiments in the hazard-identification phase of new chemicals should be carried out before full-scale manufacturing and before routine marketing.

Hazard identification and use of human subjects

Workers

Occupational medicine, if carried out at all in past centuries, was primarily aimed at the identification of the causal relationship between the occurrence of a disease and work or working conditions. If possible, the patients were medically treated, but adequate prevention through the control of the hazardous factors received less attention than nowadays. This is understandable: the nature of the hazardous factors was often poorly understood and therefore control options were difficult to identify or not available. This was particularly true for the toxic hazards.

With the development in this century of toxicology and industrial hygiene, the objective of occupational health care gradually shifted from the detection and treatment of occupational diseases to an adequate control of the risks, and the demonstration, through personal exposure monitoring, biological monitoring, health surveillance and epidemiological studies, that such controls were adequate.

The scope for an ethical use of human volunteers for occupational toxic hazard identification is more restricted than the use of human volunteers for the evaluation of a new drug. Hazard identification can be conducted in experimental animals and – to a certain extent – in *in vitro* systems and should always precede any experiments with human subjects. The possible differences in species specificity may cause problems of extrapolation from the mouse, rat, etc. to man, but these can largely be overcome by performing comparative toxicokinetic studies. In cases where the extrapolation problems have not yet been solved, there is always the option to take a worst case approach and to reduce exposures to very conservative levels. This option is not available with drugs, as strict control of exposure would result in very low, ineffective doses.

The above would imply that all toxic hazards can be detected in the animal model; this is not always the case and surprises may occur. For instance, ethylene oxide and bisphenol A (diphenylol-propane) were negative in animal tests for skin sensitization, but have caused several cases of skin sensitization in workers. The leukaemogenic properties of benzene were not detected in the animal model, but through epidemiology, and it has taken a long time to confirm these findings in the animal model. The same is true for several other human carcinogens.

In the occupational setting, exposure is not intended and can be controlled. There is therefore no cause to confirm the adverse effects found in animal studies by testing for adverse effects in humans. Toxicokinetic studies at non-toxic doses can be justified to assist in the interpretation of toxic hazards across species and for the development and validation of biological monitoring tests. The need for such studies is increasingly being recognized (Miyamoto *et al.*, 1988).

Toxicodynamic studies at non-toxic doses can be indicated for the development and validation of biochemical effect monitoring tests, such as for enzyme induction or depletion, for evaluation of predicted no-effect levels or health standards, such as TLVs, MAC, etc., or for the evaluation of safe handling or safe application procedures which are considered to provide adequate protection. Such studies may include testing for acute topical effects of a transient nature, such as: skin irritation, skin sensitization, eye irritation and upper respiratory tract irritation when the usual animal tests cannot be adequately interpreted and additional reassurance is necessary. The induction of irreversible structural or functional effects is clearly not acceptable. In this respect, extra caution is needed when skin sensitization is to be evaluated as it may be induced by testing for it. An experimental evaluation of dose(s) considered safe or of safe-use instructions in relation to any (sub)acute or chronic *systemic* effects would have to be justified very carefully because of the increased risk of serious and/or irreversible effects.

A few examples are given below.

- The need to develop biological monitoring methods using human volunteers is well demonstrated by the work done on the synthetic pyrethroid Cypermethrin. After metabolism studies in animals, a single non-toxic oral dose (as judged on the basis of adequate studies in experimental animals) was administered to four well-informed volunteers (research workers) (Eadsforth & Baldwin, 1983). Later, six well-informed male volunteers (health professionals) took non-toxic doses (two volunteers per dose level) over 5 consecutive days and collected their 24-h urine production.

Although it was demonstrated that across species (including man) Cypermethrin is broken down by ester cleavage into two metabolites, that in all tested species the urinary route is the major route of excretion, and that the urinary excretion of free and conjugated cyclopropane-carboxylic acid is also similar across species (Eadsforth *et al.*, 1988), later work – which also analysed for the other metabolite – indicated that there is a difference in the ratio between the two metabolites depending on the route of absorption: dermal or oral (Wilkes *et al.*, 1993). Without this information, actual data from exposed field workers (dermal exposure is predominant) would be difficult to interpret in terms of the equivalent of an oral dose. Only exposure expressed as equivalent oral dose can be related to the dose-effect relationships of long-term animal studies, which use the oral route for dosing.

• To determine whether dephenylation of phenyl-beta-naphthylamine (PBNA) would occur, leading to the well-known bladder carcinogen beta-naphthylamine (BNA), a non-toxic dose of 10 mg, about one-third of the amount to which workers were exposed every day (via inhalation of dust particles), was taken as an oral dose by 18 well-informed volunteers (occupational physicians and nurses). It was established that the amount of BNA in the urine was more than could be explained on the basis of its known presence as a minor impurity in PBNA. Dephenylation in the human body – probably caused by bacteria in the intestinal tract – was thereby demonstrated for the first time. This put an end to a long-lasting debate over the risk caused by the BNA as an impurity, as the newly formed BNA was obviously more important. Although the oral doses were judged to be non-toxic on the basis of the then available experimental animal data, carcinogenicity had not been adequately explored at that time and one could argue that it would be unethical to study the dephenylation in human subjects without extensive data from toxicokinetic and carcinogenicity studies in experimental animals. As PBNA was used as an antioxidant in many rubber-producing plants (and elsewhere in other manufacturing processes) and the workers were actually exposed to relatively large amounts day in, day out, the investigators were of the opinion that an immediate answer was needed once the hypothesis concerning the dephenylation had been made. This could have been achieved by comparing the inhalational exposure of dust particles (which were so large that they were cleared by the mucus stream from the respiratory tract and subsequently ingested) with the BNA in urine, but at the time the urinary monitoring of these workers was not feasible for technical and industrial-relations reasons.

At a later stage when the hypothesis was confirmed, the urine of four workers was analysed for the occurrence of PBNA and BNA and the results were consistent with those found in the studies with the volunteers (Kummer & Tordoir, 1975). The dephenylation of PBNA was also found by Moore *et al.* (1977), who conducted a study with two human volunteers who ingested doses of 50 mg PBNA and with an unspecified number of workers estimated to have inhaled 30 mg PBNA.

Subsequent toxicokinetic research in dogs (Batten & Hathway, 1977) confirmed the dephenylation of PBNA into BNA. However, the two most important carcinogenic metabolites of BNA (BNA itself is not carcinogenic) could not be detected. As a result of these studies, the use of PBNA as antioxidant was discontinued in the plant where the initial investigations had been done, and a Current Intelligence Bulletin was published by the National Institute for Occupational Safety and Health (NIOSH) in 1976 to alert for the metabolic transformation of substances, so far considered to be relatively innocuous, into well-known carcinogens. Furthermore, in this Bulletin, extensive guidelines were given on the reduction of exposure and for health surveillance. In the majority of subsequent carcinogenicity studies, no evidence of carcinogenicity was found; in some other studies there is limited evidence of a carcinogenic effect in various organs, but not in the bladder (IARC, 1978, 1987).

- To determine the relationship between an oral dose of the insecticide dieldrin taken over a prolonged period and the resulting plateau concentration of dieldrin in the blood, Hunter & Robinson (1967) and Hunter *et al.* (1969) conducted a study with well-informed subjects (research workers) who ingested, over a period of 18 months, daily doses of 0, 10, 50 or 211 μg per man per day. Each dose group consisted of three volunteers; the control group had four volunteers. At the end of the 18 months the study was continued for another 6 months in which the controls and the lowest dose group received μg per day and the other two groups continued with the previous dosages of 50 and 211 μg. Comprehensive medical examinations during the course of this rather unique experiment and after completion did not reveal any compound-related adverse health effects.

As a result of the determination of dieldrin concentrations in blood, a mathematical formula could be derived defining the relationship between the amounts of ingested dieldrin and the resulting dieldrin blood concentrations at steady state. This formula allowed an estimation of the average personal daily dose and the total personal dose of aldrin/dieldrin in a cohort of 570 workers exposed in the period 1954–90. Using the estimated total personal dose, each worker was assigned to one of three groups with high, medium or low exposures. The subsequent cancer mortality analysis could be related to a reliable estimation of total dose, which is exceptional in epidemiological studies. No statistically significant excess mortality was observed for any of the site-specific cancers examined in the exposed groups and there was no indication of a dose-response relationship (de Jong, 1991).

Consumers

Exposure of consumers may be *intended*, as is the case with cosmetics and toiletries, *incidental but avoidable*, for instance the use of cleaning agents in the house, or in practice *unavoidable* as is the case when a pesticidal strip is put into a room to control mosquitoes and flies.

- Exposure which is avoidable should be avoided by following the safe use and handling advice provided on the label. As with worker exposure, there is no justification for testing for adverse health effects in human volunteers. However, there may be scope for an evaluation of the safe use of certain consumer products (household chemicals), for instance to obtain information on the margin of safety in the case of insufficient compliance with the label instructions. Example: the degree of irritation of the upper respiratory tract when using caustic soda to clean drains.

- If exposure to consumer products is intended and results in an intense and prolonged exposure, such as with perfumes, cosmetics and toiletries, there is certainly scope for an evaluation of the safety of the prescribed use or application instructions. This evaluation should have been preceded by comprehensive animal testing and would normally be restricted to acute and transient topical effects: skin irritation, skin sensitization, eye irritation and upper respiratory tract irritation. An experimental evaluation of the adequacy of the safe-use instructions in relation to any (sub)acute or chronic *systemic* effects may be justified in exceptional cases.

Cosmetics and toiletries are routinely tested in human volunteers; there are (contract) laboratories which specialize in this and which have large numbers of volunteers available. The main reason is the inability of the well-known Draize eye and skin irritation tests to differentiate always between the absence of irritation potential and the presence of mild or slight irritation potential under practical use conditions (Schlatter & Reinhardt, 1985).

- Where exposure to consumer products is *not intended*, but in practice often un-avoidable, although sometimes controllable to a certain extent, an experimental evaluation of the safe-use instructions and the related margin of safety in case of deviation from these instructions may be required. As such exposures would often be to airborne concentrations, the evaluation of eye irritation and upper respiratory tract irritation, and the use of biochemical effect monitoring and biological monitoring may be indicated. Examples are the use of pesticide strips or pens for indoor use, air fresheners, solvents from paints, lacquers, waxes and cleaning products.

A good example is the safety evaluation of the Vapona® strip, a plastic strip which slowly releases the organophosphate dichlorvos to control flying insects indoors. Hunter *et al.* (1971) established, under carefully controlled laboratory conditions, that the degree of plasma cholinesterase reduction in human volunteers was dir-ectly related to the concentration of inhaled dichlorvos and the duration of inhala-tion. He calculated that an air concentration of 1 mg/m^3 would not affect the plasma cholinesterase concentration, independent of the length of exposure. In subsequent years several studies were carried out in various parts of the world to confirm the safety in use when the label instructions were followed. In some studies more Vapona strips were used than recommended to evaluate the margin of safety. Leary *et al.* (1974) carried out a series of home studies involving 26 families. Physical examination, haematological and clinical chemistry measurements, blood cholinesterase assays and analysis of air and food for dichlorvos were carried out.

In one group of houses the strips were used according to the label instructions, in other groups strips were renewed more frequently than recommended or were used at a two-fold rate. Control houses were also included in the study. The only exposure-related effect was a slight plasma cholinesterase depression of no toxicological significance in the inhabitants of the houses where the strips were replaced monthly instead of once in three months.

To determine the inhalatory resorption of the termiticide aldrin at low levels of exposure, well-informed volunteers (research workers) were exposed for 1 h periods to airborne concentrations of 1 $\mu g/m^3$. This is a low level when compared to the American Conference of Governmental Industrial Hygienists-Treshold Limit Value (ACGIH-TLV) of 250 $\mu g/m^3$ for 8 h per day, but it is realistic as inhabitants of houses treated with aldrin for termite control could be exposed to such levels. The resorption was about 50 per cent (Bragt *et al.*, 1985).

Members of the public

There is little scope for experiments with human volunteers to identify the health hazards for members of the public exposed to chemicals in air, drinking water or food and beverages. The hazard identification has usually been carried out in the context of risk assessment/management of occupational exposure or exposure of consumers. Nevertheless, some experimental work has been carried out, in particular in the field of air pollution.

Controlled exposure of human volunteers to air pollutants can provide definitive scientific evidence of health risks that is essential to support air quality regulatory policy decisions.

Air pollutants such as ozone and sulphur dioxide have been used in experimental studies with human volunteers to determine the short-term, mild and transient irritant effects of these air pollutants on the lung: irritation of the lower respiratory tract by ozone and bronchoconstriction by sulphur dioxide. Any longer term exposures to investigate long-term effects of a more serious nature are clearly not acceptable for practical and ethical reasons and would need to be evaluated on the basis of toxicological data from animal and epidemiology studies (Hackney *et al.*, 1984). For an overview, see Table 1.

Health monitoring

Periodic and occasional monitoring of the health of workers, consumers and members of the public exposed to chemicals, either directly, by checking for early effects or by studying morbidity or mortality patterns using epidemiological methods, or indirectly, by measuring exposure, is part of the hazard-assessment procedure and provides quality assurance. In the case of unsatisfactory results, measures have to be taken to reduce exposure. Clearly, health monitoring without possibility of intervention is pointless. Health monitoring is not an experiment and it does not conform to the characteristics of an experiment: an organized, managed and controlled sequence of staged events with controlled dosing. Any exposure is related to the use or application of chemicals and is not the result of deliberately creating a situation, as is the case in an experiment. On the other hand, one could argue that not carrying out health monitoring has the character of an uncontrolled experiment. There is then no quality assurance on the risk-assessment procedure and therefore no opportunity to refine the conclusions and to institute better risk-management procedures in the case of an unacceptable risk. To be ethically acceptable, health monitoring has to meet a number of criteria. Medical confidentiality and informed consent are the most important when living subjects are monitored. Several countries have special rules for epidemiological mortality studies.

The International Code of Ethics for Occupational Health Professionals (ICOH, 1992) provides relevant guidance which is also appropriate for situations in which the health of consumers or members of the public is monitored.

Workers

If risk assessment and risk management are carried out properly, as explained above, it is not unethical to expose workers to chemicals, nor is it unethical to use the exposed population to ascertain that exposures are within acceptable limits, as is done with personal monitoring or biological monitoring, or to carry out a medical surveillance programme (including biochemical effect monitoring). Conversely, biological monitoring and medical surveillance might be seen as making use of 'human guinea pigs' if risk assessment and risk management had not preceded these activities.

Periodical health surveillance is routine in occupational health practice and consists of specific periodical medical examinations, biological monitoring and biochemical effect monitoring. The specific medical examinations are carried out to determine whether any early health effects (ideally: non-adverse and transient) have occurred and whether any increased susceptibility to work-related hazards has developed as a result of a work- or non-work-related illness, injury or condition. In the case of unsatisfactory findings, the worker may be suspended from the relevant activity temporarily or permanently and/or exposure reduction measures should be taken. Biological monitoring to establish the internal dose following exposure at work is often performed in combination with medical examinations. By relating the internal dose to suitable standards, an insight is obtained into the adequacy of the exposure-control measures and the probability that adverse health effects will occur. Biological exposure monitoring methods have been developed for many chemicals and are often applied in a routine fashion.

Because of the major advantages of biological monitoring, it can be argued that, if at all possible, biological monitoring methods should be developed for all chemicals to which significant groups of workers/consumers/members of the public are exposed. In occupational health practice monitoring of urinary metabolites is for obvious reasons preferred over monitoring of metabolites in other media (blood, faeces, saliva, hair, exhaled air, sweat).

Many compound-specific test methods have been developed; the control of exposures has sometimes been so successful that a more sensitive method had to be developed. An example is benzene: the urinary phenol excretion is insufficiently sensitive and specific to be of much value in modern circumstances. The measurement of *S*-phenyl-mercapturic acid in urine has been proposed as a suitable biomarker for monitoring low level exposures to benzene (van Sittert *et al.*, 1993a).

Biochemical effect monitoring is carried out to determine whether, as a result of exposure, specific biochemical effects have taken place which are indicators of the exposure and also indicative for functional effects and/or structural changes. In certain areas it is a routine measure, such as the monitoring of cholinesterase levels in workers exposed to organophosphates. In other areas these methods are still in a developmental phase such as with the measurement of haemoglobin alkylation by alkylating genotoxic chemicals.

A recently published example is a 9-year follow-up study of renal effects in workers exposed to cadmium in a zinc ore refinery. Several biochemical parameters (*N*-acetyl-β-D-glucosaminidase, β_2-microglobulin, retinal binding protein, etc.) were used to assess proximal tubular and glomerular function (van Sittert *et al.*, 1993b).

The alkylation of haemoglobin in workers exposed to genotoxic chemicals provides a surrogate for the measurement of DNA adducts. As the results of such measurements indicate the time-integrated exposures (over the life span of the erythrocytes, about 120 days), unexpected personal exposures may be detected which may lead to targeted exposure control measures (van Sittert *et al.*, 1993c).

Consumers

Occasionally health effects may be studied in consumer groups as an additional reassurance that the use or application of consumer products does not cause unwanted effects. An example is the occurrence of skin irritation when using a new dishwashing liquid. Biological monitoring and biochemical effect monitoring can obviously provide the same advantages as with workers, but would be carried out only in specific situations.

Any health monitoring with consumers requires the organization of a group that is prepared to comply with the requirements and procedures of the monitoring. Because of the need to organize and manage such a group, the possibility that the monitoring will be confused with an experiment may arise.

Members of the public

Health effects studies involving members of the general public tend to be even more exceptional than with consumers. Again, a group has to be organized and managed. The scope for such studies in the general population is very limited as exposures are usually very low, as health effects in individuals cannot reliably be related to a cause and as even epidemiology is usually too insensitive an instrument to identify cause-effect relationships.

As biological monitoring and biochemical effect monitoring often provide specific and sensitive indicators, these methods are particularly appropriate for use in the general population.

Examples:

- Human fat tissues have been obtained either by a needle prick or a small excision, to study the concentration of chemicals which accumulate in the human body, such as the organochlorine pesticides (DDT, chlordane, heptachlor, aldrin, dieldrin), PCBs and dioxins. In the 1960s and 1970s dozens of studies of dieldrin in the body fat of the general population were published. Concentrations in blood and mother milk were also studied.

- Studies of lead in blood have provided data on integrated exposure from various sources (ambient air, food, beverages, dust, paint flakes, etc.). For an overview, see Table 1.

Discussion

The legislative requirements for risk assessment and risk management of new and existing chemicals laid down in Directives and Regulations of the European Commission will have an impact on the use of human subjects for hazard identification and for quality assurance of the risk-assessment process.

Increasingly, there will be a scientific interest and an economic incentive to improve the interpretation of toxic hazards identified in animal experiments by using human tissues or human subjects. It may also be expected that regulatory pressure will increase on the quality assurance aspects of the risk-assessment and risk-management procedures, hence on exposure and health monitoring of workers, consumers and members of the public.

The late Professor Wayland Hayes Jr, one of the most prominent medical toxicologists, was an outspoken advocate of (ethically acceptable) human volunteer studies. He stressed the ethical requirement for an adequate hazard identification of new products before these were introduced into the market and for existing products before these were put to new uses (Hayes, 1983). Apparently, many (medical) toxicologists hold the same views: Hayes reports in his paper on 251 studies with human volunteers in which 92 different pesticides were investigated. However, many of these studies are not experiments in the true sense of the word but were safe-use evaluations, i.e. health monitoring of persons exposed to pesticides as a result of their (non-occupational) application or use. Field studies with pesticides in the Research and Development phase provide important opportunities and are increasingly used to evaluate the safety of the handling and application procedures before a new pesticide is marketed (Tordoir, 1980).

Skin and eye irritation tests in human volunteers are routine in the development of new cosmetics and toiletries (Schlatter & Reinhardt, 1985).

All in all one may conclude that experiments with human volunteers are not exceptional and will probably increase in number. It may therefore be questioned why the currently available guidelines – with the exception of the guidelines on the use of radioactive substances – are rather general in nature. On the other hand, one could speculate that the ethical committees which have to judge ethical acceptability on a case-by-case basis apparently have had no major problems, otherwise more detailed guidelines would have been published by now.

Ethical acceptability is not only determined by the acceptability of the health effects caused by the experiment and meeting the usual requirements of informed consent, etc., but also by the added value of the experiment to the knowledge and understanding of the toxicity (van Gelderen *et al.*, 1990) and by the benefit, in terms of safety and reassurance, the experiment creates for the target population: workers, consumers or members of the public. Another aspect which deserves careful consideration is the use of staff members as volunteers. The advantages are clear: staff members are easily available, usually well motivated and have a better understanding of the purpose and risks of an experiment than 'outside' volunteers. However, their decision to participate may be influenced by concerns about their career. Additional safeguards are therefore needed to ensure their voluntary participation. To advise The Association of the British Pharmaceutical Industry on the use of staff volunteers in medical experiments, a committee issued a report on this matter and listed a number of safeguards (The Association of the British Pharmaceutical Industry, undated).

The health monitoring of workers, consumers or members of the public is not of an experimental nature and therefore less contentious. However, ethical criteria do also apply and guidance can be obtained from the Code of Ethics for Health Professionals of the International Commission on Occupational Health (1992). Although this code is written for occupational health practice, the sections on health surveillance and information to be provided to the worker would also seem relevant for health monitoring carried out with consumers and members of the public.

References

Batten, P.L., Hathway, D.H. (1977): Dephenylation of *N*-phenyl-2-naphthylamine in dogs and its possible oncogenic implications. *Br. J. Cancer* **35**, 342–346.

Bragt, P.C., Schuurbiers, C.J., Hollander, J.C.Th., Schulting, F.L. & Wolthuis, O.L. (1985): Determination of the retention of inhaled aldrin in man. *Medical Biological Laboratory TNO, MBL Report* 1985–8. Rijswijk: Netherlands Organization of Applied Scientific Research.

Council for International Organizations of Medical Sciences (CIOMS) (1993): Ethics and research on human subjects. International guidelines. *Proceedings of the XXVIth CIOMS conference,* eds. Z. Bankowski & R.J. Levine. Geneva, 5–7 Feb. 1992, Geneva: CIOMS.

Eadsforth, C.V. & Baldwin, M.K. (1983): Human dose-excretion studies with the pyrethroid insecticide, cypermethrin. *Xenobiotica* **13**, 67–72.

Eadsforth, C.V., Bragt, P.C. & van Sittert, N.J. (1988): Human dose excretion studies with pyrethroid insecticides cypermethrin and alphacypermethrin: relevance for biological monitoring. *Xenobiotica* **18**, 603–614.

European Communities (1993): Council Regulation (EEC) No. 793: On the evaluation and control of the risks of existing substances. *Off. J. Eur. Communities* L84/1–73, 5 April.

van Gelderen, C.E.M., Savelkoul, T.J.F. & Sangster, B. (1990): Safety studies in humans II: human volunteer studies. *Food Chem. Toxicol.* **28**, 775–778.

Gezondheidsraad (1980): *Advies inzake normen voor toediening van radio-actieve stoffen aan vrijwilligers,* No. 1980/14, 's-Gravenhage.

Hackney, J.D., Linn, W.S. & Avol, E.L. (1984): Assessing health effects of air pollution – the role of controlled studies of human volunteers is examined. *Environ. Sci. Technol.* **18**, 115–122.

Hayes, W.J. (1983): Ethical considerations involving studies of pesticides and other xenobiotics in man. In: *IUPAC pesticide chemistry: human welfare and environment.* Vol. 3. *Mode of action, metabolism and toxicity,* ed. J. Miyamoto, pp. 387–394. Oxford: Pergamon.

Hunter, C.G. & Robinson, J. (1967): Pharmacodynamics of dieldrin HEOD I. Ingestion by human subjects for 18 months. *Arch. Environ. Health* **15**, 614–626.

Hunter, C.G., Robinson, J. & Roberts, M. (1969): Pharmacodynamics of dieldrin HEOD II. Ingestion by human subjects for 18–24 months, and post-exposure for eight months. *Arch. Environ. Health* **18**, 12–21.

Hunter, C.G. *et al.* (1971): Dichlorvos: human inhalation studies. Abstracts of Papers for the Tenth Annual Meeting of the Society of Toxicology, Washington DC, 7–11 March. *Toxicol. Appl. Pharmacol.* **19**: 379.

International Agency for Research on Cancer (1978): Some aromatic amines and related nitro compounds – hair dyes, colouring agents and miscellaneous industrial chemicals. *IARC monographs on the evaluation of the carcinogenic risk of chemicals to man,* Vol. 16, pp. 325–341. Lyon: IARC.

International Agency for Research on Cancer (1987): An updating of IARC monographs, volumes 1–42. IARC *monographs on the evaluation of carcinogenic risk to humans,* Supplement 7, pp. 318–319. Lyon: IARC.

International Commission on Occupational Health (1992): International Code of Ethics for Occupational Health Professionals (Secretary-General: Prof. J. Jeyaratnam, Department of Community, Occupational and Family Medicine, University of Singapore, Singapore).

de Jong, G. (1991): Long-term health effects of aldrin and dieldrin. Supplement to*Toxicology Letters.* Amsterdam: Elsevier Science Publishers.

Kummer, R. & Tordoir, W.F. (1975): Phenyl-beta-naphthylamine (PBNA), another carcinogenic agent? *T. Soc. Geneesk.* **53**, 415–419.

Leary, J.S., Keane, W.T., Fontenot, C., Feichtmeir, E.F., Schultz, D., Koos, B.A., Hirsch,L., Lavor, E.M., Roan, C.C. & Hine, C.H. (1974): Safety evaluation in the home of polyvinyl chloride resin strip containing dichlorvos (DDVP). *Arch. Environ. Health* **29**, 308–314.

Miyamoto, J., Kaneko, H., Hutson, D.H., Esser, H.O., Gorbach, S. & Dorn, E. (1988): *IUPAC pesticide metabolism: extrapolation from animals to man.* Oxford: Blackwell Scientific Publications.

Moore, R.M. Jr., Woolf, B.S., Stein, H.P., Thomas, A.W. & Finklea, J.F. (1977): Metabolic precursors of a known human carcinogen. *Science* **194**, 344.

National Institute for Occupational Safety and Health (1976): Metabolic precursors of a known human carcinogen, betanaphthylamine. *Curr. Intell. Bull.* **17 December, vol. 16**, 1–6.

Royal College of Physicians of London (1986): Research on healthy volunteers. *J. R. Coll. Physicians Lond.* **20**, 4–17.

Schlatter, Ch. & Reinhardt, Ch.A. (1985): Acute irritation tests in risk assessment. *Food Chem. Toxicol.* **23**, 145–148.

van Sittert, N.J., Boogaard, P.J. & Beulink, G.D.J. (1993a): Application of the urinary *S*-phenylmercapturic acid test as a biomarker for low levels of exposure to benzene in industry. *Br. J. Ind. Med.* **50**, 460–469.

van Sittert, N.J., Ribbens, P.H., Huisman, B. & Lugtenburg, D. (1993b): A nine year follow up study of renal effects in workers exposed to cadmium in a zinc ore refinery. *Brit. J. Ind. Med.* **50**, 603–612.

van Sittert, N.J., Beulink, G.D.J., van Vliet, E.W.N. & van der Waal, H. (1993c): Monitoring occupational exposure to ethylene oxide by the determination of haemoglobin adducts. *Environ. Health Perspect.* **99**, 217–220.

The Association of the British Pharmaceutical Industry (undated): The report of the committee to investigate medical experiments on staff volunteers. London: ABPI.

Tordoir, W.F. (1980): Field studies monitoring exposure and effects in the development of pesticides. In: *Field worker exposure during pesticide application*, eds. W.F. Tordoir & E.H.A. van Heemstra, pp. 21–26. Amsterdam: Elsevier Scientific Publishing.

Wilkes, M.F., Woollen, B.H., Marsh, J.R., Batten, P.L. & Chester, G. (1993): Biological monitoring for pesticide exposure – the role of human volunteer studies. *Int. Arch. Occup. Environ. Health* **65**, 189–192.

World Medical Association (1964): Declaration of Helsinki. Recommendations guiding physicians in biomedical research involving human subjects. Adopted by the 18th World Medical Assembly, Helsinki, Finland June 1964, amended by the 29th World Medical Assembly, Tokyo, Japan, October 1975, the 35th World Medical Assembly, Venice, Italy, October 1983, and the 41st World Medical Assembly, Hong Kong, September 1989. *Proceedings XXVIth Conference*, Geneva, 1993.

Index

A

B

Q

R

U

V

W